Aminoglycoside Ototoxicity

Aminoglycoside Ototoxicity

EDITED BY
Stephen A. Lerner
Gregory J. Matz
Joseph E. Hawkins, Jr.

WITH
Elisabeth F. Lanzl

Little, Brown and Company *Boston*

First Edition

Library of Congress Catalog Card No. 81-82377

ISBN 0-316-52130-2

Printed in the United States of America

HAL

Contents

II. Studies in Human Subjects

Contributing Authors

David J. Anderson, Ph.D.
Associate Professor of Electrical and Computer Engineering and of Otorhinolaryngology, Kresge Hearing Research Institute, The University of Michigan, Ann Arbor, Michigan
Chapter 11

Matti Anniko, M.D., Ph.D.
Assistant Professor of Otorhinolaryngology, Karolinska Institutet; Consultant, Department of Otorhinolaryngology, Karolinska Sjukhuset, Stockholm, Sweden
Chapter 14

Jean-Marie Aran, Dr.Sc.
Maître de Recherche à l'I.N.S.E.R.M., Audiologie Expérimentale; Directeur, I.N.S.E.R.M. F.R.A. 39, Université de Bordeaux II, Hôpital Pellegrin, Bordeaux, France
Chapter 2

Ishan Bhattacharya, A.B.
Medical Student, The University of Chicago/The Pritzker School of Medicine, Chicago, Illinois
Chapter 25

Jeffrey W. Birns, M.D.
Clinical Instructor, Department of Surgery, UCLA School of Medicine; Attending Surgeon, Otolaryngology Division, Children's Hospital of Los Angeles, Los Angeles, California
Chapter 10

F. Owen Black, M.D., F.A.C.S.
Associate Professor and Vice Chairman, Department of Otolaryngology, University of Pittsburgh School of Medicine; Director, Division of Vestibular Disorders, Eye and Ear Hospital of Pittsburgh, Pittsburgh, Pennsylvania
Chapter 27

Robert E. Brummett, Ph.D.
Professor of Otolaryngology, Kresge Hearing Research Laboratory, and Associate Professor of Pharmacology, University of Oregon Health Sciences Center, Portland, Oregon
Chapter 4

Bernard Cohen, M.D.
Morris B. Bender Professor, Department of Neurology, Mount Sinai School of Medicine of the City University of New York; Attending Neurologist, The Mount Sinai Hospital, New York, New York
Chapter 9

Rickie R. Davis, M.S.
Graduate Research Assistant, Department of Otolaryngology, Kresge Hearing Research Laboratory, University of Oregon Health Sciences Center, Portland, Oregon
Chapter 4

Abraham Eviatar, M.D.
Professor of Otolaryngology, Albert Einstein College of Medicine of Yeshiva University; Attending Surgeon, Department of Otolaryngology, Montefiore Hospital and Medical Center, Bronx, New York
Chapters 20, 21

Lydia Eviatar, M.D.
Associate Professor of Pediatrics, State University of New York at Stony Brook Health Sciences Center School of Medicine; Pediatric Neurologist, Department of Pediatrics, Long Island Jewish/Hillside Medical Center, New Hyde Park, New York
Chapters 20, 21

Pierre Federspil, M.D.
Professor of Oto-Rhino-Laryngology, Universität des Saarlandes; Oberarzt, HNO-Universitätsklinik, Homburg (Saar), West Germany
Chapter 6

M. Angela G. Feitosa, M.A.
Graduate Student in Psychobiology and Kresge Hearing Research Institute, The University of Michigan Medical School, Ann Arbor, Michigan
Chapter 1

Terese Finitzo-Hieber, Ph.D.
Assistant Professor of Communication Disorders, Callier Center for Communication Disorders, The University of Texas Southwestern Medical School at Dallas, Dallas, Texas
Chapter 18

Kaye E. Fox, Ph.D.
Associate Professor, Department of Pharmacology, University of Oregon Health Sciences Center, Portland, Oregon
Chapter 4

Robert N. Glackin, B.S.
Instructor, Department of Laryngology and Otology, The Johns Hopkins University School of Medicine, Baltimore, Maryland
Chapter 19

Joseph E. Hawkins, Jr., Ph.D., D.Sc. (Oxon.)
Professor of Physiological Acoustics, Department of Otorhinolaryngology and Kresge Hearing Research Institute, The University of Michigan Medical School, Ann Arbor, Michigan
Chapters 12, 27

Raúl Hinojosa, M.D.
Research Associate (Associate Professor), Department of Surgery (Otolaryngology), The University of Chicago/The Pritzker School of Medicine, Chicago, Illinois
Chapter 25

Vicente Honrubia, M.D.
Professor, Department of Surgery, UCLA School of Medicine, Los Angeles, California
Chapter 10

Makoto Igarashi, M.D.
Professor and Director of Research, Department of Otorhinolaryngology and Communicative Sciences, Baylor College of Medicine, Houston, Texas
Chapter 8

David W. Jensen, Ph.D.
Assistant Professor, Department of Otorhinolaryngology and Program in Neuroscience, Baylor College of Medicine, Houston, Texas
Chapter 8

Lars-Göran Johnsson, M.D., D.D.S.
Professor of Otorhinolaryngology, Kresge Hearing Research Institute, The University of Michigan Medical School, Ann Arbor, Michigan
Chapters 12, 27

Thomas C. Kingsley, M.D.
Pathologist, Kennestone Hospital, Marietta, Georgia
Chapter 27

Clifford G. Y. Lau, Ph.D.
Adjunct Assistant Professor, Division of Head and Neck Surgery, UCLA School of Medicine, Los Angeles, California
Chapter 10

Stephen A. Lerner, M.D.
Associate Professor, Departments of Medicine and Microbiology, The University of Chicago/The Pritzker School of Medicine, Chicago, Illinois
Chapters 16, 22, 23, 25

Paul S. Lietman, M.D., Ph.D.
Wellcome Professor of Clinical Pharmacology and Professor of Medicine, Pediatrics, and Pharmacology and Experimental Therapeutics, The Johns Hopkins University School of Medicine, Baltimore, Maryland
Chapter 19

Christian Manuel, M.D.
Head, Department of Clinical Pharmacology of Antibiotics, I.N.S.E.R.M. U13, Hôpital Claude Bernard, Paris, France
Chapter 5

Gregory J. Matz, M.D.
Professor of Surgery and Chairman, Section of Otolaryngology, The University of Chicago/The Pritzker School of Medicine, Chicago, Illinois
Chapters 16, 22, 23, 25, 27

George H. McCracken, Jr., M.D.
Professor of Pediatrics, The University of Texas Southwestern Medical School at Dallas; Attending Physician, Parkland Memorial Hospital and Children's Medical Center, Dallas, Texas
Chapter 24

Cathy S. McGinn, B. S.
Research Assistant, Kresge Hearing Research Institute, The University of Michigan Medical School, Ann Arbor, Michigan
Chapter 1

Alain Meulemans
Assistant, Chef de Travaux, Laboratoire de Biophysique et de Médecine Nucléaire, Hôpital Xavier-Bichat, Paris, France
Chapter 5

David B. Moody, Ph.D.
Associate Professor, Department of Psychology; Associate Research Scientist, Department of Otorhinolaryngology and Kresge Hearing Research Institute, The University of Michigan, Ann Arbor, Michigan
Chapter 1

*Harris J. Mowry, M.S.**
Director of Audiology, Department of Surgery (Otolaryngology), The University of Chicago/The Pritzker School of Medicine, Chicago, Illinois
Chapters 16, 22

Joseph B. Nadol, Jr., M.D.
Assistant Professor of Otolaryngology, Harvard Medical School; Associate Surgeon, Department of Otolaryngology, Massachusetts Eye and Ear Infirmary, Boston, Massachusetts
Chapter 28

Jerry L. Northern, Ph.D.
Professor of Otolaryngology, University of Colorado School of Medicine; Head, Audiology Division, University Hospital, Denver, Colorado
Chapter 15

Alfred L. Nuttall, Ph.D.
Associate Professor, Department of Otorhinolaryngology and Kresge Hearing Research Institute, The University of Michigan Medical School, Ann Arbor, Michigan
Chapter 3

Leonard R. Proctor, M.D.
Associate Professor of Surgery, Department of Laryngology and Otology, The Johns Hopkins University School of Medicine; Attending Surgeon and Director, Vestibular Function Laboratory, Johns Hopkins Hospital, Baltimore, Maryland
Chapter 19

Cynthia A. Prosen, Ph.D.
F. V. Hunt Post-Doctoral Fellow in Acoustics, Northwestern University, Evanston, Illinois; formerly graduate student in Psychobiology and Kresge Hearing Research Institute, The University of Michigan Medical School, Ann Arbor, Michigan
Chapter 1

Cedric A. Quick, M.D.
Professor, Department of Otolaryngology, West Virginia University School of Medicine, Morgantown, West Virginia (Present address: Sycamore Professional Center, Petersburg, Virginia)
Chapter 26

*Deceased.

Richard T. Ramsden, F.R.C.S.
Consultant Otolaryngologist, University of Manchester; Department of Otolaryngology, Manchester Royal Infirmary, Manchester, England
Chapter 17

Theodore Raphan, Ph.D.
Research Assistant Professor of Neurology, Mount Sinai School of Medicine of the City University of New York, New York
Chapter 9

James W. Roeder, M.D.
Chief Resident in Otolaryngology, The University of Chicago/The Pritzker School of Medicine, Chicago, Illinois
Chapters 16, 22

Nancy J. Russell, Ph.D.
Research Assistant Professor, Department of Pharmacology, Kresge Hearing Research Laboratory, University of Oregon Health Sciences Center, Portland, Oregon
Chapter 4

Jochen Schacht, Ph.D.
Associate Professor of Biochemistry, Department of Otorhinolaryngology and Kresge Hearing Research Institute, The University of Michigan Medical School, Ann Arbor, Michigan
Chapter 7

Robert Seligsohn, M.D.
Fellow, Department of Pharmacological and Physiological Sciences and Department of Medicine, The University of Chicago/The Pritzker School of Medicine, Chicago, Illinois
Chapter 25

John V. Serafin, Ph.D.
Assistant Professor of Psychology, St. Vincent College, Latrobe, Pennsylvania; formerly graduate student in Psychobiology and Kresge Hearing Research Institute, The University of Michigan Medical School, Ann Arbor, Michigan
Chapter 1

Jane D. Siegel, M.D.
Assistant Professor, Department of Pediatrics, The University of Texas Southwestern Medical School at Dallas; Attending Physician, Parkland Memorial Hospital and Children's Medical Center, Dallas, Texas
Chapter 24

Craig R. Smith, M.D.
Associate Professor of Medicine, The Johns Hopkins University School of Medicine; Director, Division of Internal Medicine, Johns Hopkins Hospital, Baltimore, Maryland
Chapter 19

William C. Stebbins, Ph.D.
Professor, Departments of Otorhinolaryngology and Psychology and Kresge Hearing Research Institute, The University of Michigan, Ann Arbor, Michigan
Chapter 1

Patricia L. Thompson, M.A.
Instructor, Department of Otolaryngology, University of Colorado School of Medicine; Clinical Audiologist, Otolaryngology, University Hospital, Denver, Colorado
Chapter 15

Patrice Tran Ba Huy, M.D.
Chef de Clinique à la Faculté, C.H.U. Lariboisière-Saint-Louis, Université Paris VII; Assistant des Hôpitaux, Chaire de Clinique ORL—Hôpital Lariboisière, Paris, France
Chapter 5

Norman D. Weiner, Ph.D.
Professor of Pharmacy, The University of Michigan College of Pharmacy, Ann Arbor, Michigan
Chapter 7

Jan Wersäll, M.D.
Professor of Otorhinolaryngology, Karolinska Institutet and Karolinska Sjukhuset, Stockholm, Sweden
Chapter 13

Preface

The aminoglycosides have been important, life-saving tools in the treatment of infectious diseases, from the earliest clinical trials of streptomycin to the current worldwide use of a variety of naturally occurring and semisynthetic antibiotics of this class. However, well-justified concern about their toxic effects on both the auditory and the vestibular functions of the inner ear, and on the kidney as well, has complicated their effective use and compromised their therapeutic value. Since the toxic:therapeutic ratio of the aminoglycosides is generally low, the question of risk versus benefit must be weighed by all physicians who prescribe them. Unfortunately, the magnitude of the risk for the individual patient remains uncertain, as do the contributions of various risk factors. Consequently, physicians may refrain from giving an aminoglycoside when one is indicated or may use a lower dose than might be effective and well tolerated; or they may prescribe doses that are inappropriately high for patients who are especially susceptible to ototoxic injury.

Many investigators from a diverse range of basic and clinical disciplines have engaged in research bearing on the problems of understanding and controlling aminoglycoside ototoxicity. Their approaches have varied considerably, as might be expected from their different backgrounds and their areas of interest and expertise.

In convening the International Conference on Aminoglycoside Ototoxicity, held at the University of Chicago on September 26–28, 1979, we brought together basic and clinical scientists to present their views of aminoglycoside ototoxicity from the various perspectives of their own work. We believe that this symposium facilitated a fruitful and stimulating exchange of information, ideas, and unresolved questions among those investigators who work with patients, those who work with animals, and those who study ototoxicity in the cellular and subcellular structures of the inner ear.

As editors of this book, we have endeavored to bring the information and excitement of the conference to the scientific and medical communities that are concerned with the problem of aminoglycoside ototoxicity and are interested in the research it has generated. Most of the chapters are edited versions of papers presented at the conference. We have included chapters on topics not directly related to aminoglycosides and their toxicity, for example, inner ear physiology and methods of testing inner ear function. Such information is intended to improve our ability to detect and to study aminoglycoside ototoxicity. Each section of the book is introduced by brief editors' comments. Edited discussions have been placed after individual chapters or after groups of related chapters. For reasons both medical and legal, we have omitted specific practical recommendations on the management of patients treated with aminoglycoside antibiotics. Any statements that appear to make such recommendations represent the opinions of the individual authors.

We would like to express our wholehearted gratitude to the Schering Corporation for its generous support of the conference and of the publication of this volume. We particularly appreciate the confidence and counsel of Dr. Irving I. A. Tabachnick and Grace E. Wright.

We are indebted to Drs. César Fernández and Robert Butler of the University of Chicago for critically reviewing selected chapters. Ms. Fay Yates and Mrs. Janyce Nasgowitz have exhibited both skill and patience in the typing and retyping of all of the chapters and discussions. We appreciate the editorial support of Barbara Ward, Lois Hall, and Helane Manditch-Prottas of Little, Brown and Company.

This book stands as testimony to the editorial skill, patient understanding, wisdom, and endurance of Elisabeth F. Lanzl, Editor in the Division of the Biological Sciences of the University of Chicago, who has devoted much of the past year to its preparation. We greatly appreciate her quiet counsel and her persistence in coordinating the efforts of the many contributors and in facilitating our task as editors.

We dedicate this book to the memory of Harris J. Mowry, Director of Audiology at the University of Chicago, whose recent death abruptly ended his enthusiastic participation in clinical studies on the auditory and vestibular effects of the aminoglycosides.

S. A. L.
G. J. M.
J. E. H.

Introduction: Historical Perspective

Joseph E. Hawkins, Jr.

The phenomenon of drug ototoxicity hardly needs a formal introduction. By now all of us are more or less familiar with it, either from direct observation of patients in the clinic and animals in the laboratory, or at least from reading about it in the hundreds of publications that have appeared over the past thirty-odd years.

Historical perspectives have a tendency to be long and dry, full of dates and names of half-mad monarchs, but here I shall try to keep the names and dates to a minimum and the tale reasonably brief; it has been told in greater detail elsewhere [3,4]. One name we cannot omit is that of Waksman, the soil scientist at Rutgers, whose announcement of the isolation of streptomycin came in 1944 [9]. It was the result of his carefully planned effort to discover clinically useful antimicrobial substances elaborated by the streptomycetes of the soil. He had been hoping that his search would yield a product that would be useful in the treatment of infections caused by gram-negative and acid-fast bacteria—especially one that would be effective against *Mycobacterium tuberculosis.* He found it (and a Nobel prize) in streptomycin.

Waksman's new antibiotic almost immediately was tried out at the Mayo Clinic by Hinshaw and Feldman [5], who soon reported their successful use of streptomycin in the treatment of pulmonary and other forms of tuberculosis. At the same time they made known their wholly unexpected observation of both vestibular and cochlear toxicity in a substantial number of their patients. It soon became clear that streptomycin was so effective in the therapy of tuberculosis in forms that had been completely untreatable by any drugs in the past, notably miliary and meningitic tuberculosis, that its virtues and faults had to be evaluated on a very large scale. Something then came to pass that was previously unknown in this country—a nationwide cooperative therapeutic study organized and sponsored by the Veterans Administration. Many of the early explorations of the effectiveness and the toxicity of streptomycin and related substances were first reported at the semiannual Streptomycin Conferences of the Veterans Administration.

We should also recall the laboratory investigations of the pharmacologic properties of streptomycin by the late Hans Molitor and his associates at the Merck Institute for Therapeutic Research in Rahway, New Jersey [7]. That study showed that the acute toxicity of a given sample in mice was of little or no help in predicting its chronic ototoxicity. An interesting finding of theirs [8] was the convulsant effect of streptomycin when the drug was applied to the central nervous system, either directly to the cortex or by intracisternal injection. But this acute action, which was not unlike that of penicillin, did not appear to be in any way related to the problem of a slowly developing, chronic ototoxicity.

There was also the much-debated question of whether the effects on the auditory and vestibular systems were central or peripheral. In the beginning, most bets were on the central rather than the peripheral site, but in 1948 Caussé [1] was able to show, on the basis of his study of a handful of mice and a histologic follow-up, that there was indeed a lesion in the neuroepithelia of the inner ear, pointing clearly to a peripheral rather than a central site of action. Up to that time, I had been hoping that the ototoxicity of streptomycin might prove to be more subtle and to represent an interference with synaptic transmission in the cochlea. The whole problem of chemical mediation at synapses was still relatively new and very much in the air in those days. Unfortunately, this did not turn out to be the case, and we still do not know the identity of the afferent transmitter of the cochlea. Nevertheless, streptomycin did bring about some interesting and worthwhile experimental observations about the inner ear, vestibular dysfunction, and sensorineural deafness.

We can divide the history of the ototoxicity problem into two major periods. The first period is represented by streptomycin, which requires prolonged use in the treatment of tuberculosis and affects mainly the vestibular system. At one time as many as 90 percent of the patients being treated in the Veterans Administration study were showing vestibular disturbances [2]. Dihydrostreptomycin, which looked promising because of its lower vestibular toxicity, eventually had to be condemned because of its unpredictable effects on hearing. The second period is represented by kanamycin, which appeared in the late 1950s. This drug was too ototoxic for the prolonged treatment of tuberculosis, but it proved highly useful for short-term treatment of gram-negative infections. Its ototoxic action, like that of neomycin, which had preceded it, was predominantly on the cochlea.

The prolonged regimen required in the treatment of tuberculosis, by giving rise to vestibular disturbances in so many streptomycin-treated patients, produced an awareness of ototoxicity and taught some valuable lessons about its nature. Gradually, the drug manufacturers, as well as the rest of us, gave up the hope that the ototoxic property might be the result of some impurity that would eventually go away after additional refinements in pharmaceutical preparation.

Neomycin brought with it special difficulties and dangers, since it proved, in spite of what the initial reports had claimed, to be ototoxic regardless of the route of administration. Unfortunately, clinicians in fields other than otolaryngology were slow to recognize this danger, so that too many cases of profound deafness resulted from the use of neomycin by various other routes, after it had been recognized that the parenteral route was extremely hazardous to the patients' hearing.

Drugs developed since kanamycin include gentamicin, tobramycin, amikacin, and now netilmicin, a substance that may prove less ototoxic than some of the earlier agents. We still have two major questions facing us—first, how best to evaluate the ototoxic potential of new drugs in animals, and, second and more important, how to avoid, or at least minimize, ototoxic complications in patients. In our historical survey we should also mention the names of those who have given us clues as to the mode of action of these drugs, particularly Stupp et al. [10], Voldrich [11], and Vrabec et al. [12], all of whom demonstrated that the drugs tend to accumulate in the perilymph and to remain there longer than in the plasma. That property presumably helps to account for their selectively ototoxic action.

The basis of this action was first conceived in terms of the known antibacterial effects of aminoglycosides and was attributed to an interference with protein synthesis. We will hear from Dr. Schacht a little later in this meeting about his experiments demonstrating that it is not the protein synthesis by cells but the polyphosphoinositides of the cell membrane that seem to be primarily affected.

What have we learned from 35 years' experience with aminoglycoside ototoxicity? I hope that we have learned to respect them and their potential for both good and evil, and even to suspect other, seemingly innocent, drugs of a possible ototoxic bent. We have learned something about the barrier function in the cochlea, which seems to have been noted first by Misrahy et al. [6]. We have become much more interested than we used to be in otopharmacology and otopathology, and in the process we have also learned more about the close kinship between the ear and the kidney. In the beginning, the streptomycin problem sparked an interest in vestibular function that has paid off handsomely for otolaryngology. In fact, it helped bridge the gap between World War II, with the flurry of vestibular research arising from the problems of aviation medicine, and the space program, with its special concern for vestibular function and dysfunction. Before space flights began in earnest, equipment for the study of vestibular function in a more systematic fashion was to some extent already on hand. Unfortunately, at the time when streptomycin was in widespread use, it had not been possible to take advantage of the enormous patient material it made available for research on vestibular problems. As I look around me now at the eager, young faces of well-known investigators, I am tempted to believe that we are ready for any further challenges that the drug companies or the mold microorganisms may offer; but that may not in fact be the case, for there may still be surprises in store for us.

References

1. Caussé, R., Gondet, I., and Vallancien, B. Action vestibulaire de la streptomycine chez la souris. *C.R. Soc. Biol. (Paris)* 142:747, 1948.

2. Fowler, E. P., Jr. The effect of streptomycin on the otic mechanisms. Minutes of the Third Streptomycin Conference, Veterans Administration, St. Louis, 99:107–109, 1947.
3. Hawkins, J. E., Jr. Vestibular Ototoxicity. In R. F. Naunton (Ed.), *The Vestibular System.* New York: Academic, 1975. Pp. 321–349.
4. Hawkins, J. E., Jr. Drug Ototoxicity. In W. D. Keidel and W. D. Neff (Eds.), *Handbook of Sensory Physiology.* Berlin, Heidelberg: Springer, 1976. Vol. V/3, pp. 707–748.
5. Hinshaw, H. C., and Feldman, W. H. Streptomycin in the treatment of clinical tuberculosis: A preliminary report. *Proc. Mayo Clinic* 20:313, 1945.
6. Misrahy, G. A., Spradley, J. F., Dzinovic, S., and Brooks, C. J. Effects of intense sound, hypoxia and kanamycin on the permeability of cochlear partitions. *Ann. Otol. Rhinol. Laryngol.* 70:572, 1961.
7. Molitor, H., Graessle, O. E., Kuna, S., Mushett, C. W., and Silber, R. H. Some toxicological properties of streptomycin. *J. Pharmacol. Exp. Ther.* 86:151, 1946.
8. Molitor, H., and Kuna, S. The significance of neurotropic properties of commercial streptomycin. *Arch. Int. Pharmacodyn. Ther.* 74:334, 1947.
9. Schatz, A., Bugie, E., and Waksman, S. A. Streptomycin, a substance exhibiting antibiotic activity against gram-positive and gram-negative bacteria. *Proc. Soc. Exp. Biol. Med.* 55:66, 1944.
10. Stupp, H., Rauch, S., Sous, H., and Lagler, F. Untersuchungen über die Ursache der spezifisch ototoxischen Wirkung der basischen Streptomyces-Antibiotika unter besonderer Berücksichtigung des Kanamycins. *Acta Otolaryngol. (Stockh.)* 61:435, 1966.
11. Voldrich, L. The kinetics of streptomycin, kanamycin and neomycin in the inner ear. *Acta Otolaryngol. (Stockh.)* 60:243, 1965.
12. Vrabec, D. P., Cody, D. T. R., and Ulrich, J. A. A study of the relative concentrations of antibiotics in the blood, spinal fluid, and perilymph in animals. *Ann. Otol. Rhinol. Laryngol.* 74:688, 1965.

I. Studies in Animal Subjects

Cochlear Function

A major goal in animal studies on aminoglycoside ototoxicity is to understand its mechanism in man. Because of obvious experimental limitations in clinical studies, many investigators have used animals in various approaches to the study of toxic effects of aminoglycosides on the cochlea. This has made it possible to control parameters that cannot be controlled in human studies.

The testing of hearing in man is facilitated by the cooperation of the subject. In the absence of such cooperation, the measurement of hearing in animals has often relied on time-consuming and occasionally imprecise procedures. However, William Stebbins and his co-workers describe remarkably accurate behavioral methods of determining auditory function, analogous to audiometry in man, which they have applied to the study of ototoxicity in animals trained by operant conditioning. Nonbehavioral electrophysiologic techniques, such as measurements of the cochlear microphonic and action potentials, allow a direct assessment of cochlear function in animals and can be used in combination with histologic studies of the cochlea. These techniques are reviewed by Jean-Marie Aran.

Most electrophysiologic investigations of aminoglycoside ototoxicity involve parenteral administration of the drugs; serum levels, to say nothing of concentrations in the inner ear, are rarely controlled or even measured. Alfred Nuttall has circumvented these pharmacologic uncertainties by applying solutions of aminoglycosides in artificial perilymph directly to the cochlea.

In clinical practice, aminoglycosides are often used concurrently with loop diuretics. The latter also are potentially ototoxic by themselves, and there is a clinical impression (see Chap. 26) that loop diuretics may potentiate aminoglycoside ototoxicity. The studies by Robert Brummett and his co-workers, on electrophysiologic and histopathologic consequences of the administration of both aminoglycosides and loop diuretics to experimental animals, provide valuable data on the possible mechanism of their ototoxic interaction in man.

Studies like those by Nuttall relate the cochleotoxic effects of aminoglycosides to their concentration in perilymph. In order to apply the results of such studies in the cochlea to questions of ototoxicity in animals and in patients, we need information on the pharmacokinetics of aminoglycosides in the inner ear fluids. Patrice Tran Ba Huy and his co-workers not only have extensively reviewed earlier studies on the pharmacokinetics of aminoglycosides in the serum, perilymph, and endolymph of animals, but also have performed their own studies on the pharmacokinetics of gentamicin in the inner ear of the rat, making use of a highly sensitive assay for gentamicin. Another investigator concerned with aminoglycoside pharmacokinetics in the perilymph, Pierre Federspil, describes his work on gentamicin and several other aminoglycosides. These pharmacokinetic studies in animals can be compared with studies by Stephen Lerner et al. (see Chap. 25) on the levels of gentamicin in the perilymph of patients treated with this drug.

1. Animal Models in the Study of Ototoxic Hearing Loss

William C. Stebbins, Cathy S. McGinn, M. Angela G. Feitosa, David B. Moody, Cynthia A. Prosen, and John V. Serafin

This chapter is concerned with behavioral technique in the analysis of animal hearing and its value in the study of ototoxicity. Gone are the days when the state of the art was such that we had to ask an animal to respond to acoustic stimulation by climbing a pole to avoid electric shock, flicking its tail to prevent being roasted, twitching its ears or ceasing to shiver in a makeshift refrigerator, or even pausing in breathing or slowing the beating of its heart to indicate that it could hear. The Paleozoic era in the study of animal hearing is over. Behaviorists must provide techniques that have sufficient technical merit to match the resolving power of the microscope and the microelectrode in the study of hearing and hearing disorders. Anatomists and physiologists await the further development of such behavioral procedures, for it is only these procedures that can reveal actual hearing in the normal or impaired state. Other measures, even electrophysiologic ones, stop short of this goal, for they tap information somewhere along the route between sensory input and the final behavioral response that we refer to as hearing.

The old methods were inexpensive but hardly cost effective, since the information they provided was at best an equivocal yes or no in response to acoustic stimulation. The questions we must now ask, particularly in light of some of the interesting and more recent histopathologic findings in the inner ear of animals treated with ototoxic drugs, are considerably more complicated and demand more than simple yes or no answers. The new procedures are time-consuming and costly, yet the information they provide is valid and reliable and easily quantified. There is no ready substitute [14].

The stage was set 40 years ago with the publication of a book entitled *Behavior of Organisms* by B. F. Skinner [13]. Twenty years ago, Blough [2], in an elegant demonstration of Skinner's operant conditioning paradigm, con-

This study was supported by research and program grants from NINCDS (NS 15108, NS 05065, and NS 05785).

vinced us that we could ask questions of animals concerning their sensory experience which are every bit as complex as those we ask of human subjects. Blough's tour de force was a behaviorally determined dark-adaptation curve with a clearly demarcated rod-cone break and eventually a spectral sensitivity function for the pigeon eye. It became clear from Blough's early work, and from the subsequent work of others, that animals could be instructed in such a manner as to yield psychophysical functions equal in precision, reliability, and validity to any obtained from human subjects. Furthermore, these animals could serve as models for man in experiments on disordered sensory systems.

The advantages of the procedures lie in their power, first, to reach a variety of prospective animal models, including the guinea pig and cat, which had long been given up as recalcitrant and untestable by more traditional behavioral paradigms; and second, to encompass a wide assortment of sensory measures in addition to absolute threshold or minimum detectable intensity levels. Here, for example, we report on the monkey, guinea pig, and cat—on behaviors which measure differential resolution for sound intensity and frequency, in addition to loudness judgment, psychophysical tuning curves, and sound localization acuity. This is a sampling; more is possible. Our purpose is to argue by example for the importance of sound but versatile behavioral methodology with animals, particularly in the study of ototoxicity. With such methodology, we can begin to grapple with questions of function which arise from the work of anatomists and physiologists. Without it, we are confined to quick-and-dirty, highly variable estimates of acoustic sensitivity.

The procedures themselves require a healthy, well-motivated animal that will earn most of its daily food ration in experimental sessions by responding to some aspect of sensory stimulation. For different animal species, the procedures vary only in minor detail and take into consideration the capabilities of the animal. The guinea pig, for example, stands over a small button in the floor of the test chamber (see Fig. 1-1). Upon seeing a light signal, the guinea pig presses the button with one foot until a tone is turned on, then promptly steps off the button. Delivery of food is contingent upon this release response to acoustic stimulation. The cat stands on two pedals until a light is presented. Light plus tone calls for release of the right pedal; light alone, for release of the left pedal; correct responses are followed by food reinforcement. The monkey uses his hands to grasp a hollow tube when a light is flashing within the tube (see Fig. 1-2). Maintaining his hold and then releasing it upon hearing a sound brings a bit of food. Incorrect responses are punished not by shock, which often generates emotional behavior, but by time out from the experiment.

Measurement of hearing proceeds when the animals are well trained and their behavior has become stable in the conditioning situation. For absolute thresholds, a variant of Békésy audiometry is often used. Up-and-down, stepwise variation of sound level, or stimulus-tracking, produces a quick, efficient measure of threshold, and nine pure-tone frequencies may be tested in each ear in an hour. For differential thresholds, loudness judgment, or sound localization, different stimuli are often presented in random order (method of con-

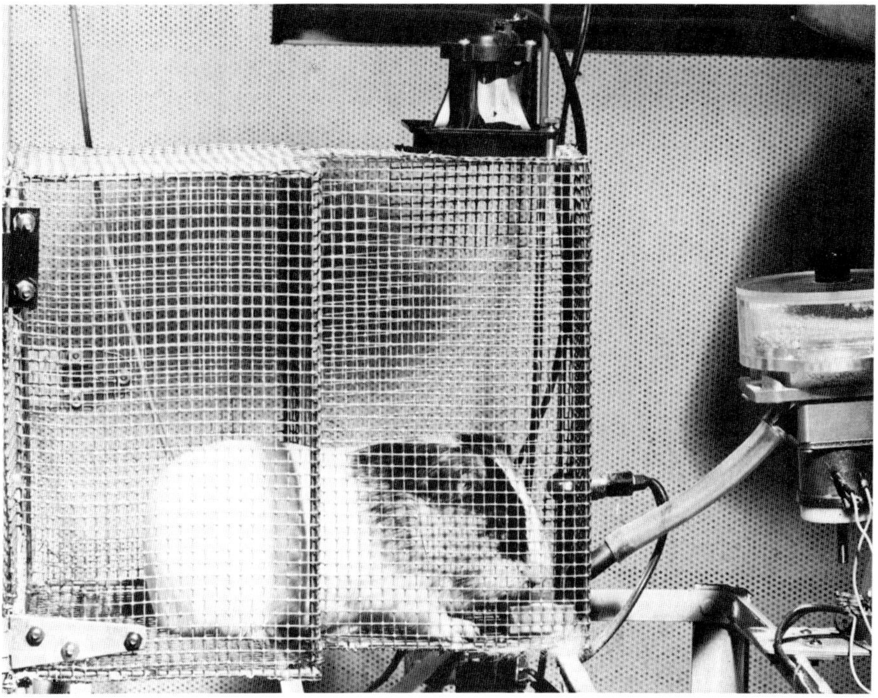

Figure 1-1. Behaviorally trained guinea pig sitting in testing apparatus. The subject shown is performing the observing response, depressing the small plastic disk located on the floor of the apparatus with its right front paw. Tonal stimuli are presented from the speaker located above the subject's head. (From C. A. Prosen and W. C. Stebbins, Ototoxicity. In P. S. Spencer and H. H. Schaumburg [Eds.], *Experimental and Clinical Neurotoxicology.* Baltimore: Williams & Wilkins, 1980. Reprinted by permission.)

stant stimuli), and the stimulus detected correctly 50 percent of the time is determined.

Error rates are carefully and continuously monitored. Stable responding, with less than 10 percent error, signifies an animal's readiness for drug treatment. The training process is slow in comparison with more traditional methods, taking 1 to 2 months for simple procedures and longer for more complex ones. There is little difference in this regard among species. We are constantly seeking methodologic variants for reducing training time. Once an animal is trained, however, the treatment and testing process moves quickly. Many of the aspects of hearing which these procedures address are simply not amenable to investigation by other methods. Because of the reliability and low variance in the behavioral data, large numbers of subjects are not required. The data are completely objective and easily quantified. For these and other reasons which we will attempt to document below, we consider these

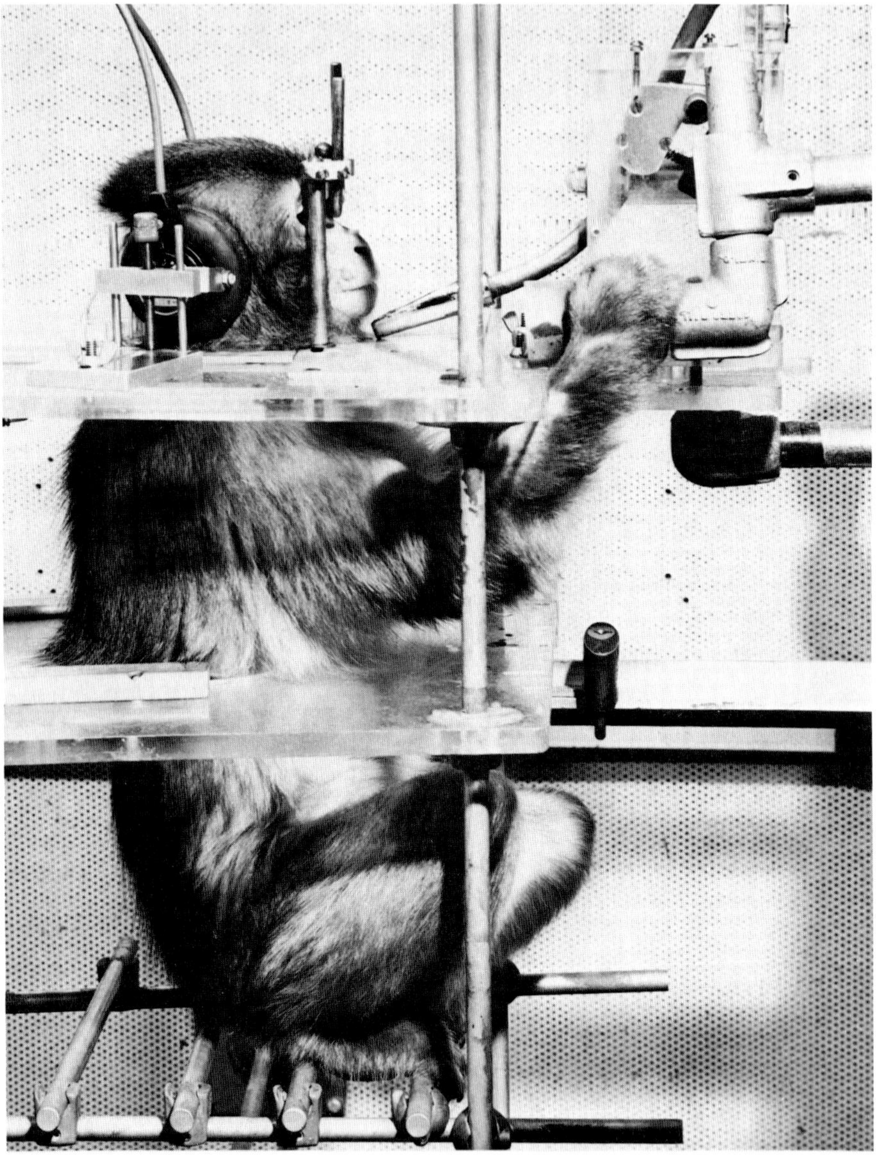

Figure 1-2. Subject (macaque monkey) seated in restraining chair for hearing testing. Earphones, cylindrical response tube, and feeder tube are shown. The monkey is in the listening position, with its hand grasping the response tube prior to tone stimulation. (From W. C. Stebbins, Hearing of the Primates. In D. Chivers and J. Herbert [Eds.], *Recent Advances in Primatology: Primate Behavior.* London: Academic, 1978. Copyright by Academic Press Inc. [London] Ltd. Reprinted by permission.)

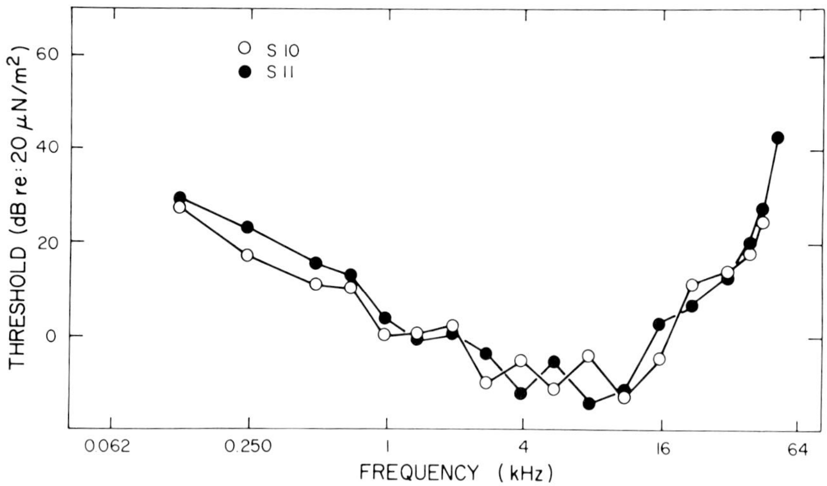

Figure 1-3. Pure-tone audiograms from two guinea pigs (S10 and S11), determined by operant methods with positive reinforcement. (From C. A. Prosen et al., Auditory thresholds and kanamycin-induced hearing loss in the guinea pig assessed by a positive reinforcement procedure. *J. Acoust. Soc. Am.* 63:559, 1978. Reprinted by permission.)

positive-reinforcement techniques to be the methods of choice, particularly in the field of ototoxicity where the issues are so complex.

Normal baseline data should fulfill several criteria. Good agreement among animals of the same species is important; such agreement is illustrated in Fig. 1-3 by the normal threshold functions for two guinea pigs. Even more important, perhaps, is within-subject reliability, as shown in Fig. 1-4 in the mean threshold function for one guinea pig; the vertical bars represent the complete range of values obtained over several test sessions.

Some investigators, such as the famous physiologist Claude Bernard [1], once cast doubt upon man's ability to extract sensory information from animal subjects; yet the consistency and reproducibility of the findings obtained when appropriate procedures are used belie such doubts. The form that the data take is insensitive to fairly drastic changes in audiometric testing procedure, as indicated by the threshold functions for one monkey in Fig. 1-5, which are relatively invariant across different procedures.

Some of the foregoing examples illustrate the necessary concern not only with stable pretreatment baselines, but also with validity, and show that, despite the skepticism expressed by Bernard and others, we are measuring what we think we are.

The use of different animal models tells us how general or perhaps how species-specific our results are. At different levels of the data, they may be either general or specific. Figure 1-6 shows the typical picture of hearing loss progressing from high to low frequencies after treatment of a cat with the drug kanamycin.

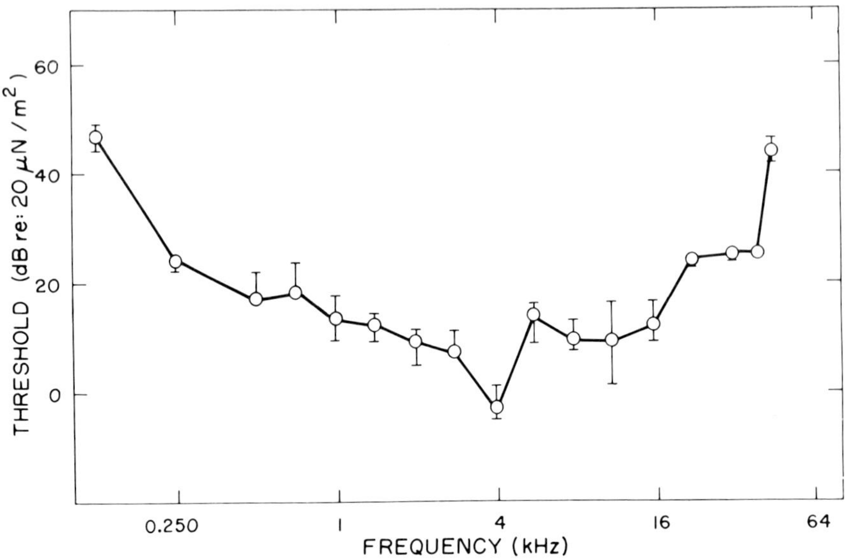

Figure 1-4. Pure-tone audiogram for one guinea pig. The vertical bars indicate the entire range of the threshold at each frequency tested during five separate determinations. (From C. A. Prosen et al., Auditory thresholds and kanamycin-induced hearing loss in the guinea pig assessed by a positive reinforcement procedure. *J. Acoust. Soc. Am.* 63:559, 1978. Reprinted by permission.)

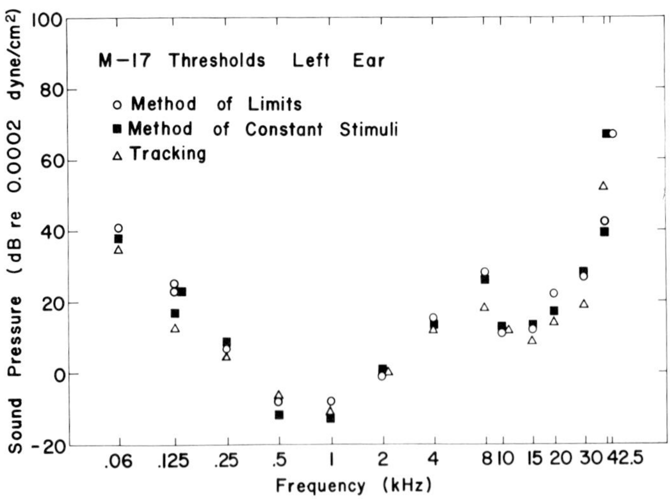

Figure 1-5. Pure-tone audiograms for one monkey tested with three different psychophysical methods. (From W. C. Stebbins, Studies of Hearing and Hearing Loss in the Monkey. In W. C. Stebbins [Ed.], *Animal Psychophysics; The Design and Conduct of Sensory Experiments.* New York: Appleton-Century-Crofts, 1970. Reprinted by permission.)

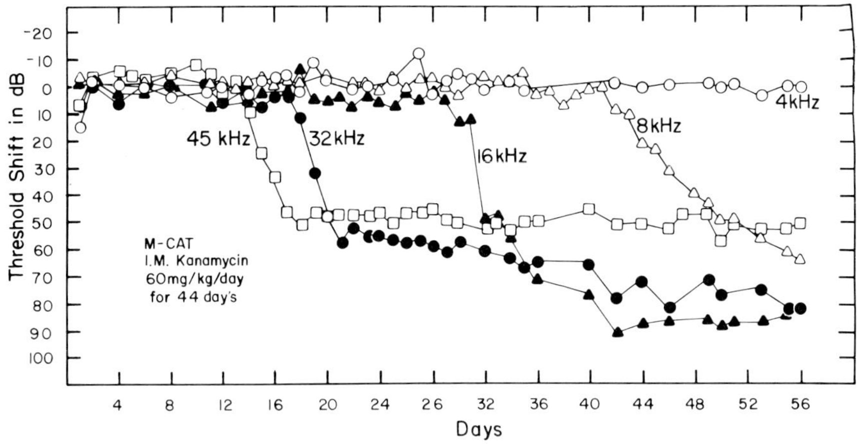

Figure 1-6. Progressive changes in auditory threshold for a cat at different frequencies during and following kanamycin treatment. The zero level represents normal hearing at all frequencies prior to drug treatment. (Day 0 = start of treatment.) (From W. C. Stebbins and D. B. Moody, Comparative behavioral toxicology. *Neurobehav. Toxicol.* 1[Suppl.]:33, 1979. Reprinted by permission.)

The sharp decline in hearing over time at the various frequencies during the course of administration of kanamycin is noteworthy. Although the dose schedules are different, the progress of the hearing loss is the same for the guinea pig (Fig. 1-7) and for the monkey (Fig. 1-8). The comparison provides a reassuring example of generality among species. Some residual hearing, however, remained at high frequencies in the guinea pig, but not in the monkey, thus furnishing an example of a difference between species.

The terminal audiogram after kanamycin administration, determined immediately before the monkey was killed, together with the cytocochleogram for the same animal, is presented in Fig. 1-9. A cochlea devoid of receptor cells in the basal turn is correlated with a high-frequency hearing loss. Hearing is normal at lower frequencies, and there appears to be a normal complement of hair cells in the apical half of the cochlea. The gradient between normalcy and impairment is steep in both cochleogram and audiogram.

A somewhat different picture is seen for the guinea pig in Fig. 1-10. Missing outer hair cells with intact, normal-appearing inner hair cells in the more basal part of the cochlea are correlated with a partial hearing loss of approximately 50 to 60 dB at the higher frequencies. These findings, which have been reported in detail elsewhere [9], substantiate those of Ryan and Dallos [11] and have generated considerable interest in the differential function of inner and outer hair cells in the normal hearing process. The finding of a difference in reaction by the guinea pig and monkey to the same drug is an interesting one, but is not yet understood.

A more remarkable difference between species is illustrated by the striking sensitivity of the patas monkey to the aminoglycoside dihydrostreptomycin

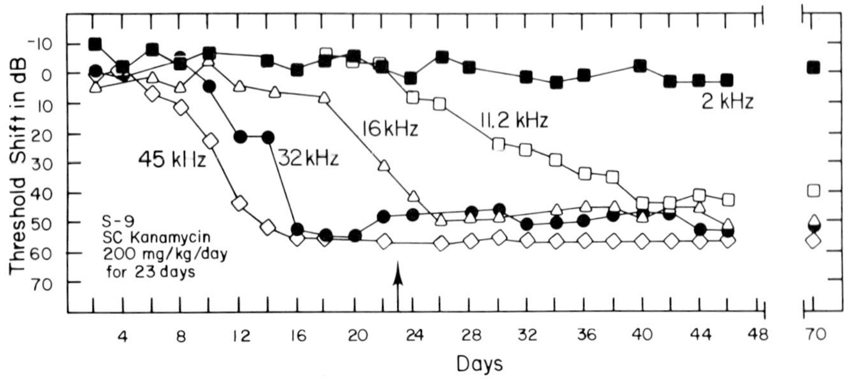

Figure 1-7. Progressive changes in threshold for a guinea pig at different frequencies during and following daily kanamycin treatment. The zero level represents normal hearing at all frequencies prior to drug treatment. (From W. C. Stebbins and D. B. Moody, Comparative behavioral toxicology. *Neurobehav. Toxicol.* 1[Suppl.]:33, 1979. Reprinted by permission.)

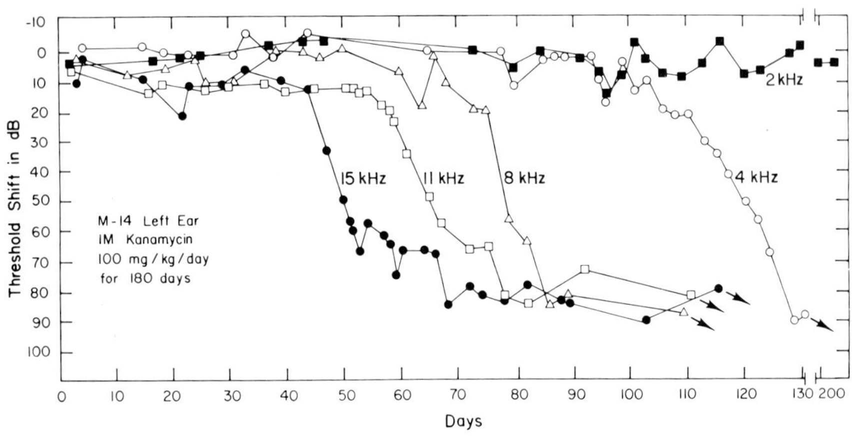

Figure 1-8. Progressive changes in threshold for a macaque monkey at different frequencies during and following daily kanamycin treatment. The zero level represents normal hearing at all frequencies prior to drug treatment. (From W. C. Stebbins et al., Ototoxic hearing loss and cochlear pathology in the monkey. *Trans. Am. Otolaryngol. Soc.* 57:110, 1969. Reprinted by permission.)

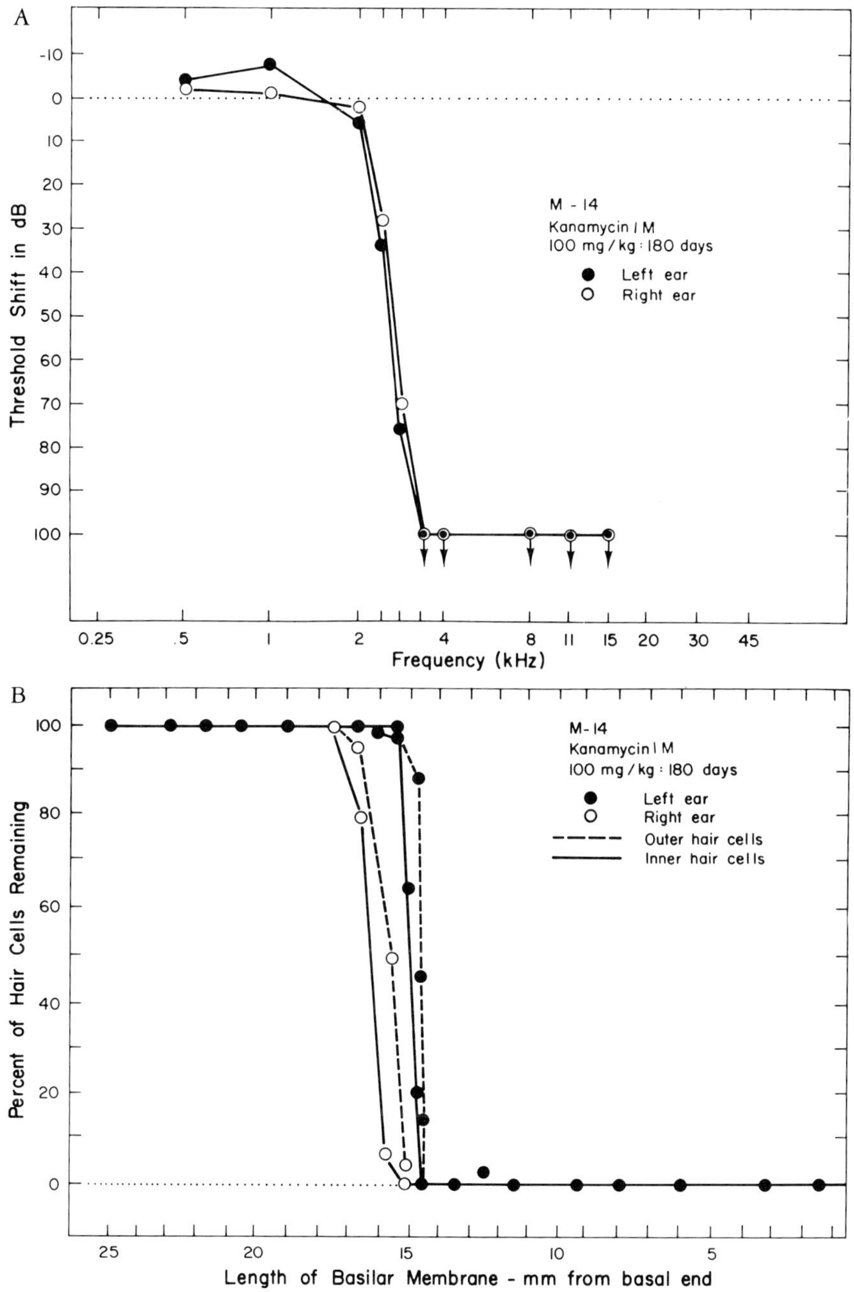

Figure 1-9. Auditory threshold shift for the monkey represented in Fig. 1-8 after 180 days of daily kanamycin treatment (A); cytocochleogram (B). (From W. C. Stebbins and S. Coombs, Behavioral Assessment of Ototoxicity in Nonhuman Primates. In B. Weiss and V. G. Laties [Eds.], *Behavioral Toxicology*. New York: Plenum, 1976. Reprinted by permission.)

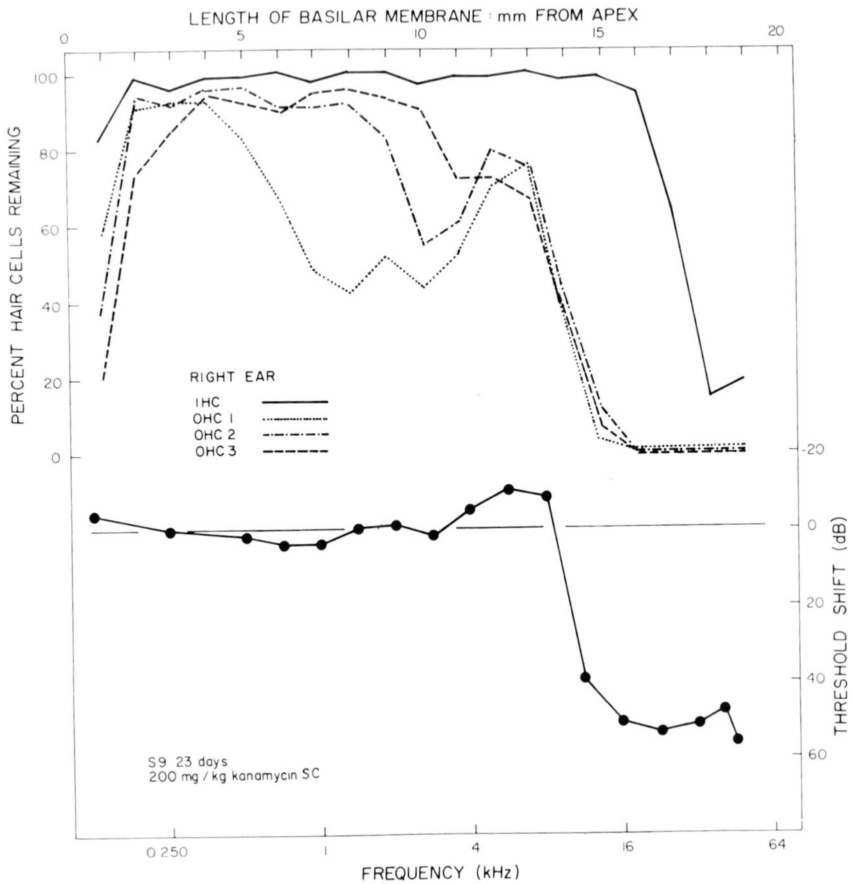

Figure 1-10. Auditory threshold shift for the guinea pig represented in Fig. 1-7, measured 5 weeks after the last treatment with kanamycin (lower panel); cytocochleogram (upper panel). (From C. A. Prosen et al., Auditory thresholds and kanamycin-induced hearing loss in the guinea pig assessed by a positive reinforcement procedure. *J. Acoust. Soc. Am.* 63:559, 1978. Reprinted by permission.)

[4]. Typical results for a single animal are shown in Fig. 1-11 in the form of a juxtaposed behavioral audiogram and cytocochleogram.

The patas monkey, in its reaction to dihydrostreptomycin, shows a marked resemblance to the guinea pig in the latter's reaction to kanamycin. Missing outer and intact, normal-appearing inner hair cells in the more basal portions of the cochlea are correlated with a 60- to 70-dB hearing loss at the higher frequencies. A significant feature of the response to dihydrostreptomycin shown here is the progressive hearing loss, which continues long after cessation of drug treatment and resembles that reported in man. In fact, the patas monkey's sensitivity to dihydrostreptomycin in doses as low as 20 mg/kg is greater than that sometimes seen when dihydrostreptomycin was used in the

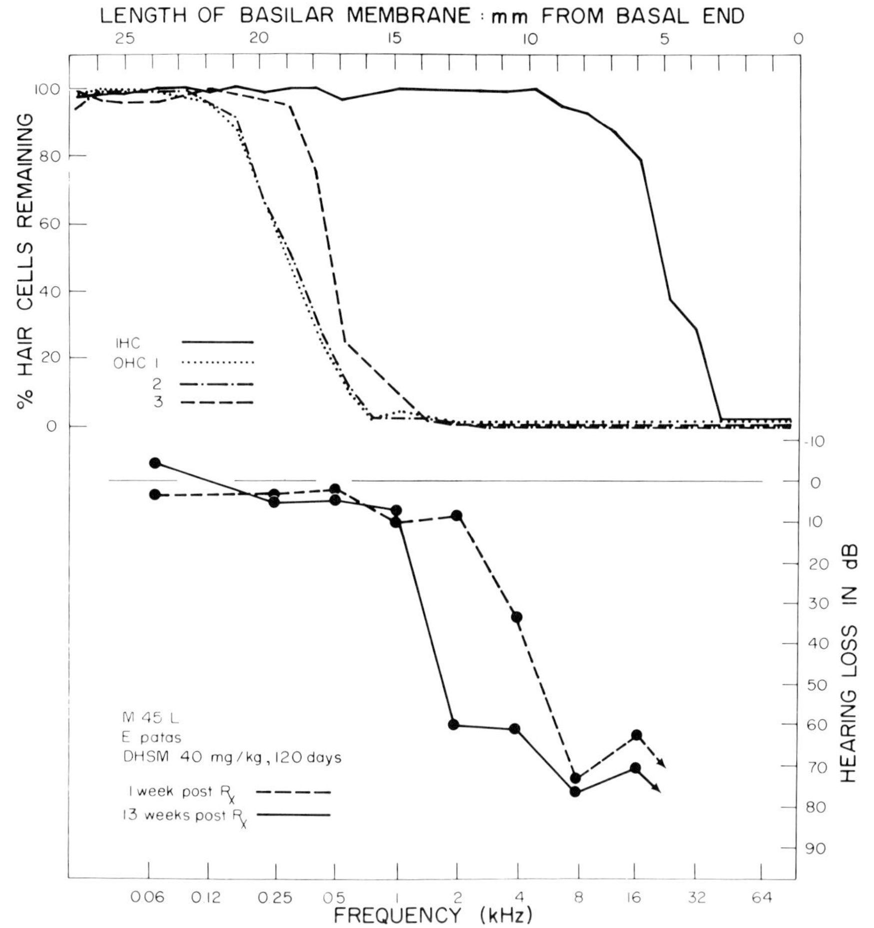

Figure 1-11. Auditory threshold shift (lower panel) and cytocochleogram (upper panel) for a patas monkey treated with dihydrostreptomycin. The dashed curve in the lower panel represents hearing loss 1 week after drug treatment was stopped; the solid curve indicates hearing loss 13 weeks later. (From J. E. Hawkins, Jr., et al., The patas monkey as a model for dihydrostreptomycin ototoxicity. *Acta Otolaryngol.* 83:123, 1977. Reprinted by permission.)

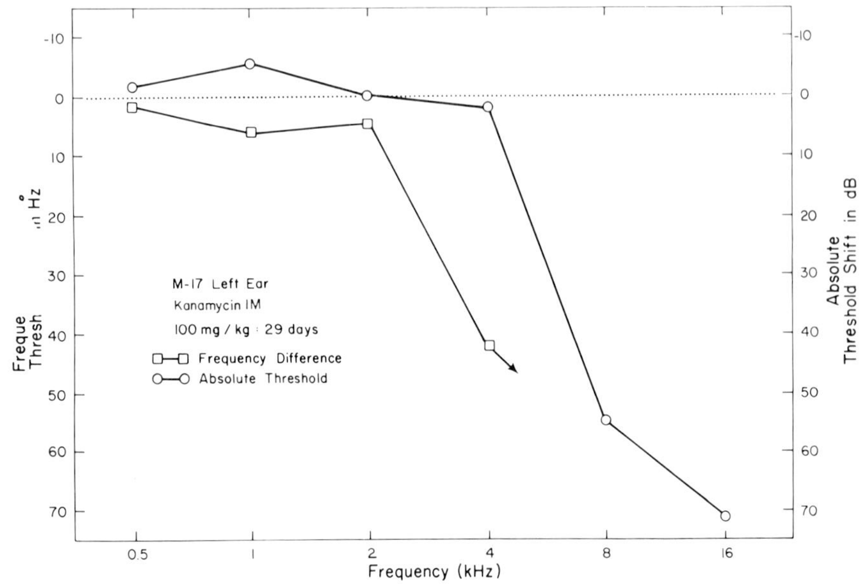

Figure 1-12. Changes in absolute auditory threshold and frequency difference threshold in a macaque monkey treated with kanamycin. (From W. C. Stebbins et al., Noise- and Drug-Induced Hearing Loss in Monkeys. In J. E. Hawkins, Jr., and M. Lawrence [Eds.], *Advances in Otorhinolaryngology: Otophysiology.* Basel: Karger, 1973. Reprinted by permission.)

treatment of human tuberculosis. This is one of the few known species-specific reactions to a drug. Closely related taxa such as the vervet, which has somewhat similar ecologic demands, show no such reaction. In macaques treated with daily doses of 100 mg/kg for as long as 8 months, hearing remained unchanged. An explanation of this unique and interesting finding has not been forthcoming [4].

Absolute threshold procedures by themselves can be expected to give only a partial account of hearing impairment, since much of our normal hearing takes place well above minimum detectable levels. Differential resolution of sound frequency and intensity, loudness perception, frequency analysis, and localization of sound sources are all different aspects of the hearing process, which may be affected quite differently by ototoxic drugs and may reveal new and complementary information about ototoxicity. Slight modifications of existing behavioral conditioning procedures permit examination of one or another of these acoustic functions. We typically measure two such functions simultaneously in a single animal.

A monkey tested for absolute pure-tone threshold and then for its ability to distinguish between two acoustic frequencies (frequency difference threshold) was treated with kanamycin and tested daily for both functions. In the course of treatment, it was noted that the breakdown in frequency resolution preceded the threshold loss. Figure 1-12 shows that, after 29 days, the frequency difference threshold when tested at 4 kHz was shifted by more than 40 Hz while the absolute threshold was still normal. This effect is currently under further investigation.

We have also measured absolute thresholds and intensity difference thresholds on the guinea pig before and after kanamycin treatment. The characteristic increase in absolute threshold after drug treatment was noted. We found, however, a very clear decrease in the differential intensive threshold [8], measured at the same sensation level before and after the shift in absolute threshold. This finding has also been reported under conditions of hearing impairment in man. If, however, the differential intensive threshold is measured at the same sound pressure level, no change is seen [8].

The inability to make normal loudness judgments in the presence of sensorineural hearing loss is known as loudness recruitment. In our laboratory, we recently developed a nonhuman primate model for measurement of loudness recruitment. Animals are trained as described previously to respond to sound; but, additionally, in order to be reinforced with food they must respond in a fraction of a second. We have noted that the dynamic range of hearing may then be represented in an animal subject by an orderly function relating latency of response to the sound pressure level of the stimulus (see Fig. 1-13). Latency or reaction time to an acoustic stimulus then provides a suitable measure for the evaluation of loudness perception, and hence of loudness recruitment, in nonverbal subjects. Pfingst and colleagues [7] have measured loudness perception in normal human subjects by traditional verbal instruction procedures as well as by the reaction time method. We have also used both procedures to measure loudness recruitment in patients with monaural (the other ear serves as a control) sensorineural hearing loss. In each instance, the two procedures yield comparable findings.

In Fig. 1-14, successive reaction time functions are plotted for a patas monkey after the termination of dihydrostreptomycin treatment. The increase in threshold at 8 kHz is clearly seen, together with the development of recruitment, as the drug continues to exert its effect long after the end of treatment. The final stable patterns of threshold and recruitment are seen in the function on the extreme right. The dynamic range has almost collapsed, and normal hearing, indicated by unchanged response latencies, remains only at the highest sound levels tested. Threshold functions immediately after the end of treatment (top function) and more than 3 months later (bottom function) are presented in Fig. 1-15. The threshold values at 8 kHz may be compared with the previous figure; both were obtained at the relatively low drug dose of 20 mg/kg, which is equivalent to that formerly used clinically. Measures of loudness together with absolute threshold yield a more complete picture of drug-induced hearing loss, particularly in its dynamic, rapidly changing phase.

Intense noise, like the aminoglycosides, can leave a permanent and devastating effect on hearing and the inner ear, depending, of course, on its level and duration. Its use in experimental animals provides an instructive comparison with the ototoxic drugs. There are similarities in the effects of noise and

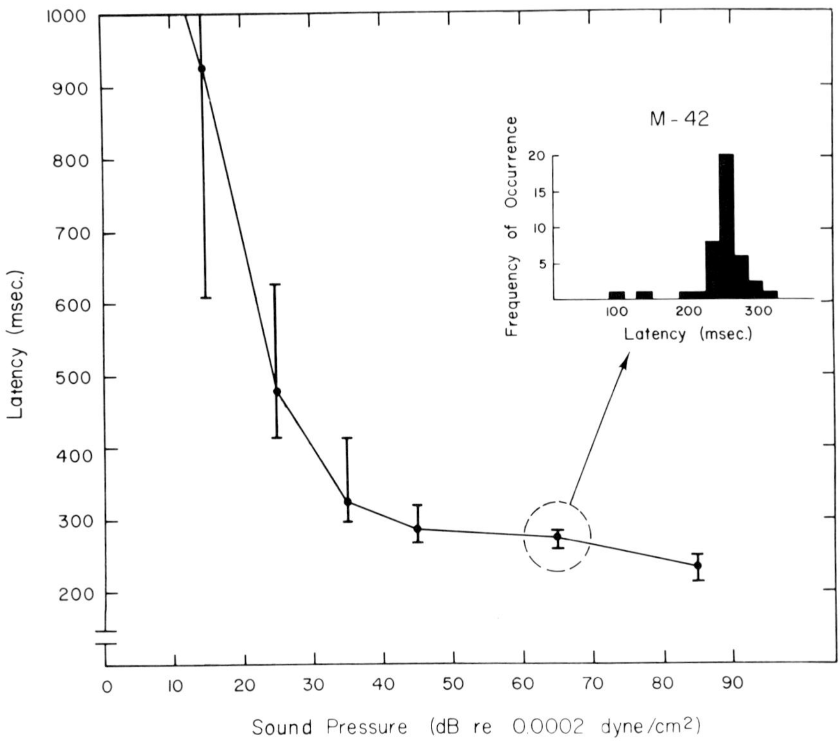

Figure 1-13. Reaction time (medians) as a function of stimulus intensity for one macaque monkey. Vertical lines indicate semi-interquartile ranges. *Inset*: Frequency distribution of reaction times at 65 dB SPL, obtained from the reaction time-stimulus intensity function. (From W. C. Stebbins et al., Sensory Processes in Animals. In I. Darian-Smith [Ed.] with J. Brookhart and V. B. Mountcastle [Section Eds.], *Handbook of Physiology, Sensory Processes* [Vol. 1]. Washington, D.C.: American Physiological Society. In press. Reprinted by permission.)

the antibiotics on hearing and the inner ear; yet differences are observed in their site of action, both with regard to the acoustic frequencies at which hearing is impaired and the site of damage to the organ of Corti. As an example, in Fig. 1-16 we see reaction time functions for a monkey after exposure to an octave band of noise centered at 2 kHz. The hearing loss is permanent and is greatest at 4 kHz, where considerable recruitment is evident. The corresponding threshold function and related cytocochleogram are shown in Fig. 1-17.

We are presently looking at other aspects of normal auditory processing with an eye toward developing new and different baselines for studies of impaired hearing in animal models. One such aspect is that of sound localization, which requires central mediation and may be relatively unaffected by agents such as drugs or noise that seem to affect primarily the auditory periphery. The ability to localize sound in space is an important characteristic

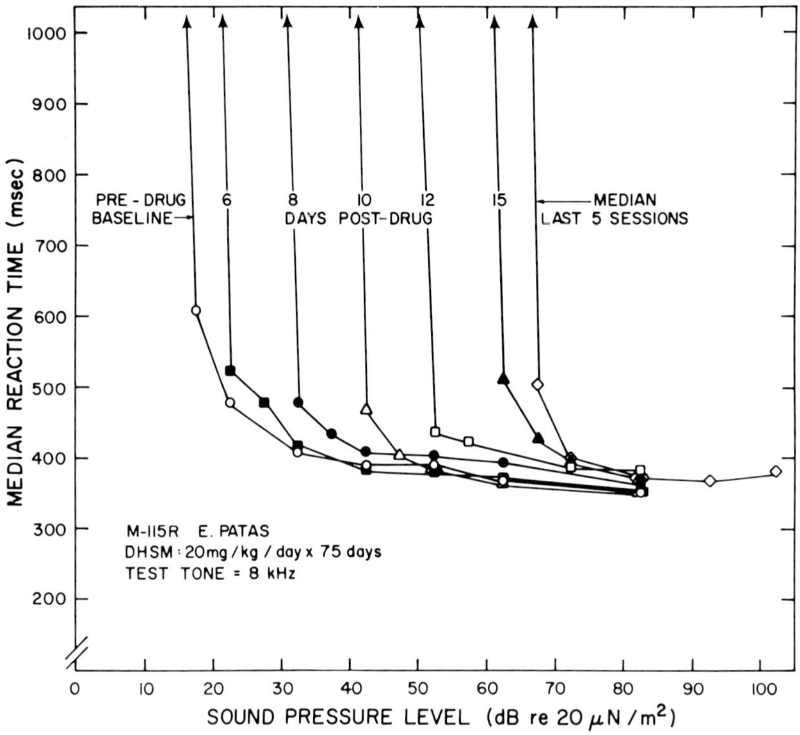

Figure 1-14. Reaction time-stimulus intensity functions at 8 kHz for a patas monkey treated with dihydrostreptomycin. The functions were obtained before and at various times after drug treatment. (From W. C. Stebbins and D. B. Moody, Comparative behavioral toxicology. *Neurobehav. Toxicol.* 1[Suppl.]:33, 1979. Reprinted by permission.)

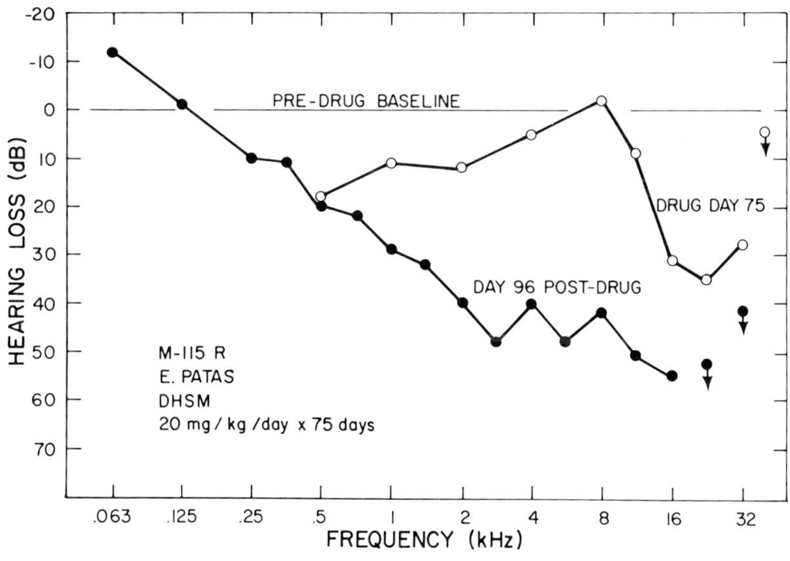

Figure 1-15. Auditory threshold shift for the monkey represented in Fig. 1-14. The upper curve shows the threshold shift at the end of drug treatment; the lower curve was obtained more than 3 months following the end of drug treatment. (From W. C. Stebbins and D. B. Moody, Comparative behavioral toxicology. *Neurobehav. Toxicol.* 1[Suppl.]:33, 1979. Reprinted by permission.)

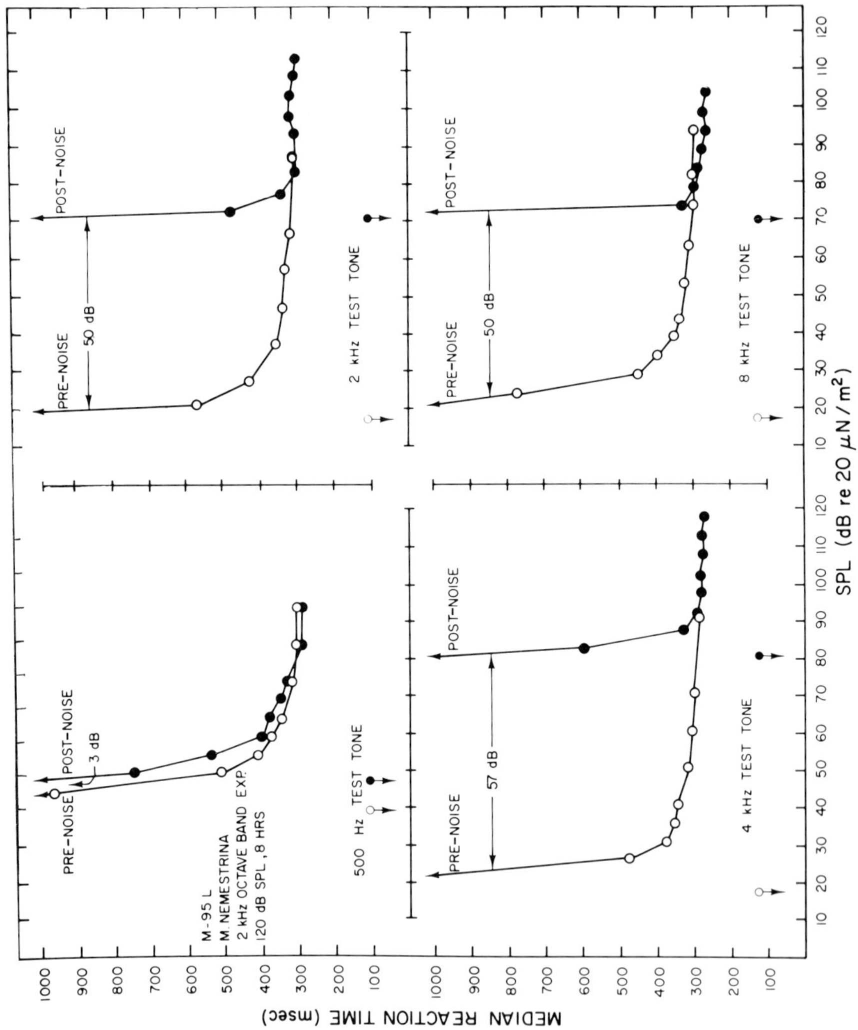
MEDIAN REACTION TIME (msec)
SPL (dB re 20 μN/m²)
PRE-NOISE
POST-NOISE
3 dB
M-95 L
M. NEMESTRINA
2 kHz OCTAVE BAND EXP.
120 dB SPL, 8 HRS
500 Hz TEST TONE
50 dB
2 kHz TEST TONE
57 dB
4 kHz TEST TONE
50 dB
8 kHz TEST TONE

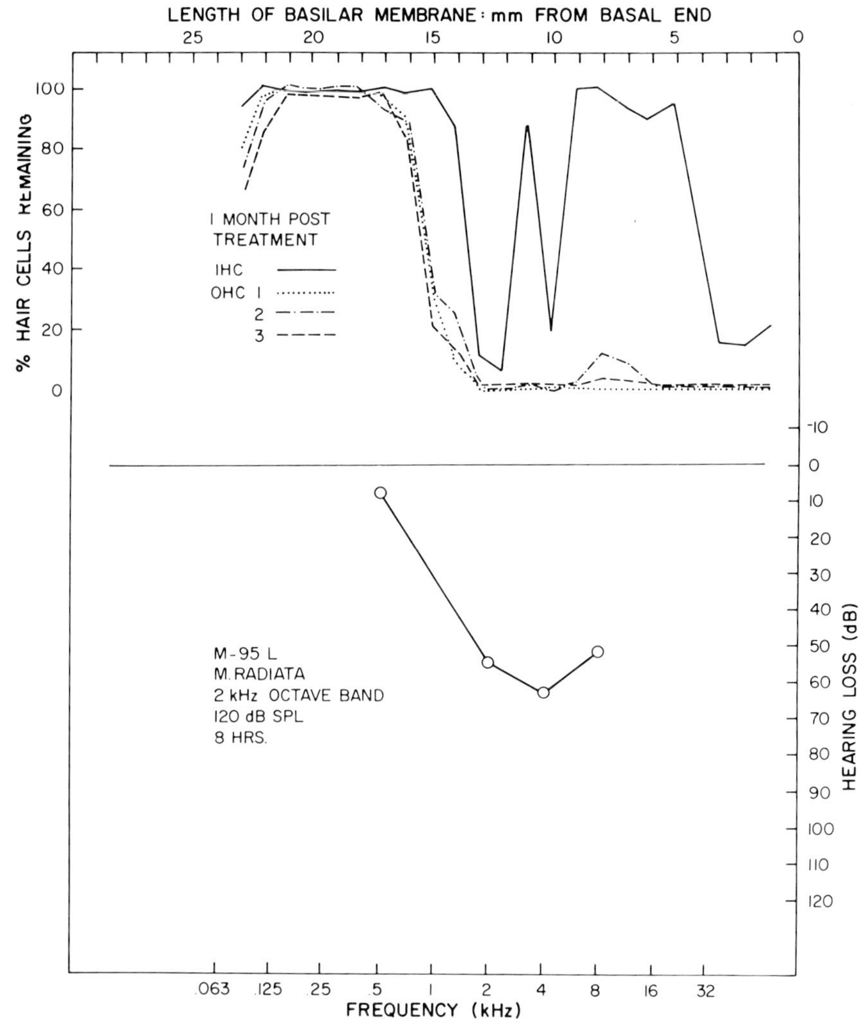

Figure 1-17. Auditory threshold shift (lower panel) and cytocochleogram (upper panel) for the monkey whose reaction time data are shown in Fig. 1-16. (From W. C. Stebbins and D. B. Moody, Comparative behavioral toxicology. *Neurobehav. Toxicol.* 1[Suppl.]:33, 1979. Reprinted by permission.)

Figure 1-16. Reaction time-stimulus intensity functions for a macaque monkey at four test tone frequencies, before and after exposure to noise. Arrows near abscissa indicate pre- and postexposure thresholds at these test tone frequencies. (From W. C. Stebbins and D. B. Moody, Comparative behavioral toxicology. *Neurobehav. Toxicol.* 1[Suppl.]:33, 1979. Reprinted by permission.)

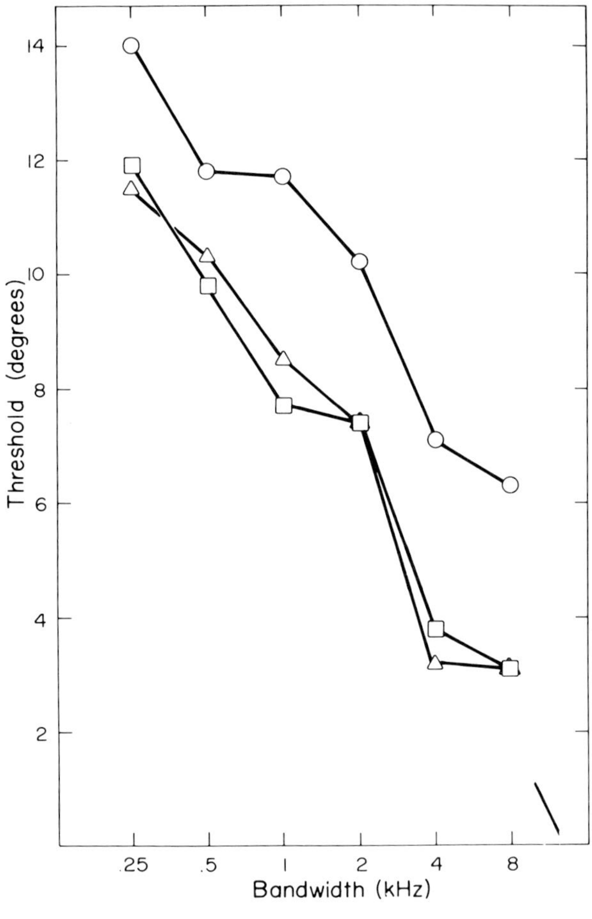

Figure 1-18. Threshold for sound localization (in degrees of arc) as a function of the bandwidth of an acoustic stimulus for three macaque monkeys. (From W. C. Stebbins, Hearing of the Primates. In D. Chivers and J. Herbert [Eds.], *Recent Advances in Primatology: Primate Behavior.* London: Academic, 1978. Copyright by Academic Press Inc. [London] Ltd. Reprinted by permission.)

of the binaural auditory system and is perhaps the most important in an evolutionary sense. It has probably been the focus of one of the most persistent selection pressures on the evolving vertebrate auditory system [5]. With little change in basic technique, animals can easily be trained to report a change in the location of a sound in space so that localization thresholds (minimum audible angle) can be determined. Localization accuracy is shown in Fig. 1-18, for three monkeys, to be a function of the bandwidth of the signal. The ability to localize sound is enhanced as the noise band is widened and the amount of spectral information is increased [3].

Physiologic tuning curves provide a measure of frequency analysis in the

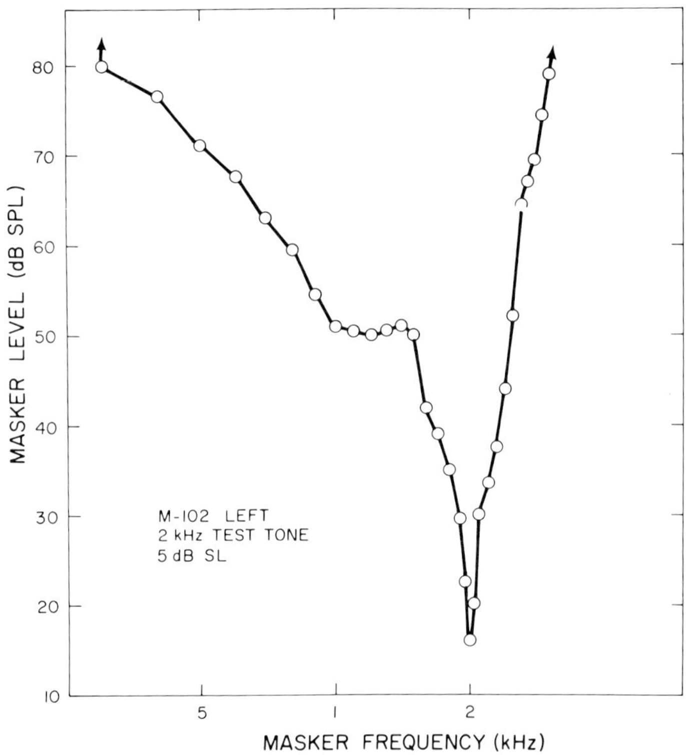

Figure 1-19. Psychophysical tuning curve for a macaque monkey. The test tone was at 2 kHz, 5 dB above threshold. (From W. C. Stebbins and D. B. Moody, Comparative behavioral toxicology. *Neurobehav. Toxicol.* 1[Suppl.]:33, 1979. Reprinted by permission.)

peripheral auditory system. Psychophysical tuning curves determined by tone-on-tone masking procedures bear a striking resemblance to physiologic tuning curves and may tell us something about the changes in this important function which occur with hearing loss as a consequence of noise exposure or drug treatment. In Fig. 1-19, a psychophysical tuning curve is presented for the macaque monkey [12]. Similar results have been reported for man [22] and for the chinchilla [6]. Such results hold considerable promise for comparison with other measures such as the frequency difference threshold in studies of hearing disorders.

Finally, in evaluating impaired hearing function after treatment with ototoxic drugs, we have tried to illustrate the efficacy and versatility of modern automated behavioral experiments with animals. There are very few significant questions regarding sensory experience that cannot be asked of properly schooled animal subjects. Histologic studies serve as a critical complement to these behavioral studies in charting the relationship between hearing loss and cochlear pathology. Although electrophysiologic measures provide an important supplement to the behavioral data, they should not be regarded as a substitute for them.

The basic conditioning techniques are adaptable to a wide variety of potential animal models and can serve in many and diverse hearing testing paradigms. They are expensive and time-consuming by traditional standards of finger-snap, Preyer reflex audiometry, but for the information they can provide there are no known available alternatives.

References

1. Bernard, C. *Introduction à l'Étude de la Médecine Expérimentale.* Paris: Baillière, 1865. (Transl. by H. C. Greene. New York: H. Schuman, 1949.)
2. Blough, D. S. A method for obtaining psychophysical thresholds from the pigeon. *J. Exp. Anal. Behav.* 1:31, 1958.
3. Brown, C. H., Beecher, M. D., Moody, D. B., and Stebbins, W. C. Localization of noise bands by old world monkeys. *J. Acoust. Soc. Am.* 68:127, 1980.
4. Hawkins, J. E., Jr., Stebbins, W. C., Johnsson, L-G., Moody, D. B., and Muraski, A. The patas monkey as a model for dihydrostreptomycin ototoxicity. *Acta Otolaryngol.* 83:123, 1977.
5. Masterton, R. B., Heffner, H., and Ravizza, R. The evolution of human hearing. *J. Acoust. Soc. Am.* 45:966, 1969.
6. McGee, T., Ryan, A., and Dallos, P. Psychophysical tuning curves of chinchillas. *J. Acoust. Soc. Am.* 50:1146, 1976.
7. Pfingst, B. E., Hienz, R., Kimm, J., and Miller, J. Reaction time procedure for measurement of hearing. I. Suprathreshold functions. *J. Acoust. Soc. Am.* 57:421, 1975.
8. Prosen, C. A., Moody, D. B., Stebbins, W. C., and Hawkins, J. E., Jr. Absolute and intensity difference thresholds in the guinea pig after cochlear injury by kanamycin and amikacin. Presented at the winter meeting of the Association for Research in Otolaryngology, St. Petersburg, Florida, 1980.
9. Prosen, C. A., Petersen, M. R., Moody, D. B., and Stebbins, W. C. Auditory thresholds and kanamycin-induced hearing loss in the guinea pig assessed by a positive reinforcement procedure. *J. Acoust. Soc. Am.* 63:559, 1978.
10. Prosen, C. A., and Stebbins, W. C. Ototoxicity. In P. S. Spencer and H. H. Schaumburg (Eds.), *Experimental and Clinical Neurotoxicology.* Baltimore: Williams & Wilkins, 1980. Pp. 62–76.
11. Ryan, A., and Dallos, P. Effect of absence of cochlear outer hair cells on behavioural auditory thresholds. *Nature* 253:44, 1975.
12. Serafin, J. V., Moody, D. B., and Stebbins, W. C. Psychophysical tuning curves in monkeys. *J. Acoust. Soc. Am.* 63:S30, 1978.
13. Skinner, B. F. *The Behavior of Organisms.* New York: Appleton-Century-Crofts, 1938.
14. Stebbins, W. C. (Ed.). *Animal Psychophysics: The Design and Conduct of Sensory Experiments.* New York: Appleton-Century-Crofts, 1970.
15. Stebbins, W. C. Studies of Hearing and Hearing Loss in the Monkey. In W. C. Stebbins (Ed.), *Animal Psychophysics: The Design and Conduct of Sensory Experiments.* New York: Appleton-Century-Crofts, 1970. Pp. 41–66.
16. Stebbins, W. C. Hearing of the Primates. In D. Chivers and J. Herbert (Eds.), *Recent Advances in Primatology: Primate Behavior.* London: Academic, 1978. Vol. 1, pp. 703–720.
17. Stebbins, W. C., Brown, C. H., and Petersen, M. R. Sensory Processes in Animals. In I. Darian-Smith (Ed.) with J. Brookhart and V. B. Mountcastle (Section Eds.),

Handbook of Physiology, Sensory Processes (Vol. 1). Washington, D.C.: American Physiological Society. In press.
18. Stebbins, W. C., Clark, W. W., Pearson, R. D., and Weiland, N. G. Noise- and drug-induced hearing loss in monkeys. *Adv. Oto-Rino-Laryngol.* (Basel) 20:42, 1973.
19. Stebbins, W. C., and Coombs, S. Behavioral Assessment of Ototoxicity in Nonhuman Primates. In B. Weiss and V. G. Laties (Eds.), *Behavioral Toxicology.* New York: Plenum, 1976. Pp. 401–427.
20. Stebbins, W. C., Miller, J. M., Johnsson, L-G., and Hawkins, J. E., Jr. Ototoxic hearing loss and cochlear pathology in the monkey. *Trans. Am. Otolaryngol. Soc.* 57:110, 1969.
21. Stebbins, W. C., and Moody, D. B. Comparative behavioral toxicology. *Neurobehav. Toxicol.* 1[Suppl.]:33, 1979.
22. Zwicker, E. On a Psychoacoustical Equivalent of Tuning Curves. In E. Zwicker and E. Terhardt (Eds.), *Facts and Models in Hearing.* New York: Springer, 1974. Pp. 132–141.

Discussion of Chapter 1

Dr. Lerner: Do you monitor renal function and check serum levels during the course of aminoglycoside treatment?

Dr. Stebbins: Yes, we have taken blood and perilymph samples, and we regularly check renal function.

Dr. Brummett: One of the interesting things about the patas monkey is its sensitivity to dihydrostreptomycin. Have you investigated whether there is any difference in the pharmacokinetics of dihydrostreptomycin in the patas and the rhesus monkey?

Dr. Stebbins: We haven't observed any obvious differences between the two species. The difference that we do see is in the amount of drug remaining in the perilymph, which is determined when the animal is killed.

Dr. Brummett: Were these drugs given for 1 day or over a period of time?

Dr. Stebbins: They were given over an extended period.

Dr. Igarashi: In my limited experience with experiments on ototoxic drugs, when we used the reward paradigm, we had a problem because the animals would become sick from the drugs and were not interested in reward or reinforcement. If you have made a comparison between the two paradigms, reward and shock avoidance, what are the advantages and what are the disadvantages? Also, I would like to know about your criterion for onset of the hearing deficit for the rhesus monkey, cat, and guinea pig. How much hearing loss is considered abnormal?

Dr. Stebbins: With regard to the problem of using food reinforcement procedures, we have had only two or three animals (out of 70) that were not testable for a brief period during drug administration. The reason we tend to stay away from shock avoidance tests is that the experimental animals become highly emotional and are very difficult to handle during shock avoidance, and sometimes they stop working in the experimental situation. Often you will read in reports on shock avoidance procedures that the experimenter had to eliminate half of the subjects because they wouldn't respond in the testing situation. It has been our experience that shock avoidance procedures yield results which are more variable than those obtained under positive reinforcement.

In answer to the question of onset time of hearing loss for the macaque monkey, cat, and guinea pig, there are fairly sizable individual differences, making it difficult to give a single figure for any species.

With regard to the degree of hearing loss considered abnormal, we would judge a 10-dB change significant. Animals are tested daily, which allows the hearing loss to be detected as soon as it occurs.

Dr. Federspil: How many patas monkeys have you studied? Have you done the comparison with rhesus monkeys simultaneously? Also, are you sure that there is not a special species sensitivity of the kidneys of these monkeys to the drugs?

Dr. Stebbins: In the particular experiment described, we treated 7 patas monkeys and 6 macaques at dose levels ranging from 20 mg/kg up to 100 mg/kg of dihydrostreptomycin. We saw a very slight hearing loss in one macaque after 8 months, but no hair cell loss. All the other macaques were unaffected by the drug. In contrast, all the patas monkeys were severely impaired.

The patas monkey is an African monkey that lives very close to the desert. His water intake is much less than that of the macaques, which live in a heavily forested, more humid environment. We thought that this ecological difference might implicate the kidneys and account for the difference in the ototoxic effects of the drug. We have since looked at the vervet monkey, which lives in circumstances very similar to those of the patas, but we haven't found the same sensitivity to dihydrostreptomycin as we observed in the patas.

Dr. Wersäll: I am very impressed by the behavioral studies you have done, especially after working with shock avoidance behavioral methods. It probably takes a good deal of time to do this kind of study. How many animals, such as guinea pigs, can you handle at a time in order to study variations of drug toxicity? A time-consuming study will limit the possibility of using large groups of animals.

Dr. Stebbins: That is a good point. These are not techniques set up for large-scale screening of ototoxic antibiotics. On the other hand, screening techniques for large numbers of animals simply do not offer the same degree of resolution, accuracy, and reliability as the positive reinforcement operant conditioning procedures.

Dr. Lietman: I am interested in the possible genetic difference of the patas monkey from other species. You really didn't answer the question about renal function. Is the kidney different in the patas monkey with regard to its susceptibility to aminoglycoside toxicity?

Dr. Stebbins: We don't know the answer to that question. It needs to be followed up by an interested renal physiologist.

Dr. Lietman: I thought you said there was a difference in the response or sensitivity to kanamycin compared to dihydrostreptomycin.

Dr. Stebbins: I was referring to the kanamycin-treated macaque compared to the dihydrostreptomycin-treated patas monkey. The typical macaque monkey's reaction to kanamycin treatment is loss of both inner and outer hair cells in equal amounts. I showed in one illustration a cochlea denuded of both inner and outer hair cells in the basal half, with normal-appearing hair cells in the apical part. In the patas monkey's reaction to dihydrostreptomycin treatment, like the guinea pig's reaction to kanamycin, there seem to be inner hair cells still remaining in much of the basal region of the cochlea, and yet the outer hair cells are completely gone.

Dr. Hawkins: The thought occurred to us that perhaps the patas monkey is the animal of choice for testing of aminoglycoside ototoxicity because of the small doses of dihydrostreptomycin required to produce ototoxic injury. This is the first animal species I know of that has shown a sensitivity greater than that of human subjects to the ototoxicity of any aminoglycoside.

We tried kanamycin in the patas monkey, and there was no difference from the reaction of the macaque. Therefore, the patas monkey has a special sensitivity, not to all aminoglycosides, but rather to dihydrostreptomycin specifically. In years of experience in attempting to develop an animal model for dihydrostreptomycin, I have never succeeded with any other species in getting any reliable reaction to dihydrostreptomycin. Cats, guinea pigs, and rats generally showed perfectly normal hearing regardless of the length of time of treatment.

2. Electrophysiology of Cochlear Toxicity

Jean-Marie Aran

Clinical observations in man [37], confirmed by behavioral measurements in animals, provided the first evidence of impaired hearing following treatment with aminoglycoside antibiotics. Histopathologic studies and electrophysiologic measurements, made as early as 1949 [13, 32], demonstrated the specific action of aminoglycosides on the structure and function of the cochlea. Such measurements are currently being used for the evaluation of newly developed aminoglycosides [9, 10, 12, 16, 20, 34, 35, 36] as well as for the study of the mechanisms involved in ototoxicity. In addition, research has focused on suitable methods of producing aminoglycosides with excellent antibacterial efficacy, but with low ototoxicity.

One of the goals in studies of the inner ear has been to find some morphologic changes and functional deficits associated with specific drug treatment. But the data indicate that hearing loss caused by ototoxic drugs follows very much the same course as sensorineural loss produced by noise or other injuries unrelated to drugs [27]. Many investigators have exploited these ototoxic agents in order to create a structural modification of the receptor, thereby producing specific functional changes which could lead to a more complete understanding of various physiologic phenomena. All of these approaches are interrelated. The histopathologic observations are discussed elsewhere in this book; we will review here some of the electrophysiologic data gathered during the past 30 years.

In 1930, Wever and Bray [55] recorded an electrical signal in the vicinity of the cochlea which reproduced the waveform of the stimulating sound. It became clear that this response, aptly named the cochlear microphonic potential (CM), originated inside the cochlea [1]. The demonstration that the CM is produced by vibration of the hair cells of the organ of Corti [22] accompanied

The author wishes to thank Y. Cazals, J-P. Erre, and A. Guilhaume for their participation in the studies presented here. The author is very grateful to Robert V. Harrison for his helpful comments. This work was supported by INSERM Grant 8ASR6—Oreille Interne.

the observation that no CM could be recorded when the hair cells were profoundly altered. It was Hawkins [32] who noticed, some 3 decades ago, that the CM was markedly reduced in cats treated with streptomycin. Davis et al., in 1958 [21], demonstrated in guinea pigs that the CM is essentially produced by the outer hair cells—a conclusion based on the observation that streptomycin damages the outer hair cells and that the CM was markedly reduced in these animals.

In a detailed study of the basic peripheral physiologic mechanisms, the selective impairment of outer hair cells obtained in different locations along the basilar membrane after specified doses of aminoglycosides [19] provided information on the contribution of populations of hair cells not only to the CM, but also to the direct current (DC) response to sound, i.e., the summating potential (SP). In 1976, Dallos and Cheatham [17] gave 400 mg/kg of kanamycin per day subcutaneously to guinea pigs for 10 and 15 days. Three weeks after treatment, these cochleas had massive loss of outer hair cells and a normal population of inner hair cells at the base; at the apex, however, there was extensive loss of inner hair cells with preservation of outer hair cells. In most of the animals, the CM and SP were normal in areas where outer hair cells were still present, even if the inner hair cells were totally destroyed; both potentials were markedly reduced in areas where only inner hair cells remained.

In evaluation of the damage caused by ototoxic drugs, CM measurements, together with observations on the Preyer reflex and histopathologic counts of hair cells, have commonly been used. The amplitude of the CM response as a function of the frequency of the stimulating pure tone, or the isopotential intensity-frequency function, has been construed to reflect the localization of hair cells along the basilar membrane. In the study of CM, a differential recording procedure (scala tympani vs. scala vestibuli) is the method of choice, since responses from restricted portions along the basilar membrane can be registered. Recording of CM by means of a single electrode on the round window membrane may be technically simpler, but the results are complicated by the fact that the microphonic potentials originate in different sites along the basilar membrane. Also, the basal coil of the cochlea, which is nearest the electrode, produces a CM response to all frequencies.

Although the loss in CM amplitude can be related to destruction of outer hair cells, little information about the inner hair cells can be obtained from CM measurements, since they contribute minimally to the CM. Thus, it would be difficult to differentiate, on the basis of CM alone, between loss of outer hair cells in the basal coil of the cochlea and more extensive loss involving both outer and inner hair cells, which occurs after intensive treatment with aminoglycosides. As is apparent from the data on neural responses, the functional conditions of the cochleas in these two cases are different.

Endocochlear Resting Potential

The endocochlear resting potential (EP) is dependent on the metabolic mechanisms inside the cochlear compartments. The EP changes rapidly, as do the neural responses, during anoxia or with ionic changes, both conditions being closely related. On the other hand, it is not affected by the absence of outer and inner hair cells brought on by drugs or in a hereditary disorder [40]. Konishi, however, reported in 1967 [41] and, in more detail, in 1979 [40] that the amplitude of the EP, which is normal in such diseased guinea pigs without hair cells, does not decline as rapidly during anoxia as it does in a normal cochlea with functioning hair cells. He also demonstrated that the K^+ and Na^+ concentrations in endolymph changed in a similar manner during anoxia whether or not hair cells were present. His observations suggested a correlation between the K^+ conductance of the organ of Corti and EP changes during anoxia. We have made a similar observation of a much slower decline of the EP during anoxia in guinea pigs severely impaired after kanamycin treatment, which we, too, related to the absence of outer hair cells [2]. The EP has also been analyzed extensively in experiments on the combined effects of aminoglycoside antibiotics and cochleotoxic diuretics such as furosemide and ethacrynic acid [11, 50]. These studies demonstrate that the transient alteration associated with administration of the diuretic alone is transformed into a severe and permanent loss of function, with extensive degeneration of hair cells when the antibiotics and diuretics are combined. Following administration of ethacrynic acid alone, both CM and EP decline, but then recover. After the combined administration of ethacrynic acid and kanamycin, however, the CM declines without recovery. The time pattern of the EP changes, on the other hand, is not modified, thus again demonstrating that the EP is not dependent on the presence of hair cells.

Compound Auditory Nerve Action Potential

Compound auditory nerve action potentials (CAP) have not been used extensively in the evaluation of drug ototoxicity. However, the transient evoked compound eighth nerve action potential, recorded with an electrode on the cochlea (usually on the round window, as for CM), appears in this instance to be a precise indicator of cochlear function.

The CAP response is made up of the complex waveform of the spike discharges (expressed at the recording site) and by the distribution in time of the discharges in all of the fibers of the auditory nerve [28]. Whereas the study of single fiber activity is fundamental in the investigation of cochlear function, the overall function of the end organ is more easily approached by the study of the CAP response, whose characteristics are closely related to the time pattern of the acoustic stimulus and to the distribution of the stimulated neurons along the basilar membrane. In my experience, this compound response is most useful in the study of drug ototoxicity for a variety of reasons. We found, for example, that this response could provide information which hitherto had been sought primarily by means of the cochlear microphonic.

It is easy to measure a frequency threshold curve for CAP by using filtered clicks, tone pips, or tone bursts. One can distinguish between the presence or absence of a CAP response, whereas the CM only measures isopotential curves. Furthermore, the origin of the CAP, near the threshold, can be inferred from measurement of the response latencies [4]. One can employ a change in latency to determine the site of an anatomic lesion. In such cases, the frequency threshold curve is less sensitive, since the responses to a given sound may originate from different regions along the basilar membrane.

Figure 2-1 shows results of measurements on two guinea pigs with antibiotic-impaired cochleas and includes frequency threshold curves, frequency-latency functions, and histocochleograms. Sixty-seven days after 14 intramuscular injections of 150 mg/kg of amikacin, guinea pig A305 (Fig. 2-1A) had massive loss of outer hair cells in the basal part of the cochlea. The frequency threshold curve shows a threshold elevation at high frequencies. For these high frequencies, the latencies are longer than those of normal animals, indicating that the responses observed at threshold originate in a remote area on the basilar membrane, toward the upper turns. The second animal (GP A297) (Fig. 2-1B), which received a higher dose of amikacin (14 × 300 mg/kg) and was studied 54 days after treatment, presents a typical pattern of hair cell loss: outer hair cells are entirely absent at the base, but there is a large proportion of surviving inner hair cells. The opposite occurs toward the apex; there is an abrupt loss of inner hair cells, with some outer hair cells remaining; in a portion of the second and third rows, near the apex, outer hair cells are also present. Although we observed a rather flat frequency threshold curve, there is an abrupt change in the latencies of the latency-frequency function from 2.0 to 2.5 kHz. Above this frequency, the latencies are constant, indicating that the responses must come from the base of the cochlea, where only inner hair cells remain.

These examples demonstrate that frequency threshold curves or latency-frequency functions alone are not sufficient to provide a meaningful indication of the condition of outer and inner hair cells in different parts of the basilar membrane. Both must be considered conjointly.

Another example is taken from guinea pigs having a very slight impairment of CAP after prolonged but low-level treatment with sisomicin (67 × 37.5 mg/kg, 1 month after the end of treatment) (Figs. 2-2 and 2-3). The impairment observed in the threshold is confined to the higher frequencies. Little change in latency is evident.

Thus, place information can be inferred from the latency of neural responses. Identical latency changes may be expected in any electrophysiologic response, whatever its origin along the auditory pathway. The variability of latency measurements, however, increases rapidly with increases in latency; that is, when the origin of the response is more centrally located in the auditory system. Small latency changes between excitation at the cochlear base and excitation at the apex (traveling wave delay), of the order of 5 msec in guinea pigs, cannot be measured accurately on late responses.

On the other hand, CAP recordings at various sound intensities are suitable for investigation of the dynamics of the ear, through the use of input-output functions for amplitude and latency. Information related to the functioning of the outer and inner hair cells can be obtained from these procedures. For example, in some experiments, it seemed plausible to relate a part of the

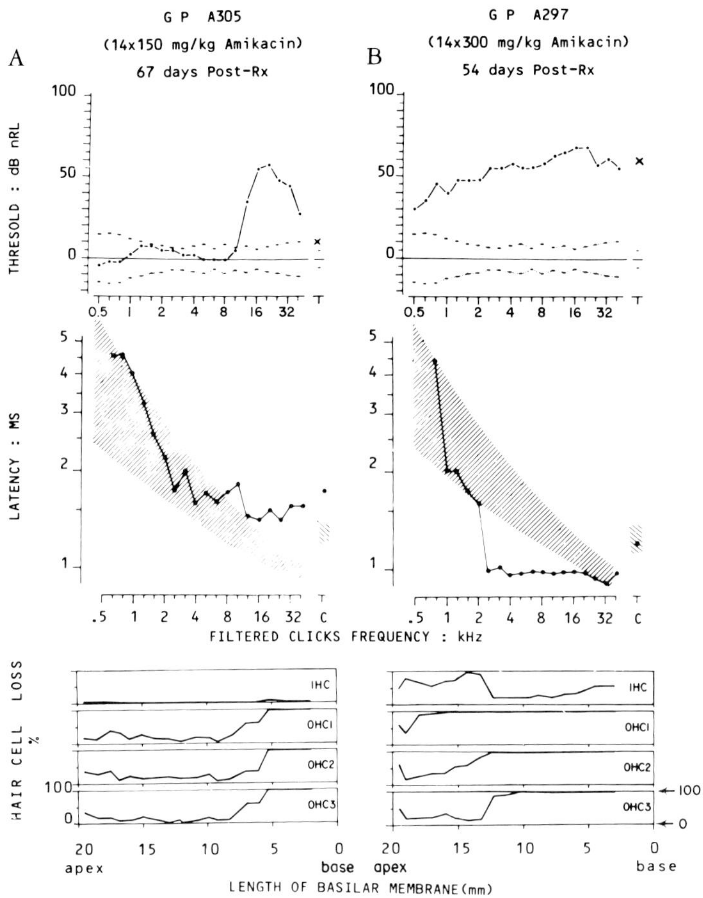

Figure 2-1. Comparison of frequency threshold curves of CAP responses to filtered clicks and to unfiltered click (C) (dashed curves enclose normal range) with latency-frequency functions of these CAP responses near threshold (hatched areas represent normal range), and with histocochleograms (% of hair cell *loss* from base [0 mm] to apex) in two guinea pigs (GP) after two different doses of amikacin. Note the good correlation among the three sets of curves for (A) GP A305 and between latency and histocochleogram for (B) GP A297.

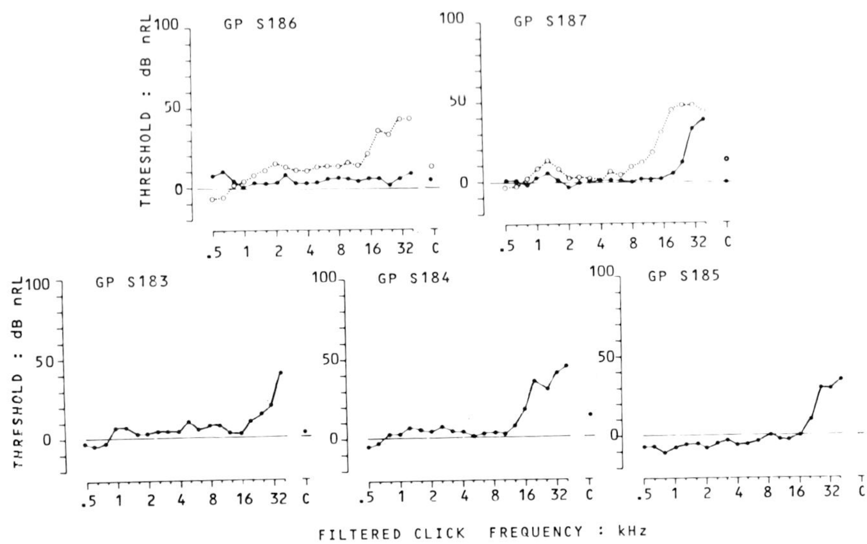

Figure 2-2. Threshold levels of CAP responses to third-octave filtered clicks and to unfiltered click (C) (frequency threshold curves) in five guinea pigs 1 month after sisomicin treatment (67 × 37.5 mg/kg). Solid lines and filled circles (•—•) are values obtained for awake animals. Dotted lines and open circles (○· · ·○), for GP S186 and S187, are values obtained at the time of electrode implantation. All of the guinea pigs except one (S186) had a permanent mild threshold elevation at frequencies above 16 kHz.

responses to outer or inner hair cells simply by observing these responses to the same stimulus, while we could assume that outer and inner hair cells were selectively and successively impaired [7] (Figs. 2-4 to 2-7). Whether those inner hair cells that sometimes remained were functioning normally at the time of the observations is being widely discussed [33].

Chronic Recordings of CM and CAP

Electrophysiologic studies, unlike histologic observations, can be repeated over time, by means of chronically implanted electrodes, thereby allowing precise monitoring of cochlear function after treatment with ototoxic agents [25, 51]. We have developed a technique [8] for recording of CM and CAP for periods up to 1 year after aminoglycoside treatment [2, 5, 7]. In addition, we have employed chronic implantation of auditory cortex and periocular electrodes. These electrodes allow us to monitor auditory function at both peripheral and central levels, and vestibular function is measured by electronystagmographic recordings [23].

We have been able to determine both acute and delayed ototoxicity following high doses of kanamycin when the electrode was implanted on the round window. With this technique, one can measure sudden changes during or

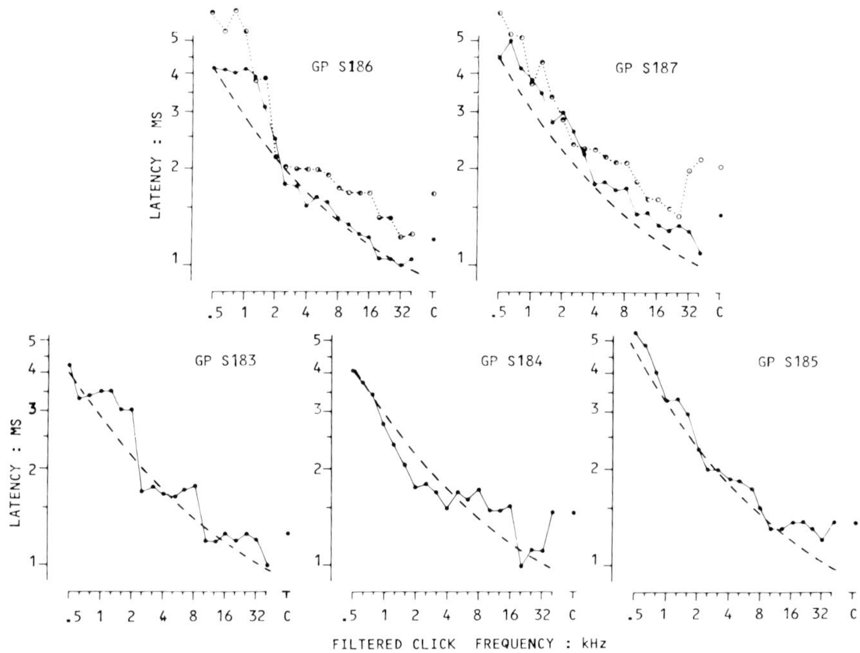

Figure 2-3. Latency-frequency functions determined near threshold in the sisomicin-treated guinea pigs of Fig. 2-2. In some cases, there is only a slight shift in latency at the very high frequencies. (Dashed curves represent normal latency-frequency function; ●—● curves represent values obtained for awake animals; ○···○ curves represent values obtained at the time of electrode implantation; C = unfiltered click).

immediately after treatment (Figs. 2-4A and 2-5A, B) as well as slow but steady alterations in the responses over several months (Figs. 2-4B and 2-5C, D). These observations are in accord with histologic data indicating that ototoxic antibiotics interfere directly with basic cellular mechanisms [29].

In short, chronic electrophysiologic recordings are most suitable for dynamic studies of cochlear toxicity and will, no doubt, serve to bring about a more complete understanding of cochlear mechanisms. They have, however, been used only sparingly, in experiments with higher than therapeutic doses of the drugs (Fig. 2-8).

Another advantage of chronic recordings is that the data are not influenced by the effects of barbiturate anesthesia. The results obtained during anesthesia do not always correlate well with behavioral data obtained on normal animals [47]. We were able to demonstrate, by means of chronically implanted electrodes, some acute deleterious effects of anesthesia and surgery [15]. Furthermore, we have observed slight, but significant, functional impairment which would have been missed had only short-term recordings under anesthesia been obtained (Figs. 2-2 and 2-3). In fact, chronic recordings allow

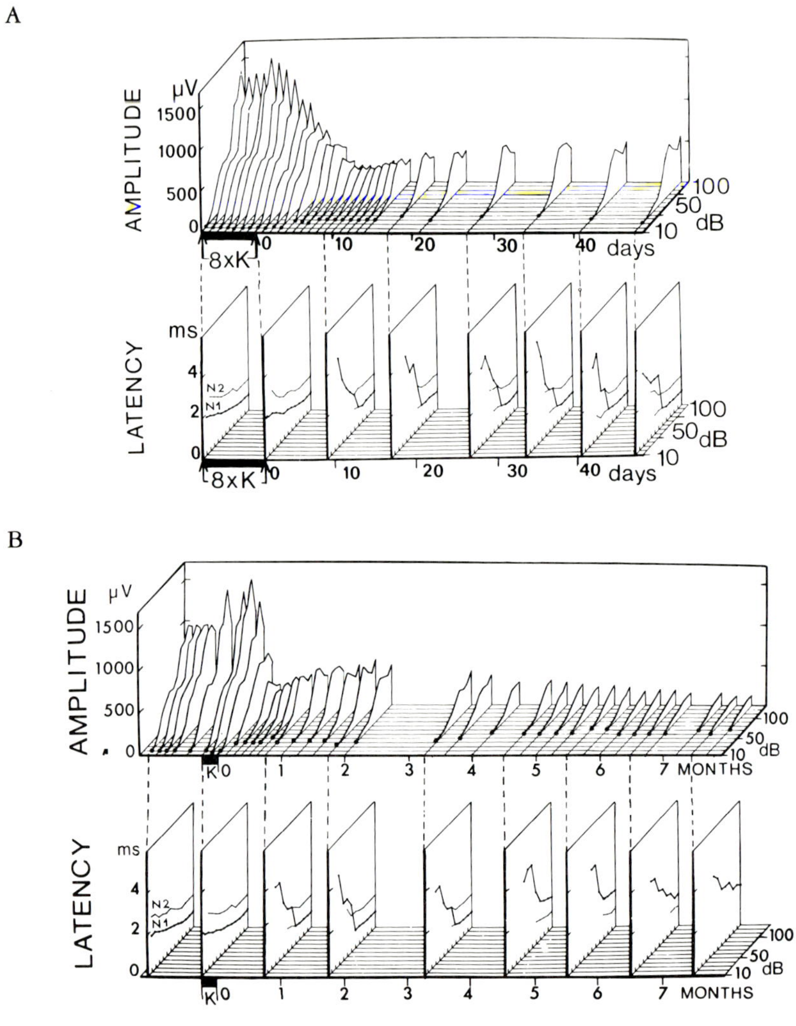

Figure 2-4. Short-term (A) and long-term (B) evolution of CAP input-output amplitude and latency functions in guinea pig 37 during and after kanamycin (K) treatment (8 × 400 mg/kg). (From J-M. Aran and J. Darrouzet, Observation of click-evoked compound VIII nerve responses before, during and over seven months after kanamycin treatment in the guinea pig. *Acta Otolaryngol. [Stockh.]* 79:24, 1975. Reprinted by permission.)

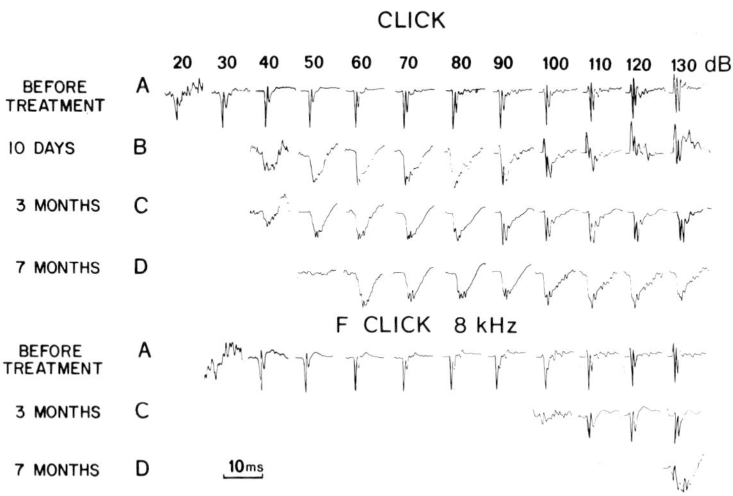

Figure 2-5. Comparison of responses to click and to high-frequency filtered (F) click (8 kHz), in left ear of guinea pig 37 (see Fig. 2-4): before kanamycin treatment (A); at the end of the rapid phase before recovery, about 10 days after treatment (B); 3 months (C); and 7 months (D) after treatment. (Negativity downward. Amplification was adjusted so that the tracings have similar amplitudes; for amplitudes in μV, see Fig. 2-6). At 3 months, outer hair cells at the base of the cochlea are expected to be destroyed, but inner hair cells should still remain [29]; there are still responses to the 8 kHz filtered click. At 7 months, inner and outer hair cells are totally missing at the base (Fig. 2-7), and there is practically no response to the 8 kHz filtered click. (From J.-M. Aran and J. Darrouzet, Observation of click-evoked compound VIII nerve responses before, during and over seven months after kanamycin treatment in the guinea pig. *Acta Otolaryngol. [Stockh.]* 79:24, 1975. Reprinted by permission.)

evaluation of minimal changes in the functional status of the cochlea, which do not seem discernible by light microscopy. These changes may be due to very slight ultrastructural impairment. Finally, such recordings, performed before, during, and after aminoglycoside treatment, serve as their own control—an essential precaution when such modest changes are evaluated.

Single-Unit Recordings

The effects of aminoglycoside treatment have been studied at the basic functional level, i.e., the single cell. These experiments, however, were not concerned primarily with the evaluation of ototoxicity or with the mechanisms involved. Instead, investigators have used the effects of these drugs in order to demonstrate fundamental properties of the cochlea. In particular, these experiments were focused on the changes in threshold and tuning of single fibers associated with outer hair cell loss [18, 30, 31, 38, 39, 49]. Although relatively few such studies have been performed, all except one [18] demonstrated that

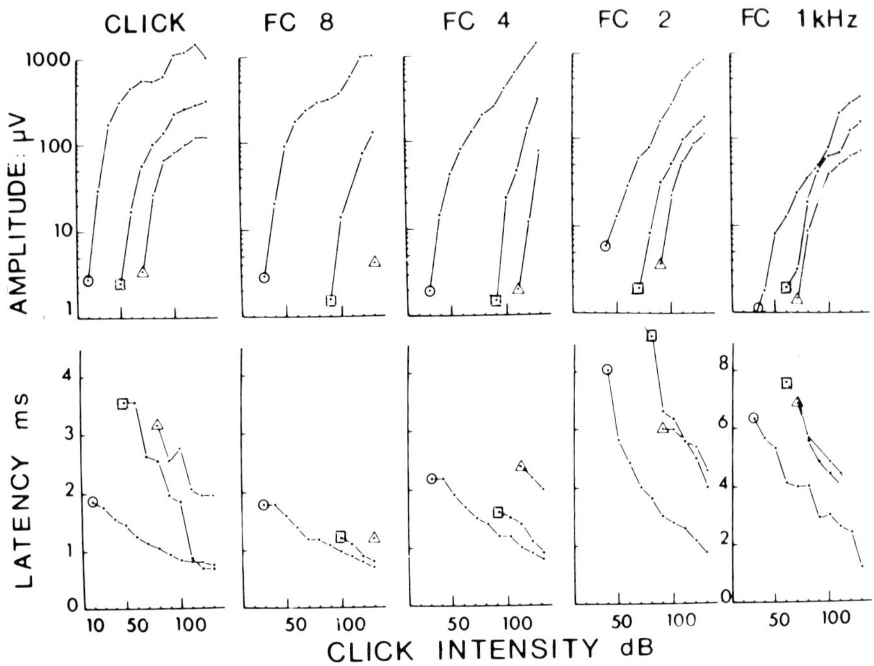

Figure 2-6. Input-output functions of amplitude (logarithmic scale) and latency of the largest negative peak (linear scale) of the responses to unfiltered click and various filtered clicks (FC) for the left ear of guinea pig 37 before (⊙), 3 months (⊡) after, and 7 months (◬) after treatment with kanamycin (see Figs. 2-4 and 2-5). The longer latency of the responses to the click after 7 months indicates that the responses are coming from an area on the basilar membrane far from the base. This correlates well with the absence of response to the 8 kHz filtered click (Fig. 2-5) and the hair cell loss at the base (Fig. 2-7). (From J-M. Aran and J. Darrouzet, Observation of click-evoked compound VIII nerve responses before, during and over seven months after kanamycin treatment in the guinea pig. *Acta Otolaryngol. [Stockh.]* 79:24, 1975. Reprinted by permission.)

the sharpness of the tuning of the fibers—their frequency selectivity—was drastically impaired when outer hair cells, in the area thought to correspond to their origin, were affected while the inner hair cells were still preserved (Fig. 2-9).

When attempts have been made to relate the frequency selectivity to outer hair cells or to conclude that this selectivity was not a characteristic of the inner hair cells, the objection has been raised that the remaining inner hair cells may not have been functioning normally but may have been altered by the drug treatment. Indeed, morphologic evidence of such alterations has been provided by Hawkins [33]. That inner hair cells disappear long after the end of short, intense series of kanamycin treatment—12 × 250 mg/kg, 140 days after treatment [29], and 8 × 400 mg/kg, 7 months after treatment [7]—suggests that they have been destroyed by the drug. One must recognize, however, that

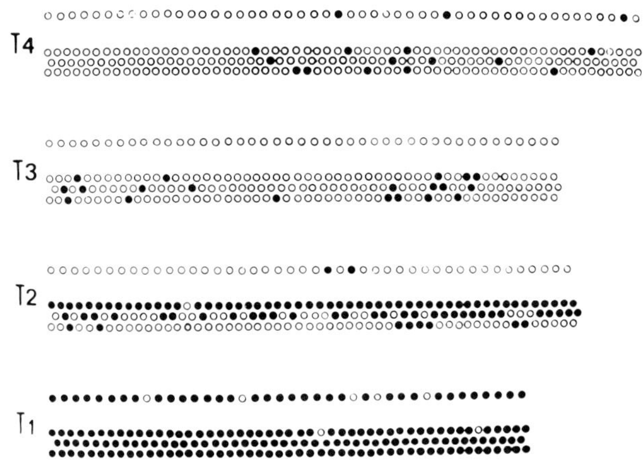

Figure 2-7. Hair cell diagrams for samples of organ of Corti (left ear) from the four turns of the cochlea in guinea pig 37, as seen in surface preparation. Note the essentially total destruction of the first turn (● = missing hair cells). (From J-M. Aran and J. Darrouzet, Observation of click-evoked compound VIII nerve responses before, during and over seven months after kanamycin treatment in the guinea pig. *Acta Otolaryngol. [Stockh.]* 79:24, 1975. Reprinted by permission.)

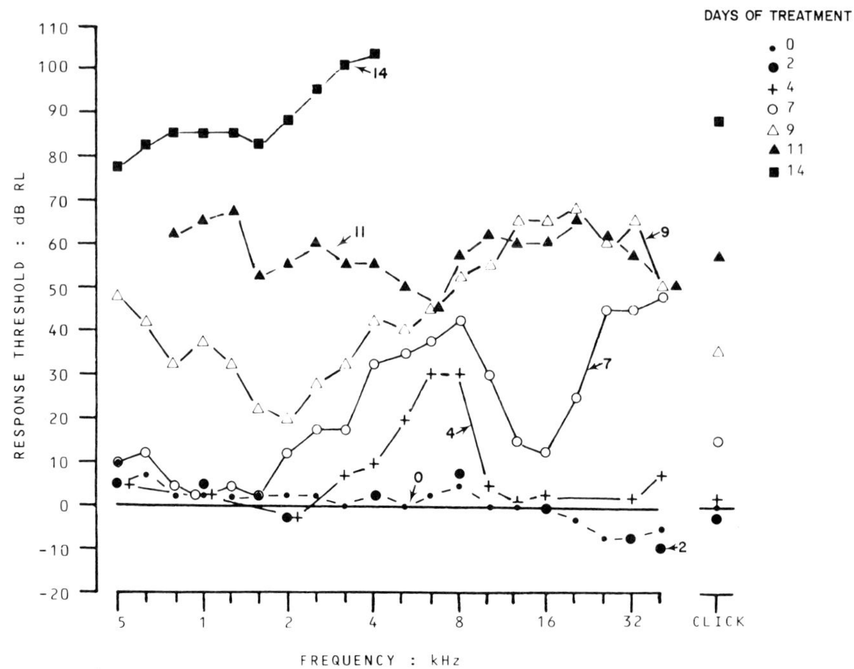

Figure 2-8. Evolution of frequency threshold curve of CAP in guinea pig 119 over 14 days during treatment with amikacin (14× daily dose of 450 mg/kg).

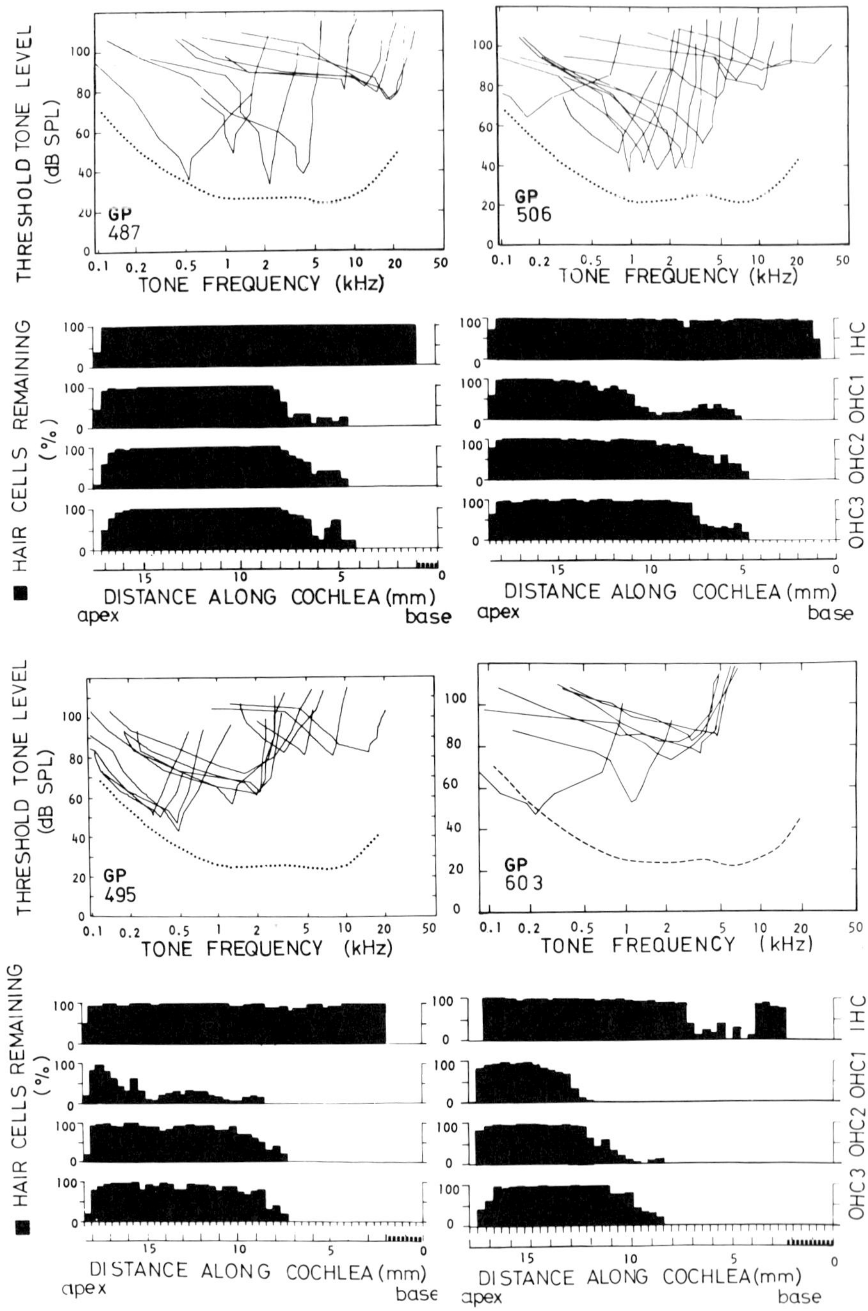

Figure 2-9. Effects of long-term kanamycin treatment (400 mg/kg × 10 days) on cochlear fiber frequency threshold curves of four guinea pigs (top half of each pair of figures). The dotted curves indicate the minimum threshold values for normal cochlear fibers. The lower half of each pair of figures is the cochleogram showing the percentage of hair cells remaining (black areas) in the cochlea at the time of the physiologic recording. (Adapted from R. V. Harrison, The effects of hair cell damage on cochlear function. University of Keele [England] Ph.D. Dissertation, 1978. Used with permission.)

before they disappear, the inner hair cells can respond to acoustic stimuli even though they may have been affected by the ototoxic antibiotic. The neural responses (either CAP or single-unit responses) when outer hair cells are destroyed differ drastically depending on the presence or absence of light-microscopically normal inner hair cells (see Figs. 2-5, 2-6, 2-7). This difference may range—for example, in CAP—from large and easily detectable responses to high-intensity sounds to no response at all (Fig. 2-5).

The pattern of single-unit responses observed in outer hair cell loss has been identical whether this loss was the consequence of antibiotic treatment or of acoustic trauma [42]. The same holds true for CAP [45], and after excessive current has been applied to the cochlea [3]. Similar, but transient, changes in the single-fiber response and CAP have also been demonstrated during various types of short-term treatment (anoxia, diuretics, etc.), which temporarily and preferentially affect outer hair cell function [24, 48]. Losses in threshold sensitivity and frequency selectivity of cochlear fibers, which correlate with alteration of outer hair cells, have been associated with the phenomenon of loudness recruitment. Recruitment is associated with aminoglycoside treatment in patients [43]; its presence has been inferred from electrocochleographic observations in man [46] and electrocochleographic as well as reaction time measurements in animals [48].

Recent experiments have provided further fundamental and puzzling information on the frequency analysis performed by the damaged cochlea. Results obtained in animals with outer hair cell loss caused by antibiotic treatment have been reported by Robertson and Johnstone [49]. They indicate not only that the threshold and the selectivity of the fibers depend on outer hair cell function, but also that the characteristic frequency of the fibers is profoundly modified. An octave shift toward the low frequencies, in neurons whose origin on the basilar membrane can be determined precisely, has been noted in areas where outer hair cells are definitely absent. Whether this change in characteristic frequency is caused by loss of sensitivity to the higher frequencies or is a true functional shift remains undetermined.

Comments

We have not attempted to review all of the electrophysiologic studies concerned with aminoglycoside ototoxicity. Instead, we have limited ourselves to studies on the peripheral responses that could be directly related to the functioning of the cochlear receptor, where the drugs presumably act. Brainstem responses or the response of the auditory cortex are also useful in the evaluation of hearing impairment of any origin [44].

It would be of interest to compare the cochleotoxicity of the aminoglycoside antibiotics with their vestibulotoxicity, since these two effects may not occur in parallel. Both have been studied histopathologically, but electrophysiologic studies on the vestibular system are much more difficult to perform. As a consequence, relatively few data from electrophysiologic studies on the vestibular system are available, and those that are available in the

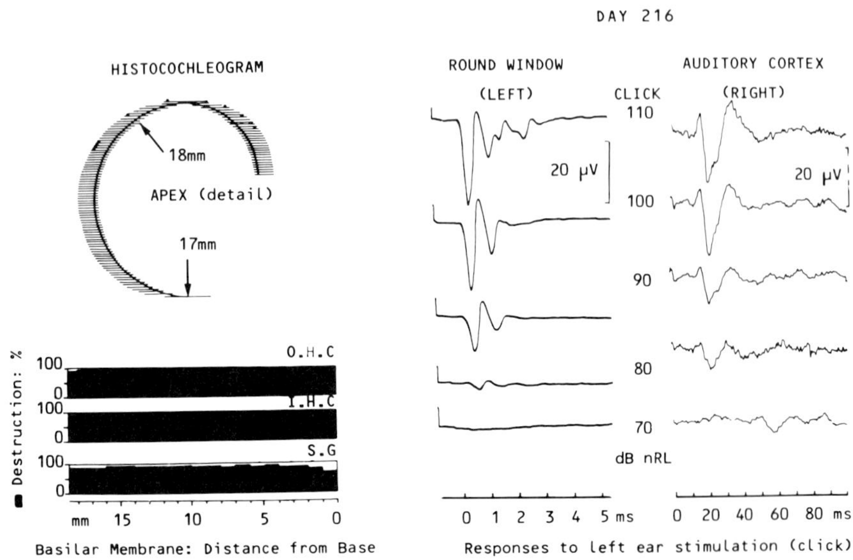

Figure 2-10. From left to right: Histocochleogram of the left ear (obtained from serial sections) and responses to click stimulation from the round window of the left ear and from the right auditory cortex, recorded just before killing of guinea pig 124 two hundred sixteen days after the beginning of amikacin treatment (14 × 450 mg/kg followed, 38 days later, by 20 × 450 mg/kg). This guinea pig, like many others after similar treatment, had total loss of inner hair cells, nearly complete loss of outer hair cells, and 90 to 95 percent degeneration of spiral ganglion neurons (black areas on the cytocochleogram). Clear round window and auditory cortex responses to acoustic clicks, however, were observed at 80 to 110 dB above the normal threshold. (dB nRL = normal response level.) (From J-M. Aran et al., Electrophysiological monitoring of the cochlea during and after total destruction of the organ of Corti. *Acta Otolaryngol. [Stockh.]* 89:376, 1980. Reprinted by permission.)

literature are largely drawn from studies on nonmammalian vestibular receptors [26, 54]. This aspect of the problem is discussed elsewhere in this book. The specific affinity of the drugs for the cochlea and vestibule is an interesting problem, however, particularly in view of the functional relationship between these two parts of the inner ear.

For example, we recently reported the presence of click-evoked responses, recorded at both the round window and the auditory cortex, from guinea pigs whose hair cells and spiral ganglion cells were almost totally destroyed [5, 6, 14]. The animals had been subjected to prolonged exposure to amikacin. Figure 2-10 illustrates the status of the cochlea, together with the evoked responses to high-intensity clicks, in one of these amikacin-treated guinea pigs. To account for this anomalous finding, we suggested that the response was initiated within the vestibular receptors, and we singled out those in the saccule as the probable source of the activity.

A recent approach to the problem of ototoxicity of aminoglycoside antibiotics that warrants mention is the study of the effects of such treatment on the developing inner ear. The potential toxic effect on the ear of the fetus can be evaluated when these drugs are administered to the pregnant female [52, 53]. Especially interesting is a study with rats in which a period of particularly high susceptibility to damage was found to exist between 11 and 15 days after birth [44]. This interval coincides with the period during which many structural and functional modifications occur. Other such studies could further elucidate the mechanisms underlying aminoglycoside ototoxicity.

References

1. Adrian, E. D. The microphonic action of the cochlea: an interpretation of Wever and Bray's experiments. *J. Physiol.* 71:28, 1931.
2. Aran, J-M. Contrôles électro-physiologiques du fonctionnement de l'organe de Corti après intoxication et après action de quelques autres agents. In M. Portmann (Moderator), Round Table: La Cellule Sensorielle de l'Organe de Corti. *Acta Otolaryngol. (Stockh.)* 63:40, 1967.
3. Aran, J-M. Neural correlates of electrically-induced cochlear dysfunction. *Clin. Otolaryngol.* 2:305, 1977.
4. Aran, J-M., and Cazals, Y. Electrocochleography: Animal Studies. In R. F. Naunton and C. Fernández (Eds.), *Evoked Electrical Activity in the Auditory Nervous System.* New York: Academic, 1978. Pp. 239–257.
5. Aran, J-M., Cazals, Y., Charlet de Sauvage, R., Guilhaume, A., and Erre, J-P. Electrophysiological monitoring of the cochlea during and after total destruction of the organ of Corti. *Acta Otolaryngol. (Stockh.)* 89:376, 1980.
6. Aran, J-M., Cazals, Y., Erre, J-P., and Guilhaume, A. Conflicting electrophysiological and anatomical data from drug-impaired guinea pig cochleas. *Acta Otolaryngol. (Stockh.)* 87:300, 1979.
7. Aran, J-M., and Darrouzet, J. Observation of click-evoked compound VIII nerve responses before, during and over seven months after kanamycin treatment in the guinea pig. *Acta Otolaryngol. (Stockh.)* 79:24, 1975.
8. Aran, J-M., and Erre, J-P. Long-term Recording of Cochleoneural Potentials in the Guinea Pig. In H. A. Beagley (Ed.), *Auditory Investigation: The Scientific and Technological Basis.* Oxford Medical Engineering Series. Oxford: Clarendon, 1979. P. 233.
9. Bernard, P. A., Bourret, C., Clermont, A., and Jequier, J. C. Anatomophysiological Correlations in Deoxystreptamine Ototoxicity, Their Value in the Evaluation of New Antibiotics. In M. Portmann and J-M. Aran (Eds.), *Inner Ear Biology.* Colloques INSERM (Paris) 68:359, 1977.
10. Bernard, P. A., Pechere, J-C., and Jequier, J. C. Detection of tobramycin- and netilmicin-induced ototoxicity in guinea pigs with evoked action potentials. *J. Infect. Dis.* 139:418, 1979.
11. Brummett, R. E., Brown, R. T., and Himes, D. L. Quantitative relationships of the ototoxic interaction of kanamycin and ethacrynic acid. *Arch. Otolaryngol.* 105:240, 1979.
12. Brummett, R. E., Himes, D. L., Saine, B., and Vernon, J. A comparative study of the ototoxicity of tobramycin and gentamicin. *Arch. Otolaryngol.* 96:505, 1972.
13. Caussé, R. Action toxique vestibulaire et cochléaire de la streptomycine au point de vue expérimental. *Ann. Otol. Rhinol. Laryngol.* 66:518, 1949.
14. Cazals, Y., Aran, J-M., Erre, J-P., and Guilhaume, A. Acoustic responses after total destruction of the cochlear receptor: brainstem and auditory cortex. *Science* 210:83, 1980.

15. Cazals, Y., Aran, J-M., and Hawkins, J. E., Jr. Threshold elevation at high frequencies of the auditory nerve action potential in acute versus chronic recordings in guinea pigs. *Hear. Res.* 2:95, 1980.
16. Christensen, E. F., Reiffenstein, J. C., and Madissoo, H. Comparative ototoxicity of amikacin and gentamicin in cats. *Antimicrob. Agents Chemother.* 12:178, 1977.
17. Dallos, P., and Cheatham, M. A. Production of cochlear potentials by inner and outer hair cells. *J. Acoust. Soc. Am.* 60:510, 1976.
18. Dallos, P., Ryan, A., Harris, D., McGee, T., and Ozdamar, O. Cochlear Frequency Selectivity in the Presence of Hair Cell Damage. In E. F. Evans and J. P. Wilson (Eds.), *Psychophysics and Physiology of Hearing.* London: Academic, 1977. P. 249.
19. Dallos, P., and Wang, C. Y. Bioelectric correlates of kanamycin intoxication. *Audiology* 13:277, 1974.
20. Darrouzet, J., and Guilhaume, A. Ototoxicité cochléaire comparée de trois antibiotiques: kanamycine, gentamicine, tobramycine. Étude histologique et ultrastructurale. *Rev. Laryngol. Otol. Rhinol.* 97:655, 1976.
21. Davis, H., Deatherage, B. H., Rosenblut, B., Fernandez, C., Kimura, R., and Smith, C. A. Modification of cochlear potentials produced by streptomycin poisoning and by extensive venous obstruction. *Laryngoscope* 68:596, 1958.
22. Davis, H., Derbyshire, A. J., Lurie, M. H., and Saul, L. J. The electric response of the cochlea. *Am. J. Physiol.* 107:311, 1934.
23. Erre, J-P., Cazals, Y., and Aran, J-M. Monitoring of cochlear, auditory cortex and electronystagmographic responses in chronically implanted guinea pigs. In preparation.
24. Evans, E. F. The sharpening of cochlear frequency selectivity in the normal and abnormal cochlea. *Audiology* 14:419, 1975.
25. Farkashidy, J., Black, R. G., and Briant, T. D. R. The effect of kanamycin on the internal ear: an electrophysiological and electron microscopic study. *Laryngoscope* 73:713, 1963.
26. Gallais, A., Caston, J., and Zittoun, A. Vestibular effects of antibiotics introduced in the inner ear. Behavioral and electrophysiological studies in the frog. *Acta Otolaryngol. (Stockh.)* 87:517, 1979.
27. Glorig, A. Clinical manifestations of ototoxicity and noise. *Adv. Oto-Rhino-Laryngol.* 20:2, 1973.
28. Goldstein, M. H., and Kiang, N. Y-S. Synchrony of neural activity in electric responses evoked by transient acoustic stimuli. *J. Acoust. Soc. Am.* 30:107, 1958.
29. Gonzalez, G., Miller, N., and Wasilewski, V. Progressive neuro-ototoxicity of kanamycin. *Ann. Otol. Rhinol. Laryngol.* 81:127, 1972.
30. Harrison, R. V. The effects of hair cell damage on cochlear function. University of Keele (England) Ph.D. Dissertation, 1978.
31. Harrison, R. V., and Evans, E. F. The Effects of Hair Cell Loss (Restricted to Outer Hair Cells) on the Threshold and Tuning Properties of Cochlear Fibers in the Guinea Pig. In M. Portmann and J-M. Aran (Eds.), *Inner Ear Biology.* Colloques INSERM (Paris) 68:105, 1977.
32. Hawkins, J. E., Jr. Cochlear signs of streptomycin intoxication. *J. Pharmacol. Exp. Ther.* 100:38, 1950.
33. Hawkins, J. E., Jr. Condition of the Inner Hair Cells after Aminoglycoside Intoxication. In M. Portmann and J-M. Aran (Eds.), *Inner Ear Biology.* Colloques INSERM (Paris) 68:327, 1977.
34. Hawkins, J. E., Jr., Johnsson, L-G., and Aran, J-M. Comparative tests of gentamicin ototoxicity. *J. Infect. Dis.* 119:417, 1969.
35. Hawkins, J. E., Jr., and Lurie, M. H. The ototoxicity of streptomycin. *Ann. Otol. Rhinol. Laryngol.* 61:789, 1952.
36. Hawkins, J. E., Jr., and Lurie, M. H. The ototoxicity of dihydrostreptomycin and neomycin in the cat. *Ann. Otol. Rhinol. Laryngol.* 62:1128, 1953.

37. Hinshaw, H. C., and Feldman, W. H. Streptomycin in the treatment of clinical tuberculosis: A preliminary report. *Proc. Mayo Clin.* 20:313, 1945.
38. Kiang, N. Y-S., Liberman, M. C., and Levine, R. A. Auditory-nerve activity in cats exposed to ototoxic drugs and high-intensity sounds. *Ann. Otol. Rhinol. Laryngol.* 85:752, 1976.
39. Kiang, N. Y-S., Moxon, E. C., and Levine, R. A. Auditory Nerve Activity in Cats with Normal and Abnormal Cochleas. In G. E. W. Wolstenholme and J. Knight (Eds.), *Sensorineural Hearing Loss.* London: Churchill, 1970. P. 241.
40. Konishi, T. Some observations on negative endocochlear potential during anoxia. *Acta Otolaryngol. (Stockh.)* 87:506, 1979.
41. Konishi, T., Kelsey, E., and Singleton, G. T. Negative potential in scala media during early stage of anoxia. *Acta Otolaryngol. (Stockh.)* 64:107, 1967.
42. Liberman, M. C., and Kiang, N. Y-S. Acoustic trauma in cats. Cochlear pathology and auditory-nerve activity. *Acta Otolaryngol. (Stockh.)* [*Suppl.* 358], 1978.
43. Lidén, G. Loss of hearing following treatment with dihydrostreptomycin or streptomycin. *Acta Otolaryngol. (Stockh.)* 43:551, 1953.
44. Osako, S., Tokimoto, T., and Matsuura, S. Effects of kanamycin on the auditory evoked responses during postnatal development of the hearing of the rat. *Acta Otolaryngol. (Stockh.)* 88:359, 1979.
45. Portmann, M., Aran, J-M., and Coste, C. Vérification expérimentale sur l'animal de quelques aspects électro-cochléographiques de la pathologie humaine. *Acta Otolaryngol. (Stockh.)* 75:132, 1973.
46. Portmann, M., Aran, J-M., and Lagourgue, P. Testing for recruitment by electrocochleography. Preliminary results. *Ann. Otol. Rhinol. Laryngol.* 82:36, 1973.
47. Prosen, C. A., Petersen, M. R., Moody, D. B., and Stebbins, W. C. Auditory thresholds and kanamycin-induced hearing loss in the guinea pig assessed by a positive reinforcement procedure. *J. Acoust. Soc. Am.* 63:559, 1978.
48. Pugh, J. E., Moody, D. B., and Anderson, D. J. Electrophysiological Studies of Loudness Recruitment. In R. J. Ruben, C. Elberling, and G. Salomon (Eds.), *Electrocochleography.* Baltimore: University Park Press, 1976. P. 471.
49. Robertson, D., and Johnstone, B. M. Aberrant tonotopic organization in the inner ear damaged by kanamycin. *J. Acoust. Soc. Am.* 66:466, 1979.
50. Russell, N. J., Fox, K. E., and Brummett, R. E. Ototoxic effects of the interaction between kanamycin and ethacrynic acid. *Acta Otolaryngol. (Stockh.)* 88:369, 1979.
51. Simmons, F. B., Galambos, R., and Albrite, J. P. Serial studies of the onset and progression of drug-induced cochlear damage in cats. A new electrophysiologic method. *Arch. Otolaryngol.* 72:233, 1960.
52. Uziel, A., Romand, R., and Gabrion, J. Intrauterine Ototoxicity of Kanamycin in the Guinea Pig. In M. Portmann and J-M. Aran (Eds.), *Inner Ear Biology.* Colloques INSERM (Paris) 68:347, 1977.
53. Uziel, A., Romand, R., and Marot, M. Electrophysiological study of the ototoxicity of kanamycin during development in guinea pigs. *Hear. Res.* 1:203, 1979.
54. Vallancien, B., Effets de quelques toxiques sur les potentiels d'action du vestibule de la grenouille. *Pract. Otorhinolaryngol.* 17:157, 1955.
55. Wever, E. G., and Bray, C. W. Auditory nerve impulses. *Science* 71:215, 1930.

Discussion of Chapter 2

Dr. Lerner: When you are treating guinea pigs chronically either with various doses of one aminoglycoside or comparing one aminoglycoside with another, do you monitor renal function, and do you measure serum aminoglycoside levels in these animals? If so, do you adjust dosages to maintain a set serum level?

Dr. Aran: No, we do not monitor renal function. This is a study of cochlear function, without systemic measurement of the action of the drug.

Dr. Federspil: How often have you noticed otitis media in the guinea pigs that are tested?

Dr. Aran: Very few guinea pigs had detectable otitis media.

Dr. P. A. Bernard (Laval University, Quebec): Did you find modifications in the CAP waveform during treatment with high doses of aminoglycosides?

Dr. Aran: We found changes in the CAP waveform after high doses. We designed the experiments to see how aminoglycoside administration modifies the waveform, but this was difficult to analyze. We had to measure the summating potential, which became difficult to measure during acute changes.

Dr. Wersäll: In your animals, you showed a loss of hair cells associated with the preservation of some ganglion cells. In the majority of our treated animals surviving for more than 1 month, the ganglion cell population was well below 50 percent. In some animals, 30 to 40 percent of the ganglion cells remained. It is of interest to ask what is the mechanism of stimulation of these nerve endings, since many of these nerves do not have remaining sensory hair cells. I think this indicates that we have to make a very careful study of the mode of stimulation at high stimulus intensities. Dr. Ylikoski's study* of the actual passage of nerve fibers through the spiral lamina is

*J. Ylikoski, Guinea-pig hair cell pathology from ototoxic antibiotics. *Acta Otolaryngol. (Stock.)* [*Suppl.* 326]:5, 1974.

essential, since it enables us to determine whether the nerve fibers are intact.

Dr. Aran: We have been looking at the spiral ganglion and the habenula perforata and examined how far the nerve fibers go in the remnant of the organ of Corti. We saw a few nerve fibers, but no trace of inner hair cells; we could easily see the remaining outer hair cells at the apex, however. The CAP response remains completely stable from 1 month up to 1 year after treatment, while the spiral ganglion degenerates slowly but progressively [Chap. 2, ref. 5].

Dr. Honrubia: Have you obtained information about the value of measuring the resting potentials in the cochleas of these guinea pigs that lack hair cells, but produce action potentials? Have you been able to record any change in the resting potentials during stimulation?

Dr. Aran: We did not measure the resting potential in these guinea pigs. We do know that it is present in other experiments after kanamycin treatment, when the hair cells are destroyed [Chap. 2, refs. 2 and 41].

3. Perfusion of Aminoglycosides in Perilymph

Alfred L. Nuttall

The perfusion of antibiotics into the spaces of the inner ear is a useful technique for studies of the ototoxicity of these drugs, chiefly because with this method a constant concentration of the test agent can be held within the ear. An additional benefit of this model is its relatively fast assessment of the drug action on the basis of physiologic variables indicating the function of the inner ear.

Perfusion of the perilymphatic or endolymphatic scalae of the cochlea is, in essence, the topical application of solutions directly to the sensory tissue. It bypasses the vascular system of distribution, which may be affected by declining concentrations in serum caused by renal clearance and delivery of the drug to the large fluid compartments of the body. Also bypassed is the blood-perilymph (or endolymph) barrier, which may be of great importance in determining the ototoxicity when the drug is given systemically. For proper evaluation of drug action with this local application method, sufficiently high perfusion rates must be used so that the drug concentration remains constant within the inner ear in spite of natural drug clearance and metabolism.

The perfusion technique has been used in one variation or another by a number of investigators studying cochlear metabolism, the physiology of inner ear fluids, or the relationships among the cochlear potentials [5, 6, 11, 8–10, 17, 19–21, 25]. Ototoxic drug effects resulting from local application have only recently begun to receive attention. Perhaps the earliest example of the assessment of aminoglycoside toxicity (on hair cells) is the report of the reversible action of streptomycin on the cochlear microphonic in the lateral line organ of the fish [27]. In more recent years, several investigators perfused the

The author gratefully acknowledges the assistance of Mr. Michael J. LaRouere in the collection of data for this report and the generosity of Eli Lilly and Company for their gift of the tobramycin used in this study. Special thanks are extended to Dr. Merle Lawrence for comments on the manuscript and to Ms. Janet Fisk for the secretarial work. This study was supported by Public Health Service Grants NS 05785, NS 11731, and NS 15107.

cochlea in order to study aminoglycoside ototoxicity [8, 16, 18]. Perfusion has been reported by Schacht and his colleagues [12, 23] as a tool for the study of basic mechanisms of inner ear biochemistry as well as the biochemistry of the aminoglycosides.

This chapter has a threefold purpose. First, I wish to review our perfusion method in its current state of development. Second, I shall address two methodological questions: (1) whether the results obtained during drug perfusion with solutions at room temperature are an appropriate estimate of those that would be derived from experiments carried out at physiologically normal temperatures; and (2) whether the use of CM as the physiologic indicator of primary drug action is appropriate. Third, this report compares the toxicity of two aminoglycosides, one of which has not been tested previously by the local application technique.

Methods

Albino guinea pigs, weighing between 200 and 400 g, were anesthetized with 0.8 ml/kg body weight of Dial* anesthetic, administered intraperitoneally. They were artificially ventilated, and heart rate and body temperature were monitored throughout the experiment. A heating pad, along with a blanket covering the body, was used to maintain the rectal temperature at 37° to 38°C. Curare, 0.3 mg administered intramuscularly, eliminated middle ear muscle movement and created an electrically quiet recording environment for observation of the whole-nerve action potential (AP) on an oscilloscope.

Perfusion System

A ventral surgical approach gave access to the cochlea with preservation of the middle ear mechanism. The perfusion technique used was a modification of that described by Nuttall et al. [16]. The head of the animal was securely fastened in a head holder to prevent any significant movement during the course of the perfusion. Figure 3-1A illustrates the attachment of the perfusion capillaries to the first turn of the cochlea. One capillary was fitted into a hole (0.1-mm diameter) drilled into the scala tympani, and it served as the inlet for the perfusate. A similar hole in the scala vestibuli of the first turn, fitted with a second capillary, served as the outlet for the perfusate. The capillaries were made of glass tubing drawn to a fine tip with an electrode puller. They were cemented in position so that a leak-free system was created. Polyethylene tubing connected the glass capillaries to the reservoir and the receiving vessel. Flow was established by syphon action when the outlet capillary was lowered below the level of the supply reservoir, thereby creating a hydrostatic pressure head.

This technique is essentially a constant-pressure method. In contrast to constant-flow methods, it has the advantages of minimizing pressure-created leaks and of maintaining the CM at a more constant level, since inner ear

*Each ml of Dial contained allobarbital, 100 mg; urethane, 400 mg; monoethylurea, 400 mg.

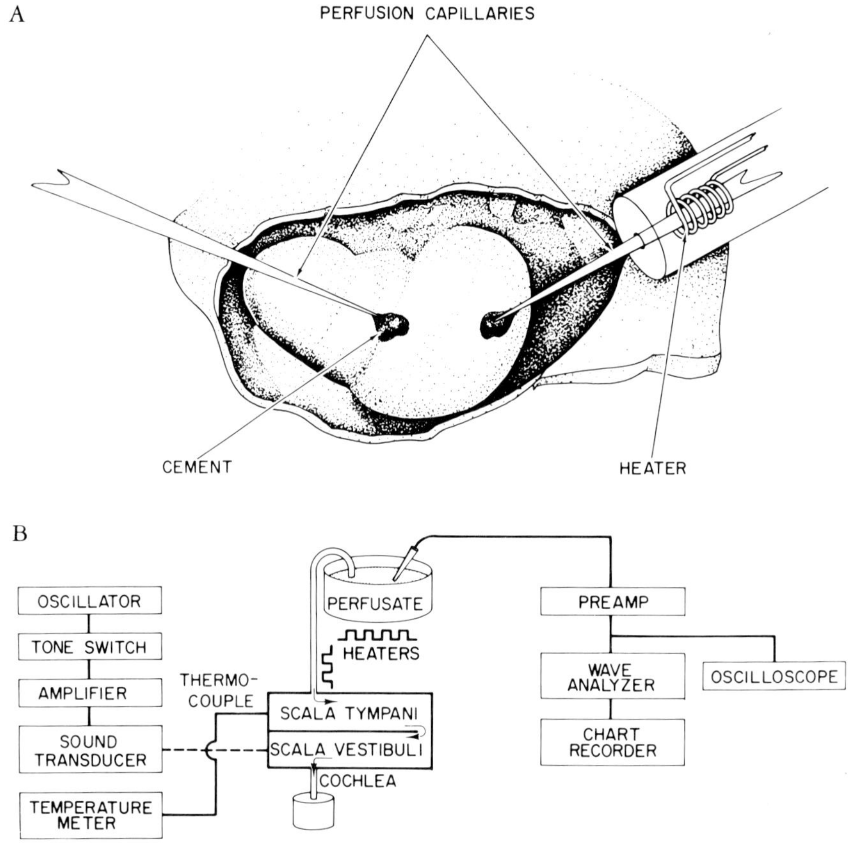

Figure 3-1. A. Position and placement of the perfusion capillaries in the first turn of the cochlea. Inlet for perfusate is in scala tympani, and outlet is from the scala vestibuli. A heater coil around the inlet capillary provided the mechanism for control of cochlear temperature. B. Schematic representation of the perfusion system and of the stimulating and recording systems. Note the thermocouple on the round window membrane for monitoring of temperature.

biopotentials are quite sensitive to perfusion pressure changes. The flow rates used ranged between 20 and 50 μl per minute. The method also maintains the middle ear in a "dry" condition, preventing artifactual CM or AP changes caused by fluctuations in middle ear sound conduction or by electrical shunting of the signals.

Figure 3-1A shows a heating element which was incorporated into the capillary holder close to the cochlea on the perfusate inlet side. Direct current was applied to the heater coil in variable amounts for control of the temperature of the perfusate entering the cochlea. An actual measurement of the cochlear temperature was made possible by placement of a K-type (Chromel-Alumel) thermocouple onto the round window membrane. The thermocouple was constructed from insulated 0.075-mm thermocouple wires and was positioned and cemented in place before attachment of the perfusion capillaries. By appropriate choice of the heater current and of the perfusate flow rate, the round window temperature could be raised from its resting value of 29° to 30°C, measured during perfusion with room-temperature perfusate (22°C), to approximately 37°C (see Nuttall and LaRouere [15] for a discussion of the experimental determination of cochlear temperature). The complete system is diagrammed schematically in Fig. 3-1B.

Perfusion Fluids

The artificial perilymph had the following composition: 130 mM NaCl, 10 mM $NaHCO_3$, 4 mM KCl, 1 mM $MgCl_2$, 1.5 mM NaH_2PO_4, 20 mM HEPES buffer. The pH was adjusted to between 7.4 and 7.8 with HCl or NaOH. The aminoglycoside antibiotics were added at two concentrations (10^{-2} and 10^{-3}M) to the artificial perilymph. In the present study, gentamicin (gentamicin sulfate, 41.5% C_1, 17.6% C_{1a}, 41.2% C_2, Sigma Co.) and tobramycin (Eli Lilly Co.) were tested for their relative effects on the CM and AP when they were perfused at room temperature and at 37°C.

When perfusions were carried out at the higher temperature, the perfusate was preheated and maintained in the supply reservoir at 40°C during the perfusion period. This procedure partially degasses the perfusate, preventing bubble formation. Control perfusions were also conducted with the degassed artificial perilymph.

Stimulation and Recording

Acoustic stimuli consisted of pure tones at 4 kHz and click-type sounds, which were delivered to the external auditory meatus with a closed-field sound system. A 1-inch condenser microphone produced the sounds. Clicks were created by one cycle of an 8-kHz sinusoid, delivered at a rate of five clicks per second.

All inner ear electrical signals were recorded from the inlet capillary, used as a single-ended recording electrode. The reference electrode was silver wire placed in the masseter muscle on the contralateral side. The CM was measured at the 4-kHz stimulation frequency on a wave analyzer and traced on a chart recorder. The starting level was approximately 8 μV; this corresponded to a stimulus intensity of 70 to 75 dB sound pressure level (SPL). The AP level, i.e., the peak magnitude of the N_1 component of the waveform as measured on an oscilloscope, was determined at varying intervals during the time course of the perfusion. The AP signal was extremely sensitive to the perfusion hydrostatic pressure, and therefore a convenient level between 80 and 200 μV was chosen for each animal. This AP signal level was obtained with a peak acoustic stimulus of between 80 and 100 dB SPL.

Results

When the perilymphatic space of the cochlea is first perfused with artificial perilymph, a consistent decrease in the levels of CM and AP is observed. An instantaneous fall, which is directly related to the perfusion hydrostatic pressure, is followed by a further gradual downward drift. After several minutes, the levels of CM and AP stabilize and, if a control perfusion is allowed to proceed for 1 hour, the potentials will remain remarkably steady. Control studies have indicated that, at most, a 10 percent decrease in cochlear output can be expected; however, some perfusions will show no loss at 60 minutes. Animals in which the potentials did not stabilize within 10 percent of baseline were excluded from the study.

After perfusate flow has been established and the cochlear temperature is raised (as measured by the round window thermocouple), there is usually a further transient shift in the potentials. This results from both a transient alteration of the perfusion hydrostatic pressure (caused by the heater) and a possible physiologic shift in the cochlear electrical output in response to the increase in temperature (see Butler et al. [2]). As with the room-temperature perfusate, the output signals then became stable. For all results reported below, a stable level was obtained from 10 to 15 minutes before the application of a drug to the cochlea began.

Loss functions of CM against time are presented in Fig. 3-2. The initial CM in most experiments was arbitrarily set between 6 and 10 μV root mean square (most commonly 8 μV). In order to normalize these curves and to facilitate comparison with past and future experiments, the CM loss is presented as percent of decrease from baseline. The four panels of Fig. 3-2 include data for the two aminoglycosides tested (gentamicin and tobramycin) at two cochlear temperatures and at two concentrations of the drugs (only one temperature is given for 10^{-3}M gentamicin in Fig. 3-2D). It seems that there is an early fast CM loss, followed later by a shallower slope or a saturating function.

The ototoxicity of the drugs can be quantified in several ways, based on parameters of these physiologic loss functions. Two reasonable estimates would be the percentage loss at 30 minutes and the linear approximation of the slope of the function between the initial application of the drug and the 30-minute time point. These estimates would have the advantage of measuring the portion of the loss functions with the greatest change and would avoid possible cumulative physiologic error from prolonged perfusion. In this model, high concentrations of the gentamicin mixture clearly appeared to be more toxic than similarly high concentrations of tobramycin.

For an answer to the question of the importance of temperature in testing of aminoglycosides by perfusion, the mean values of data from Fig. 3-2 are replotted in Fig. 3-3. Figure 3-3A demonstrates that, when the cochlear temperature is raised to physiologic levels, there is a large increase in the cochleotoxic activity of tobramycin. However, the relative effect of tobramycin concentration remains the same at both temperatures, i.e., the curves for 10^{-2}M and 10^{-3}M tobramycin are shifted upward by a similar amount with increased temperature. According to Fig. 3-3B, the temperature shift appears to be similar for tobramycin and gentamicin, and gentamicin appears more ototoxic than tobramycin at both temperatures.

The AP and CM losses are compared in Fig. 3-4, which represents the pooled data from all guinea pigs in which AP was measured. All combinations

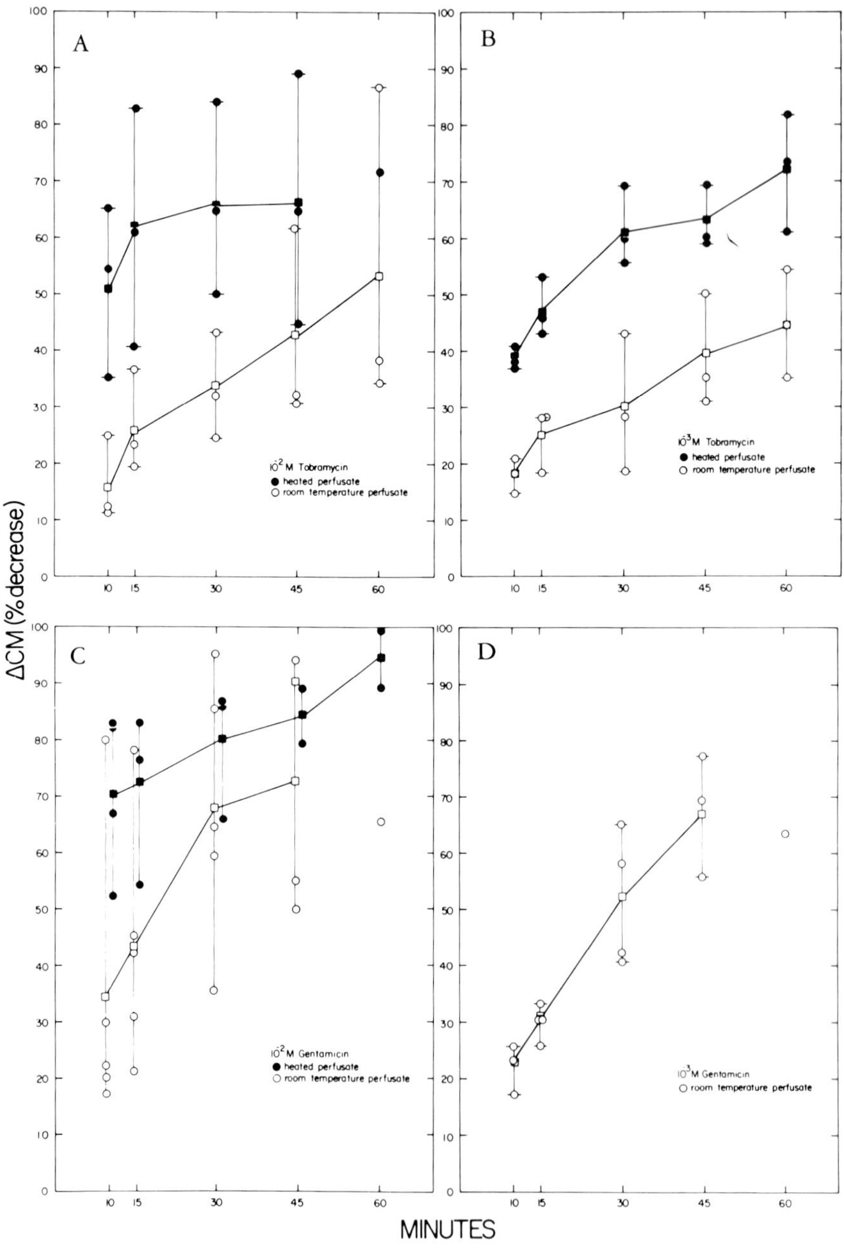

Figure 3-2. CM loss functions, with mean values (■, □) and range bars, are presented for two drugs at two concentrations and for two perfusion temperatures. The perfusions were conducted with room-temperature perfusate (20°–22°C) and with heated perfusate such that the cochlear temperature was 37° to 38°C. The room-temperature perfusate resulted in a cochlear temperature of 29° to 30°C (see text). (●, ○ = data points.) A, B. Tobramycin perfusion results. C, D. Gentamicin perfusion results.

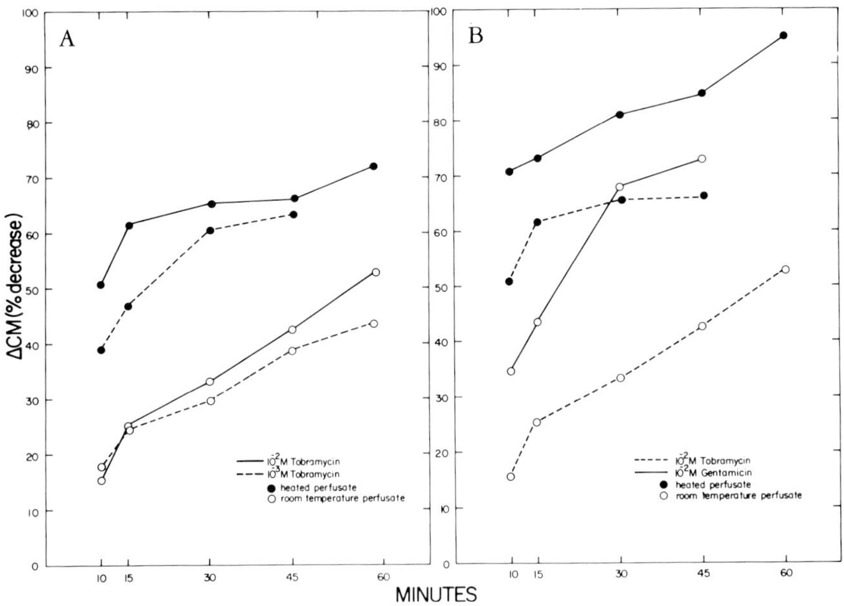

Figure 3-3. A. Effect of concentration on the loss of CM with time for tobramycin perfusion and the shift in the functions that resulted from the experimental control of perfusion temperature. Mean losses of CM are plotted from Fig. 3-2. B. The CM loss functions comparing the relative ototoxicity of tobramycin and gentamicin and the shift in these loss functions that resulted from the experimental control of perfusion temperature. Mean losses of CM are plotted from Fig. 3-2.

of temperature (30° or 37°C), drug (gentamicin or tobramycin), and concentration (10^{-3}M or 10^{-2}M) are represented, with at least four data points for each animal. There is a clear correlation between AP and CM changes during drug perfusion.

Comments

Acute perilymphatic perfusion is a useful tool for the assessment of aminoglycoside ototoxicity. The results showed that perfusion of the cochlea over minutes can produce loss of CM output. In the present study and in previous reports [8, 12, 16], the relative toxicity of several aminoglycosides and other ototoxic agents has been determined by means of perfusion. The rapid response of the inner ear potentials to the drug is related to the actual concentration within the cochlea, which was kept constant in these experiments. Voldrich [26] reported that, after a schedule of daily injections of neomycin (150 mg/kg), the concentration of the neomycin in the perilymph was close to those used here. After a single subcutaneous injection (100 mg/kg) of neomycin, Stupp [24] found that neomycin in the perilymph reached a concentration of just over 10^{-4}M. The actual drug concentration in the inner ear fluctuates as

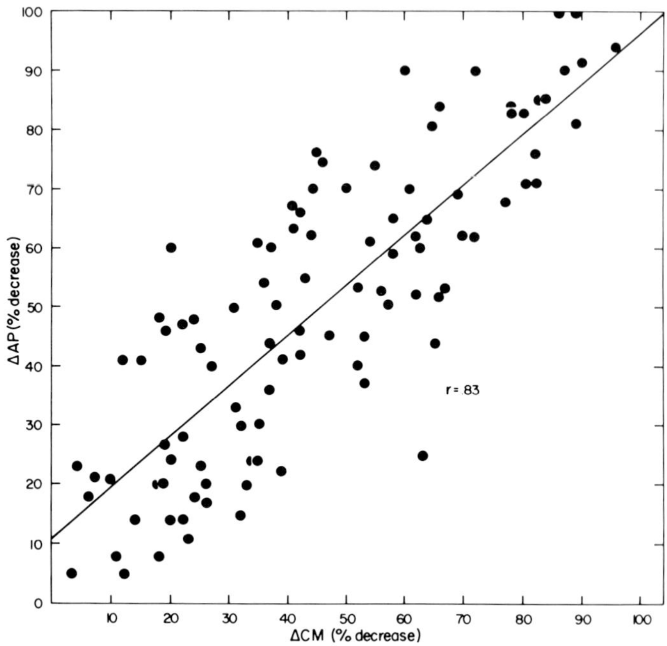

Figure 3-4. Decrease of CM plotted against the decrease of whole-nerve action potential (AP) for all perfusions in the present study in which AP change was determined. The regression line illustrates the high correlation of loss between these auditory electrical signals during perfusion.

a function of accumulation and clearance of the agent from the ear and the body. The relative order of toxicity among aminoglycoside antibiotics, determined from changes in cochlear potential during aminoglycoside infusion in perilymph, is supported by similar findings in long-term studies of systemic administration in which cochlear potential, morphologic changes [4], and behavioral effects [22] were measured. The fact that the decline of CM potential is highly correlated with changes in membrane phospholipid metabolism during the early phase of drug action [12, 23] suggests that CM is a sensitive predictor of the first (early) component of aminoglycoside toxic action within the inner ear.

Figure 3-2 shows the effect of cochlear temperature on the results of this experiment. Temperature is a potential variable of the perfusion technique that was not explicitly investigated in the earlier studies [12, 16, 23]. Previously, all of the perfusion studies were performed with the perfusate at room temperature. Since the room-temperature perfusate is at only 20° to 23°C, any significant cooling of the cochlea must be considered. If the perfusion were conducted at physiologic temperatures, would the results differ only by parallel shifts, which could in turn be accounted for by the expected shift caused by the chemical reaction rate?

Nuttall and LaRouere [15] have determined that the cochlear temperature in the guinea pig after opening of the bulla falls from the normal level (38°C) to a steady value between 30° and 32°C. Perfusion with room-temperature perfusate reduces the cochlear temperature further, to a value between 29° and 30°C. Apparently, the heat content of the guinea pig's head effects considerable warming of the perfusate.* On the other hand, the net loss in cochlear temperature is as much as 8°C and could be expected to produce a measurable shift in the activity of the antibiotic.

The perfusion at 38°C did, in fact, produce a dramatic increase in the loss functions for both of the drugs tested at either concentration. The increase shown in Fig. 3-3 is within the range that would be predicted from temperature effects on biochemical reaction rates. The important information obtained is that the loss functions shift predictably and in parallel for both drug types and concentrations. Therefore, in comparing the ototoxicity of aminoglycoside antibiotics, one is justified in carrying out the perfusion experiment at a lower than physiologic temperature as long as the temperature is held constant.

The determination of the appropriate physiologic variable to be measured as a response to the drug action was a further objective in the present study. Several previous investigators had measured the CM [12, 16, 23]; Konishi [8] also determined the reduction in endocochlear potential (EP) and AP during perfusion. One may argue that the CM is a peripheral response and that, since the aminoglycoside is acting on the sensory epithelium, CM is the appropriate signal to be measured. On the other hand, the AP, as an output signal from the whole system, should provide information on the entire transduction-transmission process. (There could, of course, be a direct effect of the drug on nerve fiber response, since aminoglycosides have been shown to cause convulsions if they are applied directly to the central nervous system [13, 14].) Whereas Hawkins [3] noted an apparent differential effect of chronic kanamycin ototoxicity on CM and AP in the cat, the present study (Fig. 3-4) demonstrates good correspondence between the CM and the AP signals as indicators of toxicity. This would suggest that either signal could be used as a measure of toxicity. The AP, however, is highly labile and is more difficult to evaluate than the CM.

One might ask, why employ perilymphatic rather than endolymphatic perfusion? The present study does not offer any experimental evidence to favor one over the other. The recent work of Konishi [8] indicates that the CM and AP were suppressed to a greater extent during endolymphatic perfusion with aminoglycosides than during perfusion of the perilymphatic spaces. On the basis of this finding, Konishi interpreted the site of likely action of the drugs to be the hair-bearing end of the receptor cells. The EP is also much more susceptible to the drugs when these are given topically in the endolymph rather than

*The decrease in cochlear temperature during perfusion is, of course, highly dependent on the flow rate of the perfusate, which, for the present study, ranged between 20 and 50 μl/min. These high flow rates, compared to those used in previous studies, are necessary for the temperature manipulation of the cochlea. They also ensure a constant drug concentration and do not appear to be particularly detrimental to the electrical response of the inner ear.

by systemic application. The reason for the greater effects of aminoglycoside perfusion within the scala media is not known. One possible explanation is that there could simply be a much-reduced concentration of the drug in endolymph when perfusion of the perilymphatic space is carried out or when systemic application is used. The effect on EP cannot, without further study, be attributed to an action of the drug directly on the stria vascularis because it is possible that the effect is secondary to damage to the organ of Corti. For example, if membrane barriers of the organ of Corti were compromised by the aminoglycoside, this would lower the electrical resistance of one wall bounding the scala media space and would have the effect of short-circuiting the EP.

Balogh et al. [1] have found that, after systemic administration of dihydrostreptomycin, this drug reached a higher concentration in the perilymph than in the endolymph. Accumulation possibly occurred by the pathway of the superstrial vessels of the spiral ligament above Reissner's membrane. Thus, in the use of the perilymphatic perfusion method, there may be a delay and possibly a reduced effect while a drug diffuses to the appropriate site(s) of action, which may be several fluid compartments away from the perilymphatic space. Intervening metabolic and clearance factors could reduce the effective concentration at these sites.

Nevertheless, the additional difficulties of attempting to perfuse the scala media, which include damage to the spiral ligament and stria vascularis with resulting microhemorrhage, as well as the need for an open perfusion system, would militate against the use of such a procedure unless there were specific physiologic or biochemical reasons for doing so. The relative toxic activity of similar drugs would be expected to remain unchanged with either perfusion method.

References

1. Balogh, K., Hiraide, F., and Ishii, D. Distribution of radioactive dihydrostreptomycin in the cochlea: An autoradiographic study. *Ann. Otol. Rhinol. Laryngol.* 79:641, 1970.
2. Butler, R. A., Konishi, T., and Fernández, C. Temperature coefficients of cochlear potentials. *Am. J. Physiol.* 199:688, 1960.
3. Hawkins, J. E., Jr. The ototoxicity of kanamycin. *Ann. Otol. Rhinol. Laryngol.* 68:698, 1959.
4. Hawkins, J. E., Jr. Drug Ototoxicity. In W. D. Keidel and W. D. Neff (Eds.), *Handbook of Sensory Physiology.* New York: Springer, 1976. Vol. V/3, p. 707.
5. Honrubia, V., Johnstone, B. M., and Butler, R. A. Maintenance of cochlear potentials during asphyxia. *Acta Otolaryngol.* 60:105, 1965.
6. Jung, W. Zur pH-Abhängigkeit des Mikrofonpotentials der Meerschweinchen-Cochlea. *Arch. Klin. Exp. Ohren- Nasen-Kehlkopfheilkd.* 199:473, 1971.
7. Kuijpers, W. Cation transport and cochlear function. *Acta Otolaryngol.* 67:200, 1969.
8. Konishi, T. Effects of local application of ototoxic antibiotics on cochlear potentials in guinea pigs. *Acta Otolaryngol.* 88:41, 1979.
9. Konishi, T., and Kelsey, E. Effect of sodium deficiency on cochlear potentials. *J. Acoust. Soc. Am.* 43:462, 1968.

10. Konishi, T., Kelsey, E., and Singleton, G. T. Effects of chemical alteration in the endolymph on the cochlear potentials. *Acta Otolaryngol.* 62:393, 1966.
11. Konishi, T., Kelsey, E., and Singleton, G. T. Negative potential in scala media during early stage of anoxia. *Acta Otolaryngol.* 64:107, 1967.
12. Lodhi, S., Weiner, N. D., Mechigian, I., and Schacht, J. Ototoxicity of aminoglycosides correlates with their action on monomolecular films of polyphosphoinositides. *Biochem. Pharmacol.* 29:597, 1980.
13. Molitor, H., and Kuna, S. The significance of neurotropic properties of commercial streptomycin. *Arch. Int. Pharmacodyn. Ther.* 74:334, 1947.
14. Molitor, H., and Kuna, S. Pharmacologic study of the neurotoxic properties of streptomycin. *Arch. Int. Pharmacodyn. Ther.* 78:197, 1949.
15. Nuttall, A. L., and LaRouere, M. Depression of the guinea pig cochlear temperature caused by anesthesia and ventral-approach ear surgery. *J. Acoust. Soc. Am.* 68:489, 1980.
16. Nuttall, A. L., Marques, D. M., and Lawrence, M. Effects of perilymphatic perfusion with neomycin on the cochlear microphonic potential in the guinea pig. *Acta Otolaryngol.* 83:393, 1977.
17. Prazma, J. Active ion transport from the scala vestibuli into the scala media. *Acta Otolaryngol.* 67:631, 1969.
18. Schindler, K. Die Abschätzung der unmittelbaren Innenohrtoxizität von Furosemid und Mefrusid beim Meerschweinchen. *Arch. klin. exp. Ohr.-, Nas.- u. Kehlk.-Heilk.* 205:261, 1973.
19. Schnieder, E-A. Die Entstehung des Schalltraumas. Ein Beitrag über die Physiologie der Perilymphe. University of Würzburg Thesis, 1970.
20. Sellick, P. M., and Bock, G. R. Evidence for an electrogenic potassium pump as the origin of the positive component of the endocochlear potential. *Pfluegers Arch.* 352:351, 1974.
21. Sellick, P. M., and Johnstone, B. M. Changes in cochlear endolymph Na^+ concentration measured with Na^+ specific microelectrodes. *Pfluegers Arch.* 336:11, 1972.
22. Stebbins, W. C., Miller, J. M., Johnsson, L-G., and Hawkins, J. E., Jr. Ototoxic hearing loss and cochlear pathology in the monkey. *Ann. Otol. Rhinol. Laryngol.* 78:1007, 1969.
23. Stockhorst, E., and Schacht, J. Radioactive labeling of phospholipids and proteins by cochlear perfusion in the guinea pig and the effect of neomycin. *Acta Otolaryngol.* 83:401, 1977.
24. Stupp, H-F. Untersuchung der Antibiotikaspiegel in den Innenohrflüssigkeiten und ihre Bedeutung für die spezifische Ototoxizität der Aminoglykosidantibiotika. *Acta Otolaryngol.* [*Suppl. 262*], 1970.
25. Tasaki, I., Davis, H., and Eldredge, D. H. Exploration of cochlear potentials in guinea pigs with a microelectrode. *J. Acoust. Soc. Am.* 26:765, 1954.
26. Voldrich, L. The kinetics of streptomycin, kanamycin, and neomycin in the inner ear. *Acta Otolaryngol.* 60:243, 1965.
27. Wersäll, J., and Flock, A. Suppression and restoration of the microphonic output from the lateral line organ after local application of streptomycin. *Life Sci.* 3:1151, 1964.

Discussion of Chapter 3

Dr. Brummett: If you give an aminoglycoside such as kanamycin parenterally or subcutaneously every 6 hours, you get perilymph concentrations that rise rapidly and remain high while the concentration in the blood falls off very rapidly. Thus, if you give the dose every 6 hours, you will gradually increase the concentration in the perilymph, with little accumulation in the blood. Even with high doses that will produce cochlear damage several weeks later, we don't see any changes in the cochlear microphonic or the N-1 response within 2 hours after the end of treatment, when perilymph concentrations have reached a peak of about 80 μg/ml.

Dr. Nuttall: Your data on differential aminoglycoside concentration between blood and perilymph seem to correspond to the results of Stupp [Chap. 3, ref. 24] and Voldrich [Chap. 3, ref. 26], who found similar variations. The quick-acting effect of our perfusions on the cochlear microphonic and the compound action potential may be related to the somewhat higher and more constant drug concentrations than achieved by your injections. In our studies, lower concentrations take longer to have a measurable effect.

Dr. Schacht: I would like to remind Dr. Nuttall of some experiments we did a long time ago. It is not necessary to use an aminoglycoside concentration of 10^{-2}M, because you also get an effect at 10^{-3}M. At 10^{-4}M no effect is observed, but this may be related to the short (30- to 60-minute) time period of observation.

Dr. Federspil: I think it is important to do these studies with low concentrations.

Dr. Lietman: I have two related questions. One: Do you know whether the aminoglycoside has to enter the cells? This might account for the delay in response that you see if the drug had to get into a second, intracellular compartment.

The second related question is: If you cease perfusing with the aminoglycosides, but continue to perfuse with the control substance, is the effect on the cochlear microphonic reversible? If so, does the time course of this reversal correlate with the decrease in the drug concentration?

Dr. Nuttall: To answer your second question, I can report that we do not usually see a recovery of cochlear microphonic when attempting to wash out the aminoglycoside. However, there may be a change in the rate of decline or a stabilization of the reduced microphonic level. Shorter perfusion times, which produce less loss, would be appropriate for investigation of reversibility.

On the question of fluid compartments, it must be pointed out that, with the method of perilymphatic perfusion, the drug may be passing through multiple compartments to reach the place of action. I would cite the recent study by Konishi [Chap. 3, ref. 8], who perfused aminoglycosides into the scala media and found that the toxic effect was greater there. This suggested to him that the drug was acting at the stereocilia ends of the hair cells. If that is the case, we would expect a diffusion delay in the method of perilymphatic perfusion.

Dr. Brummett: A couple of years ago, Kaye Fox and I did some experiments with cultured mammalian thymocytes to determine the effect of ethacrynic acid and kanamycin on cell growth. We were looking for an in vitro model of our interaction experiments, and we found that concentrations of kanamycin of the order of 10^{-2}M stopped the thymocytes from growing in vitro.

I don't doubt that this type of cytotoxicity affects the cochlea, but I wonder whether this is as specific an effect as you see when drugs are administered parenterally and then selectively destroy hair cells. Maybe, when you perfuse at these high concentrations, this represents an effect on all the cells of the cochlea.

Dr. Nuttall: The results of short-term exposure to high aminoglycoside concentrations may not be comparable to those of long-term exposure on cell growth. Your question is whether a 10^{-2}M concentration of kanamycin can affect all the cells of the cochlea. We have not been able to determine if this is the case. After a 1-hour perfusion, we do not see any morphologic changes as assessed by light microscopy. I cannot comment, at present, on the possible physiologic effects of the drug on nonsensory cells.

Dr. Wersäll: The question of reversibility, of course, is extremely interesting. Dr. Flock and I reported a few years ago on the lateral line organ, where we could demonstrate that 10 μg/ml streptomycin inhibited the microphonic [Chap. 3, ref. 27]. When we increased the concentration to 100 μg/ml, we could not achieve full reversibility of the microphonic of the lateral line organ.

We also found, in recent experiments with gentamicin, that we inhibited not only the microphonic of the lateral line organ, but also the action potentials of the innervating nerves. Even that was reversible at lower concentrations, but with increased concentrations the reversibility decreased.

According to your findings, you would expect to get rid of the gentamicin in the cochlear fluids by perfusing with artificial perilymph. However, we could never reduce the effects of antibiotics with artificial perilymph. We had to add either polysaccharides or potassium at high concentration. In our experiments, we were able to eliminate the microphonic with drug concentrations as low as 10 μg/ml. Have you tried to vary the ionic content of your solution to see whether you can increase or decrease the effects of the drug?

Dr. Nuttall: No, we have not.

4. Interaction Between Aminoglycoside Antibiotics and Loop-Inhibiting Diuretics in the Guinea Pig

Robert E. Brummett, Kaye E. Fox, Nancy J. Russell, and Rickie R. Davis

The first loop-inhibiting diuretic, ethacrynic acid, was introduced into clinical medicine in the middle 1960s. Soon after its introduction, reports began appearing in the clinical literature that ethacrynic acid could produce temporary [28] as well as permanent hearing loss [23]. After the advent of furosemide, it became evident that this new potent diuretic was also capable of producing loss of hearing [29]. With both of these drugs, the hearing loss occurred with a very short latency following intravenous administration. In animal experiments it was shown that the interval between the time of administration of an intravenous dose and the detection of cochlear effects was only a few minutes [18].

By the end of the 1960s, clinical reports strongly suggested that permanent hearing loss resulting from the use of these potent diuretics occurred especially in patients who were simultaneously receiving an aminoglycoside antibiotic [1, 17]. The time course of the hearing loss in man resulting from concomitant therapy with an aminoglycoside antibiotic and a loop-inhibiting diuretic was well described in a clinical report by Johnson and Hamilton [14]. A patient with acute tubular necrosis was given a single 1-g dose of kanamycin intramuscularly for treatment of gram-negative sepsis. Two hours later, the patient was given a single 50-mg dose of ethacrynic acid intravenously. Thirty minutes after the injection, the patient complained of loss of hearing. Subsequently it was determined that he had a 60- to 70-dB hearing loss at all frequencies tested. This hearing loss was still present when the patient was discharged from the hospital. The patient's hearing was not evaluated before the drugs were administered; however, a 60- to 70-dB hearing deficit would render the patient unable to communicate. Since there was no mention of any difficulty in speech communication before the drugs were given, it can be assumed that the drug treatment had produced the severe hearing loss. The time course of the onset of hearing loss in this patient, resulting from the interaction between kanamycin and ethacrynic acid, is very similar to that in

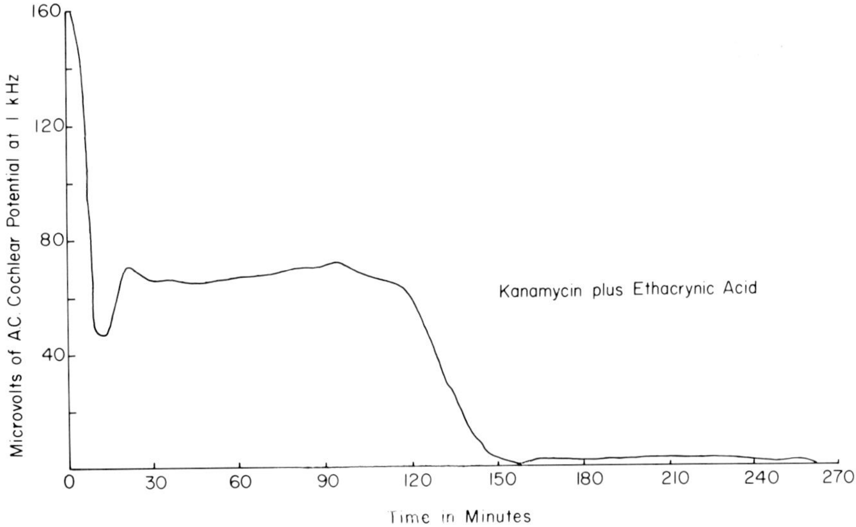

Figure 4-1. Time course of the AC cochlear potential at 1 kHz for a guinea pig treated with a single subcutaneous dose of 400 mg/kg kanamycin, followed in 2 hours (0 time on graph) by a single 400-mg/kg intravenous dose of ethacrynic acid.

the guinea pig model developed by West et al. [31]. In this animal model, a single 400-mg/kg dose of kanamycin is administered subcutaneously, and 2 hours later, a single 40-mg/kg dose of ethacrynic acid is administered intravenously. The progression of the ototoxicity is followed by the continuous monitoring of the AC cochlear potential in response to a continuous tone (Fig. 4-1).

After the administration of ethacrynic acid, there is a latency period of 3 to 5 minutes before the AC cochlear potential begins to fall. The potential falls rapidly, reaching a minimum in approximately 15 minutes; it then rises to a plateau. About 2 hours later, there is a second drop in the AC cochlear potential, with no apparent recovery. Guinea pigs treated in this manner still had a severely depressed capacity to generate the AC cochlear potential 30 days later, and histopathologic examination showed a pronounced loss of both inner and outer hair cells. It is clear that this dose regimen results in permanent cochlear damage. In animals treated with kanamycin followed by saline, there is no effect; in animals treated with saline followed by ethacrynic acid, only the initial temporary effect is seen.

This interaction will occur if kanamycin is given as long as 8 hours before and up to 2 hours after ethacrynic acid. The maximum effect is obtained when kanamycin is given within the time period of 4 hours before or simultaneously with the injection of the ethacrynic acid. This timing requirement coincides with the maximal concentration of kanamycin in the perilymph following a single subcutaneous dose [2]. For this reason, Brummett and Fox [3] have postulated that the magnitude of the interaction effect is proportional to the

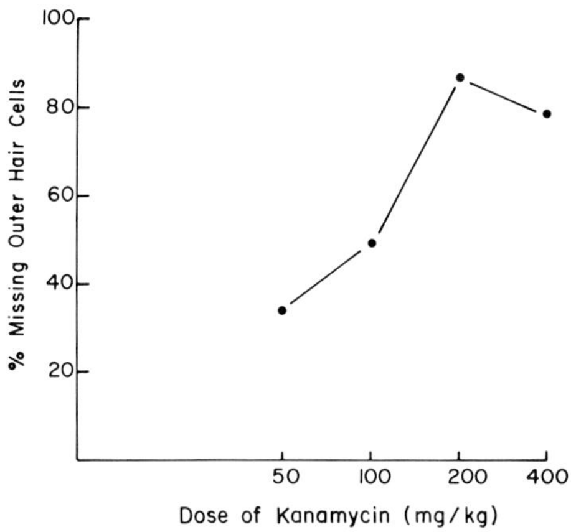

Figure 4-2. Dose-effect curve for guinea pigs treated with a single 40-mg/kg dose of ethacrynic acid 2 hours after the indicated dose of kanamycin. Outer hair cells were evaluated by phase-contrast microscopy of surface preparations 30 days after drug treatment.

amount of kanamycin in the perilymph at the time the ethacrynic acid reaches the cochlea.

The dose-effect relationship of the interaction is seen in Figs. 4-2 and 4-3. All of the data in Fig. 4-2 are from guinea pigs treated with a 40-mg/kg dose of ethacrynic acid 2 hours after the indicated doses of kanamycin. There is some effect even at doses as low as 12.5 mg/kg of kanamycin (not shown), which is smaller than the total daily human therapeutic dose. Figure 4-3 shows data for guinea pigs treated with a 400-mg/kg subcutaneous dose of kanamycin 2 hours prior to the indicated doses of ethacrynic acid. The dose-effect curve for ethacrynic acid is remarkably steep, in contrast to that in Fig. 4-2. The marked difference in the shape of the two dose-effect curves is of particular interest. If both drugs were exerting their ototoxic effect by the same mechanism, the slopes of the curves should be the same. The difference in the curves for kanamycin and ethacrynic acid suggests, however, that the drugs exert their effects by different mechanisms.

In many investigations on the mechanism of biologic effects of drugs, it is useful to develop an in vitro model in which the effects can be isolated from complicating influences. Fox and Brummett [11] used mammalian thymocytes grown in vitro as a possible model for the study of the toxic interaction that occurs with kanamycin and ethacrynic acid. Each drug alone was toxic to this cell system. The concentration of kanamycin required to produce a 50 percent reduction in growth of the cells was 1.4×10^{-2}M (7 mg/ml); for ethacrynic acid, it was 2.3×10^{-5}M (0.007 mg/ml). When the two drugs were used in combination, no evidence of interaction was found. Fox and Brummett [11] concluded that this in vitro system was not a suitable model for the interaction effects of the drugs. They also pointed out that the toxicity of these drugs for

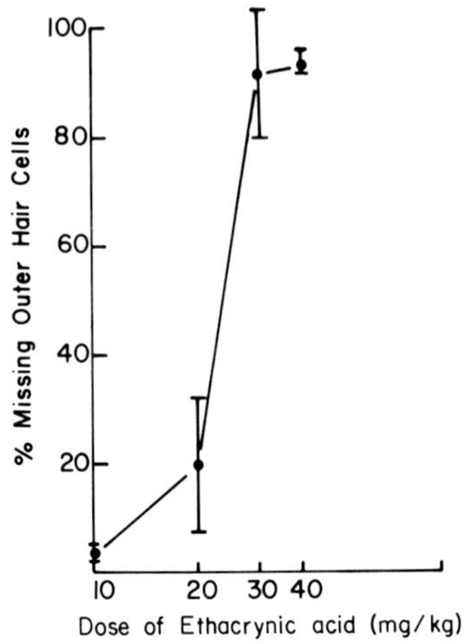

Figure 4-3. Dose-effect curve obtained for guinea pigs treated with a 400-mg/kg dose of kanamycin 2 hours before the indicated dose of ethacrynic acid. Hair cell loss was evaluated as in Fig. 4-2.

mammalian cells not involved with cochlear function makes it difficult to explain their selective toxicity for cochlear hair cells. The concentrations of kanamycin required to produce the toxic effect on thymocytes, however, were orders of magnitude higher than the levels of drug in the perilymph of animals that developed ototoxicity after subcutaneous administration of kanamycin and intravenous administration of ethacrynic acid [11]. Aminoglycosides as well as loop-inhibiting diuretics have been perfused into the cochlea in attempts to investigate the biochemical events that lead to the development of ototoxicity [16, 22, 30]. The drug concentrations required to produce effects after cochlear perfusion with either drug are similar to those found to produce effects on cultured thymocytes. Therefore, the biochemical effects proposed as the mechanisms by which these drugs exert their cochlear effects must be considered with caution, as they may not represent the mechanism by which the drugs produce selective hair cell toxicity.

Russell et al. [24–27] investigated the mechanism by which hair cell destruction occurs as a result of the combined administration of kanamycin and ethacrynic acid. They conducted a series of experiments in which they tried to discover which cellular structures are damaged by the combined administration of these two drugs. The observed alterations in ultrastructure were correlated with functional changes in cochlear electrophysiology. The most striking effects were seen in the hair cells and the stria vascularis. In the hair cells, clumping of the nuclear chromatin and loss of the subsurface cisternae were seen as early as 1 hour after the administration of ethacrynic acid, when it was preceded 2 hours earlier by kanamycin. The changes were much more pronounced at 2 hours after ethacrynic acid, and by 4 to 6 hours, the outer hair cells appeared to be dying. They were grossly swollen, the mitochondria were distorted, the cilia had fused, the nucleus was swollen, and the nuclear chromatin was clumped. There was pronounced thinning of the subsurface cisternae. Russell et al. [25] postulated that this thinning results from fusion of the subsurface cisternae with the plasma membranes. At present, it is not possible to determine whether the changes seen in the plasma membrane or those in the nucleus occur first. Since cells can remain alive for some time without a nucleus, the changes in the plasma membrane would be expected to result in cell death faster than changes occurring in the nucleus. Thus, it would seem that plasma membrane changes represent the initial event leading to the death of the cells. At the time the outer hair cells were dying, the supporting cells appeared quite normal. None of these changes was found in control animals treated with kanamycin or ethacrynic acid alone. All evaluations were made blindly with respect to which treatment the animals had received.

Ethacrynic acid also produces marked swelling and edema of the stria vascularis [26]. The duration of this strial edema appears to be prolonged by a couple of hours by the presence of kanamycin. A relationship between the prolongation of the strial changes and the death of the hair cells remains unknown. There appears to be little, if any, permanent change in the stria vascularis as a result of the interaction between ethacrynic acid and kanamycin.

While ethacrynic acid by itself is altering the AC cochlear potential, there is a simultaneous change in the DC endolymphatic potential [27]. In fact, the observed change in the AC cochlear potential can easily be accounted for by the reduction in the DC potential. However, when the AC cochlear potential drops for the second time 2 hours after ethacrynic acid in animals pretreated with kanamycin, there is no corresponding change in the DC potential [27]. This observation led Russell et al. [27] to postulate that the initial drop in the AC cochlear potential is the result of changes in the stria vascularis that are responsible for maintaining the DC endolymphatic potential, whereas the second drop is the result of changes in the hair cells.

A possible explanation for the enhanced ototoxicity resulting from the combined use of the two drugs is that one drug facilitates the entry of the other into the cochlea. Russell et al. [27] have found that ethacrynic acid does not increase the concentration of kanamycin in the perilymph. Likewise, Fox and Brummett [10] were unable to demonstrate any significant amounts of ethacrynic acid in the perilymph. In a separate experiment it was found that kanamycin did not alter these results [unpublished observation]. It appears that altered drug concentrations in the perilymph do not play any significant role. It is possible, however, that alterations in the distribution of drugs in the endolymph or within the hair cells are involved.

As pointed out above, this type of interaction is not specific to kanamycin and ethacrynic acid, but is seen also with other aminoglycoside antibiotics and loop-inhibiting diuretics. Brummett et al. [8] were unable to demonstrate such an interaction in guinea pigs treated with kanamycin and osmotic, thiazide, or mercurial diuretics. It does occur, however, with kanamycin and all loop-inhibiting diuretics that have been tested clinically. In an unpublished study, we found that the experimental loop-inhibiting diuretic MK-196, which is a structural analog of ethacrynic acid, apparently does not cause hair cell death within 48 hours, even when extremely large doses are used in combination with kanamycin (Fig. 4-4). The MK-196 also has little effect on cochlear electrophysiology when it is used alone in near-lethal doses (Figs. 4-5 and 4-6). Although they differ in chemical structure, various loop-inhibiting diuretics alter cochlear function. Thus one could postulate that their cochleotoxic and diuretic effects are caused by similar mechanisms. This is further suggested because of the previous observation that only the loop-inhibiting diuretics, even though they differ in chemical structure, are capable of altering cochlear function. The lack of effect of MK-196, a potent diuretic, on cochlear function casts some doubt, however, on the hypothesis that loop-inhibiting diuretics exert their effects on the ear by a mechanism similar to that by which they affect the kidney.

The potential of the different loop-inhibiting diuretics to produce an augmented ototoxic effect when they are used in combination with kanamycin has been determined [2, 7]. Figure 4-7 shows the dose-effect relationships for ethacrynic acid and furosemide. Ethacrynic acid is much more potent than furosemide; there is no overlap between the two curves. These data are supported by clinical reports; there are numerous cases in which this interaction involves ethacrynic acid, but few in which furosemide is involved [1, 15, 19, 20, 21, 24, 26]. The dose-effect curves of the new loop-inhibiting diuretics bumetanide and piretanide appear to be very similar to that of ethacrynic acid. Although there are marked differences in the ototoxic potential of various loop-inhibiting diuretics, there are also differences in their diuretic potency. For example, ethacrynic acid and furosemide have similar diuretic potencies, but marked differences in ototoxic potential. The diuretic potency of ethacrynic acid seems to be about 1/40 that of bumetanide, but the ototoxic potential appears to be approximately equal. One may reason that, if the therapeutic dose of bumetanide is 1/40 that of ethacrynic acid, the likelihood of ototoxicity brought on by this interaction with bumetanide should also be about 1/40 that of ethacrynic acid. Confirmation of this prediction must await the more widespread clinical use of bumetanide. Similar differences exist in the potential of the different aminoglycoside antibiotics to interact with ethacrynic acid. The ED_{50} (i.e., the dose required to produce loss of 50 percent of the outer hair cells) interpolated from Fig. 4-8 is 27 mg/kg for gentamicin, 32 mg/kg for tobramycin, 45 mg/kg for netilmicin, and 62 mg/kg for kanamycin. These differences in ototoxic potential are essentially those that have been reported for these drugs elsewhere [4, 5, 7, 12].

Loop-inhibiting diuretics interact in this model system with all of the aminoglycoside antibiotics that are available for testing. It does not involve only the aminoglycoside antibiotics, however. Davis and Brummett [9] have reported that the same type of interaction can take place with the nonaminoglycoside antibiotics viomycin, polymyxin B, and capreomycin. In a more recent unpublished experiment, it has been found that the loop-inhibiting diuretics ethacrynic acid, furosemide, and bumetanide will all interact with *cis*-platinum to produce an augmented ototoxic effect. Interaction of loop-

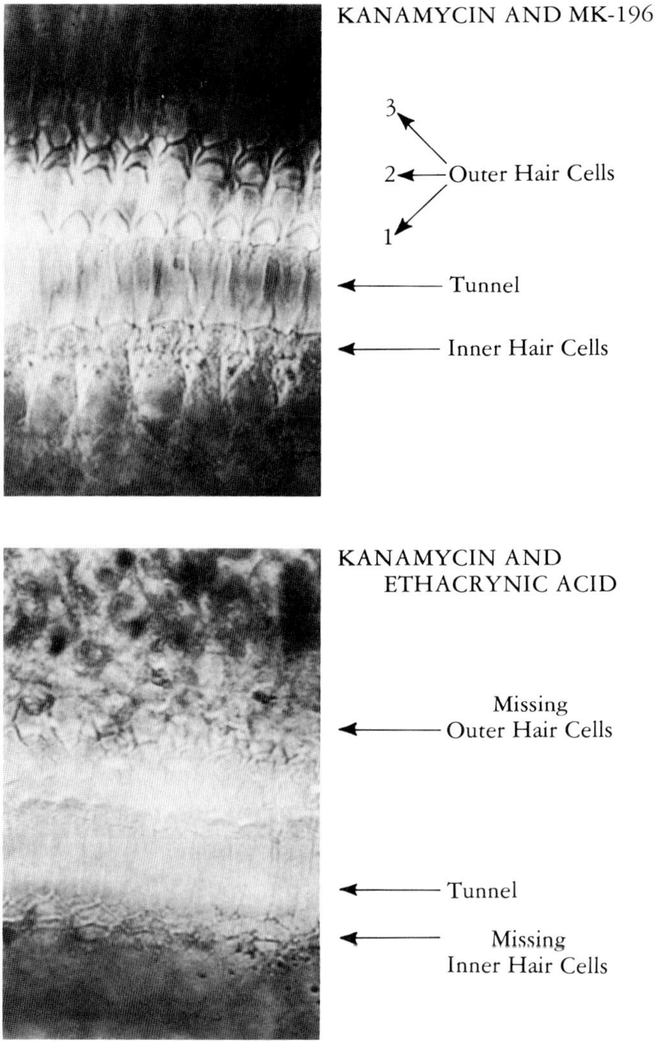

Figure 4-4. Surface preparations of cochleas obtained from the second turn of the cochlea of guinea pigs 48 hours after treatment with kanamycin, 400 mg/kg, and MK-196, 100 mg/kg; or kanamycin, 400 mg/kg, and ethacrynic acid, 40 mg/kg.

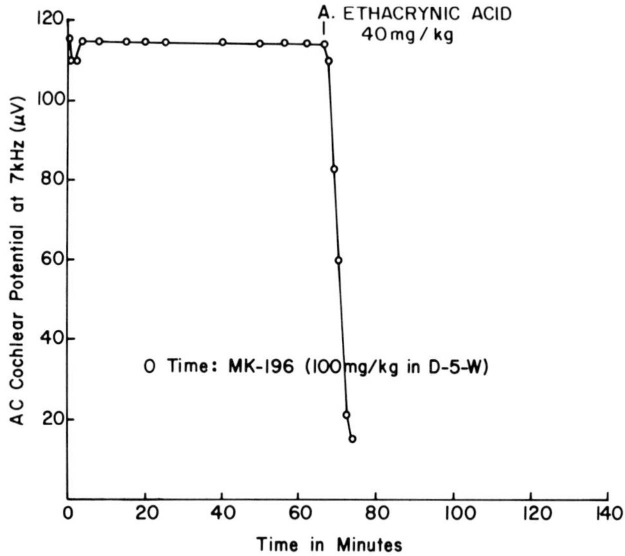

Figure 4-5. AC cochlear potential for a guinea pig treated with a single intravenous dose of MK-196 at 0 time. A single intravenous dose of ethacrynic acid was given at A to show that the animal could respond to the standard ototoxic loop-inhibiting diuretic.

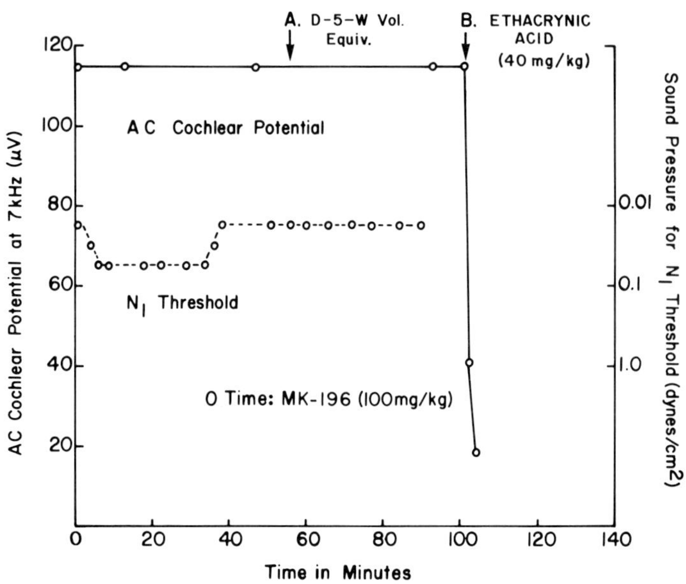

Figure 4-6. AC cochlear potential and N_1 threshold responses for a guinea pig treated with a single dose of MK-196 at 0 time. At A, a single dose of 5% dextrose in water (D-5-W) was administered intravenously to show that the diluent for MK-196 had no effect. At B, a single dose of ethacrynic acid was given intravenously to show that the animal was capable of responding to it. In this experiment, the AC cochlear potential and N_1 responses could not be recorded simultaneously.

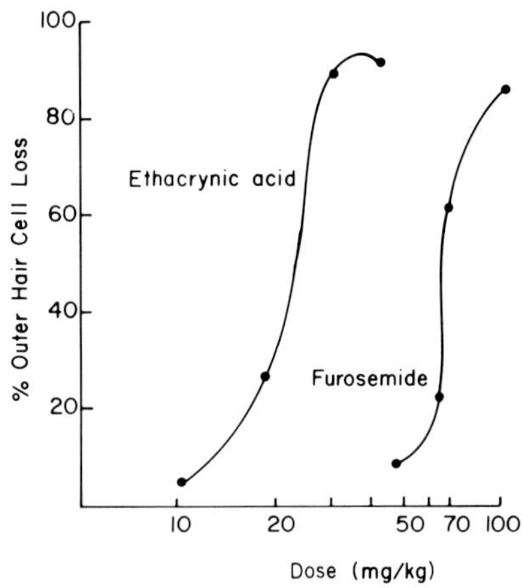

Figure 4-7. Dose-effect curves for guinea pigs treated with a single 400-mg/kg dose of kanamycin 22 hours before the indicated doses of diuretic. Hair cell loss was evaluated as in Fig. 4-2.

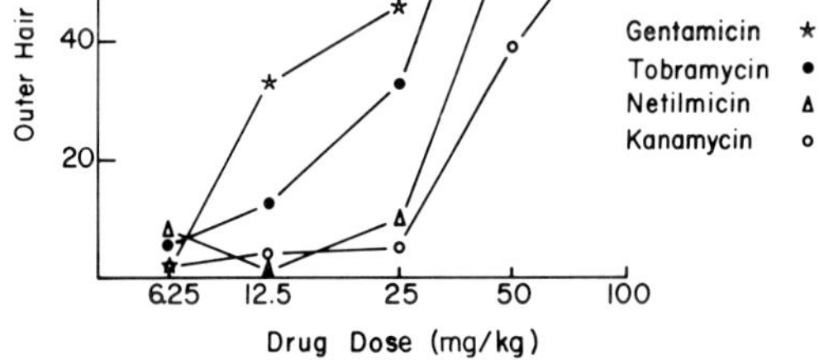

Figure 4-8. Dose-effect curves for guinea pigs treated with 40 mg/kg of ethacrynic acid 2 hours after the indicated doses of aminoglycoside anitibiotics. Hair cell loss was evaluated as in Fig. 4-2.

inhibiting diuretics does not occur with other antibiotics such as polymyxin E, chloramphenicol, vancomycin, or amphotericin B. The possibility of such an interaction should be kept in mind when the loop-inhibiting diuretics are used in combination with any potentially ototoxic drug.

References

1. Brown, C. B., Ogg, C. S., Cameron, J. S., and Bewick, M. High dose furosemide in acute reversible intrinsic renal failure. *Scott. Med. J.* 19 [Suppl. 1]:35, 1974.
2. Brummett, R. E., Brown, R. T., and Himes, D. L. Quantitative relationships of the ototoxic interaction of kanamycin and ethacrynic acid. *Arch. Otolaryngol.* 105:240, 1979.
3. Brummett, R. E., and Fox, K. E. Studies of Aminoglycoside Ototoxicity in Animal Models. In A. Whelton and H. C. Neu (Eds.), *The Aminoglycosides: Microbiology, Clinical Use and Toxicologic Complications.* New York: Marcel Dekker. In press.
4. Brummett, R. E., Fox, K. E., Bendrick, T. W., and Himes, D. L. Ototoxicity of tobramycin, gentamicin, amikacin and sisomicin in the guinea pig. *J. Antimicrob. Chemother.* 4:73, 1978.
5. Brummett, R. E., Fox, K. E., Brown, R. T., and Himes, D. L. Comparative ototoxic liability of netilmicin and gentamicin. *Arch. Otolaryngol.* 104:579, 1978.
6. Brummett, R. E., Himes, D., Saine, B., and Vernon, J. A comparative study of the ototoxicity of tobramycin and gentamicin. *Arch. Otolaryngol.* 96:505, 1972.
7. Brummett, R. E., Traynor, J., Brown, R., and Himes, D. Cochlear damage resulting from kanamycin and furosemide. *Acta Otolaryngol.* 80:86, 1975.
8. Brummett, R. E., Traynor, J., Manor, N., and West, B. Ototoxic interaction between aminoglycoside antibiotics and diuretics. *Toxicol. Appl. Pharmacol.* 29:97, 1974.
9. Davis, R. R., and Brummett, R. E. Cochlear destruction resulting from an interaction of some non-aminoglycoside antibiotics and ethacrynic acid. *Pharmacologist* 21:144, 1979.
10. Fox, K. E., and Brummett, R. E. Tissue distribution of ^{14}C-ethacrynic acid and its ^{14}C-cysteine adduct during depression of the cochlear potential in guinea pigs. *Pharmacologist* 16:283, 1974.
11. Fox, K. E., and Brummett, R. E. The relationship between the cytotoxicity of kanamycin and ethacrynic acid for mammalian cells in vitro and their ototoxicity in vivo. *Acta Otolaryngol.* 87:72, 1979.
12. Fox, K. E., Brummett, R. E., Brown, R., and Himes, D. A comparative study of the ototoxicity of gentamicin and gentamicin C_1. *Arch. Otolaryngol.* 106:44, 1980.
13. Hinshaw, H. C., and Feldman, W. H. Streptomycin in treatment of clinical tuberculosis: A preliminary report. *Proc. Staff Meetings Mayo Clin.* 20:313, 1945.
14. Johnson, A. H., and Hamilton, C. H. Kanamycin ototoxicity—possible potentiation by other drugs. *South. Med. J.* 63:511, 1970.
15. Jones, H. C. Intrauterine ototoxicity. *J. Natl. Med. Assoc.* 65:201, 1973.
16. Kusakari, J., Ise, I., Comegys, T. H., Thalmann, I., and Thalmann, R. Effect of ethacrynic acid, furosemide and ouabain upon the endolymphatic potential and upon high energy phosphates of the stria vascularis. *Laryngoscope* 88:12, 1978.
17. Mathog, R. H., and Klein, W. J. Ototoxicity of ethacrynic acid and aminoglycoside antibiotics in uremia. *N. Engl. J. Med.* 280:1223, 1969.
18. Mathog, R. H., Thomas, W. G., and Hudson, W. R. Ototoxicity of new and potent diuretics. *Arch. Otolaryngol.* 92:7, 1970.
19. Matz, G. J., and Beal, D. D. Ototoxicity of ethacrynic acid. *Arch. Otolaryngol.* 90:152, 1969.
20. Meriwether, W. D., Mangi, R. J., and Serpick, A. A. Deafness following standard intravenous dose of ethacrynic acid. *J.A.M.A.* 216:795, 1971.

21. Muth, R. G. Furosemide in severe renal insufficiency. *Postgrad. Med. J.* 47 [April Suppl.]:21, 1971.
22. Nuttall, A. L., Marques, D. M., and Lawrence, M. Effects of perilymphatic perfusion with neomycin on the cochlear microphonic potential in the guinea pig. *Acta Otolaryngol.* 83:393, 1977.
23. Pillay, V. K. G., Schwartz, F. D., Ami, K., and Kark, R. M. Transient and permanent deafness following treatment with ethacrynic acid in renal failure. *Lancet* 1:77, 1969.
24. Russell, N. J., Brummett, R. E., and Fox, K. E. Morphologic, electrophysiologic and pharmacokinetic correlates of the ototoxic interaction between kanamycin and ethacrynic acid. *Fed. Proc.* 36:412, 1977.
25. Russell, N. J., Brummett, R. E., and Fox, K. E. Interaction of kanamycin and ethacrynic acid: Early cochlear hair cell damage. *Pharmacologist* 21:253, 1979.
26. Russell, N. J., Fox, K. E., and Brummett, R. E. Alterations in the stria vascularis of the guinea pig cochlea after treatment with kanamycin/ethacrynic acid and ethacrynic acid alone. *Soc. Neurosci. Abs.* 4:10, 1978.
27. Russell, N. J., Fox, K. E., and Brummett, R. E. Ototoxic effects of the interaction between kanamycin and ethacrynic acid: Cochlear ultrastructure correlated with cochlear potentials and kanamycin levels. *Acta Otolaryngol.* 88:369, 1979.
28. Schneider, W. J., and Becker, E. L. Acute transient hearing loss after ethacrynic acid therapy. *Arch. Intern. Med.* 117:715, 1966.
29. Schwartz, G. H., David, D. S., Riggio, R. R., Stenzel, K. H., and Rubin, A. L. Ototoxicity induced by furosemide. *N. Engl. J. Med.* 282:1413, 1970.
30. Stockhorst, E., and Schacht, J. Radioactive labeling of phospholipids and proteins by cochlear perfusion in the guinea pig and the effect of neomycin. *Acta Otolaryngol.* 83:401, 1977.
31. West, B. A., Brummett, R. E., and Himes, D. L. Interaction of kanamycin and ethacrynic acid: Severe cochlear damage in guinea pigs. *Arch. Otolaryngol.* 98:32, 1973.

Discussion of Chapter 4

Dr. Wersäll: Have you done similar studies with gentamicin and netilmicin? If so, that would indicate whether your experimental model would serve as a good screening method.

You get a very high concentration of kanamycin right at the site of the cell, with an immediate killing effect. There is a difference between the effects of streptomycin and gentamicin on the cochlear physiology when a therapeutic dose of, say, 3 μg/ml is applied to the round window. Does this difference depend on the fact that you increase the penetration of your antibiotics to the extent that you get a very sharp increase in kanamycin in the endolymph, which acts as a killing agent on the cell? Did you measure endolymph concentrations?

Dr. Brummett: We have not measured the concentration in the endolymph, but are planning to do this. We have measured the concentrations in the perilymph and, surprisingly, we don't find any difference.

I want to comment on the specificity of the interaction with loop diuretics, which occurs with all aminoglycosides. All of the loop diuretics, including ethacrynic acid and furosemide, have ototoxic augmentation with aminoglycosides. Furosemide causes this augmentation only at high doses, and the other loop diuretics, at low doses. Ototoxic augmentation with loop diuretics also occurs with nonaminoglycosides such as viomycin, polymyxin B, and capreomycin. It does not occur with spectinomycin, vancomycin, or amphotericin B.

Dr. Schacht: We have been interested in this problem of potentiation. Our hypothesis of aminoglycoside action suggests that the aminoglycosides break down the permeability barriers of the cell, so that ethacrynic acid may cause increased toxicity. This was tested by measuring cochlear ethacrynic acid concentrations by radioautography after application of ethacrynic acid alone or in combination with neomycin. The presence of the aminoglycoside caused a three- to five-fold increase of ethacrynate in the cochlea.*

Dr. Brummett: We have considered that concept, but have not been able to confirm it with autoradiography. Also, aminoglycosides cause nuclear chromatin clumping, which is an early finding. We have noted changes in the plasma membrane as well, but we have not been able to detect whether these or nuclear chromatin clumping occurs first.

Dr. Schacht: The morphologic changes in the stria vascularis that you showed point to an augmentation of the ethacrynic acid effect, which fits very nicely with what we are seeing in terms of concentrations of the drug in the cochlea.

Dr. Hawkins: Gary Wright and I injected ethacrynic acid, furosemide, and other similar drugs into the middle ear and found that the ototoxicity was much greater than that of gentamicin and other aminoglycosides. A single dose of less than 0.1 mg of ethacrynic acid injected into the middle ear space is sufficient to produce permanent destruction of the organ of Corti.

Dr. Brummett: We found that 10^{-5}M concentrations of ethacrynic acid killed cultured thymocytes very quickly. This same effect could take place when the cochlea is perfused with ethacrynic acid. The cytotoxicity of ethacrynic acid is greater than that of most of the cancer chemotherapy drugs.

Dr. Anniko: An interaction with ethacrynic acid seems to occur also with drugs other than aminoglycosides. For example, we have used atoxyl with ethacrynic acid and obtained similar results.

*A. Orsulakova and J. Schacht, *Acta Otolaryngol.* In press.

5. Kinetics of Aminoglycoside Antibiotics in Perilymph and Endolymph in Animals

Patrice Tran Ba Huy, Christian Manuel, and Alain Meulemans

The aim in any pharmacokinetic study is to define the absorption, distribution, and excretion of a drug. For a given dosage, this determines the concentration of the drug at its site of action, and hence the intensity of its effect as a function of time. Such studies are necessary for more accurate prediction of potential drug toxicity. The well-known ototoxicity of aminoglycoside antibiotics (AAB) affects sensory structures in the inner ear. The unique access of a drug to these structures is by way of the fluid compartments, perilymph and endolymph. Thus, the study of AAB toxicity implies precise knowledge of drug kinetics in perilymph, endolymph, and tissues of the inner ear, and the mechanism of drug-binding to these tissues. In this chapter, we review the literature on the kinetics of parenterally administered AAB in the inner ear fluids of animals and discuss some methodologic problems in these studies. We also report the findings of our kinetics studies and comment on their toxicologic and therapeutic implications.

Review of the Literature

The data available from the literature on the kinetics of AAB in inner ear fluids are summarized in Table 5-1. The emphasis on concentrations in the perilymph may be explained by the relative ease of collecting this fluid. It must be emphasized that the conclusions drawn from such studies may not fully reflect ototoxicity, since there is no proof that perilymph is the main route of AAB to the organ of Corti. Despite considerable variation in pharmacokinetic parameters such as levels and half-lives in plasma and perilymph, it is possible to draw some general conclusions:

1. Most of the studies on kinetics have been conducted on perilymph. Microbiologic assays were used for measurement of drug concentrations after administration of high doses in single or repeated intramuscular or subcutaneous injections.

Table 5-1. Literature Review of Pharmacokinetics of AAB in Animals

Study	Animals	AB Assay*	Limit of Sensitivity (μg/ml)†	Sample Volume (μl)	AAB‡	Dose (mg/kg)	Route	Time of Sampling (Hours after last dose)	Concentration in Plasma (μg/ml)	Concentration in Perilymph (μg/ml)	Time of Highest Concentration in Perilymph (Hours after last dose)	Concentration in Endolymph (μg/ml)	Half-Life in Perilymph (Hours)
Vrabec et al. [23]	Cat	Bio	0.0156	?	SM	30	IM	5	7	6	5		
								11	3.8	4.5			
						30, twice daily for 2 days				10–15			
Voldrich [22]	GP	Bio	?	9	SM	200	IM	4		13	4		
								24		0			
				2	KA	150		4		10	4		
								8		4.5			
								24		1.5			
				2	NEO	150		3–6	800	7–8	4		
								24		2.5			
						150, daily for 4 days				20			
Stupp [19]	GP	Bio	0.5	5	SM	20	SC	2	25	10			
								5	20	25	5		
						250		1		18			
								5		20	5		
								18		13			
			0.5	5	DhSM	250		1		55	1		9
								5		40			
								18		15			
	GP	Bio	5	5	NEO	25		1	25	111	1		8.5
								5	3.5	45			
								18	0.1	20			
								25	0.1	10.6			
			5	5	NEO	100		1		100	1		
								5		80			
								18		45			

			0.5	5	KA	25		1	10	2.5	1		15
								5		2			
								18		1.8			
						250		1	510	18	1		
								2		19			
								5	19	18		18	
								18	0.7	9		11	
								25		6			
Watanabe et al. [25]	GP	Bio	0.003/μg total	1–2	KA	400	IM	1	1,000	25		ND	8
								4		30	4	ND	
								8		20		ND	
								12		15		ND	
								24		5		ND	
						400, daily for 1 week				22.5		ND	
						400, daily for 2 weeks				21		3	
						400, daily for 3 weeks				10.5		3.5	
						400, daily for 4 weeks				12		10	
Wagner et al. [24]	Rab	Bio	?	3	SM	200	IM	2	300	6	2		3.38
								6	25	3			
von Ilberg et al. [11]	Rab	Bio	?	3	SM	200	IM	2		20	2		
								6		6			
Strauss et al. [18]	GP	Bio	0.625	1	GE	2	IM	2	10	2			
						4		6	13	5			
Quante et al. [15]	GP	Bio	0.625	1	GE	16	IM	7	47	14			
Federspil et al. [2, 10]	GP	Bio+ ^{14}C-GE	?	?	GE	50	SC	1	140	8			12
								2	100	10	2		
								5	9	9			
								18	0	4			
		Bio	?		TO	50		1	130	5.5			11
								2	90	10	2		
								5	20	9			
								8	4	4			
								18	0	3.7			
		Bio	?		AM	50		1	800	18			10
								2	500	30			
								5	30	9.6	5		

Table 5-1 (Continued)

Study	Animals	AB Assay*	Limit of Sensitivity (μg/ml)†	Sample Volume (μl)	AAB‡	Dose (mg/kg)	Route	Time of Sampling (Hours after last dose)	Concentration in Plasma (μg/ml)	Concentration in Perilymph (μg/ml)	Time of Highest Concentration in Perilymph (Hours after last dose)	Concentration in Endolymph (μg/ml)	Half-Life in Perilymph (Hours)
Tachibana et al. [20]	GP	Bio	0.01	?	KA	400, daily for 10 days	IM	1	361	21			
								3	84	28			
								6	34	40	6		
								12	2	40			
								24	0.65	2.6			
Toyoda et al. [21]	GP	Bio	0.5	?	KA	400	IM	6	8	41	6		
								24	0.7	2.7			
						400, daily for 10 days		6		51			
								24		23			
Ohtani et al. [14]	Rab	Bio	?	?	KA	200	IP	4	254	27	4		
								24	0	3.6			
Christensen et al. [8]	Cat	Bio	?	10	AM	45, daily for 2 months	SC		73	3.16			
						90, daily for 2 months			183	14.45			
					GE	9, daily for 2 months			36	26.7			
						18, daily for 2 months			42	2			
Brummett et al. [7]	GP	REA	0.5	?	GE	150	IM	1	250	8			9.5
								2	143	20	2		
								4	25	10.5			
								6		13			
								12		7			
						50, daily for 4 weeks		2	40	5.5			
						100, daily for 4 weeks		2	98	17.1			
						150, daily for 4 weeks		2	402	32.7			

		REA	0.5		NET	150		1	250	2	2	11.4
								2	140	10		
								4	25	8.5		
								6	7	7.5		
								12		7		
						50, daily for 4 weeks		2	12	3.2		
						100, daily for 4 weeks		2	45	4.2		
						150, daily for 4 weeks		2	98	12.5		
Russell et al. [17]	GP	REA	0.5	?	KA	400	IM	3		107	3	10
								4		72		
								6		63		
								24		6.1		
Tran Ba Huy et al.§	Rat	RIA	0.1	0.1	GE	4	IM	0.5	8.31	0.099		3.20
								1	5.45	0.103		
								1.5	2.61	0.133		
								2	1.23	0.121		
								3	0.70	0.143	3	
								4	0.2	0.099		
								5	0.11	0.056		
								6	0.098	0.063		
								7	0.044	0.056		
								8	0.054	0.042		
								9	0.029	0.033		

*Antibiotic assay.

†Volumes submitted for AB assay.

‡Aminoglycoside antibiotics

§Tran Ba Huy, P., Manuel, C., Meulemans, A., Sterkers, O., and Amiel, C. Pharmacokinetics of gentamicin in perilymph and endolymph of the rat as determined by radioimmunoassay. *J. Infect. Dis.* 143:476, 1981.

GP = guinea pig; Rab = rabbit; Bio = biologic; ^{14}C-GE = ^{14}C-gentamicin tracer; REA = radioenzymatic assay; RIA = radioimmunoassay; SM = streptomycin; KA = kanamycin; NEO = neomycin; DhSM = dihydrostreptomycin; GE = gentamicin; TO = tobramycin; AM = amikacin; NET = netilmicin; IM = intramuscular; SC = subcutaneous; IP = intraperitoneal; ND = not done.

Source: The data presented in this table were compiled specifically for this chapter and have been obtained directly from the listed references or calculated from the authors' figures.

2. The time required for AAB to reach maximal values is greater in perilymph than in plasma. With gentamicin, Federspil et al. [9, 10] and Brummett et al. [7] found a peak in perilymph at 2 hours. With other compounds, the perilymphatic peak time varies between 1 and 6 hours, depending on the drug, the dose, and the sampling time.
3. After administration of doses that produce peak levels in serum similar to those achieved in man, maximal levels of AAB in the perilymph are 10 to 25 μg/ml with streptomycin (dose, 20 mg/kg) [19], 2.5 to 5.0 μg/ml with kanamycin (dose, 25 mg/kg) [19], and 0.14 μg/ml with gentamicin (dose, 4 mg/kg) [our study].
4. Most half-lives of AAB in perilymph given by the authors or calculated from their three or four experimental values range from 8 to 15 hours. A 3.38-hour value, however, was reported by Wagner et al. [24] for streptomycin. For gentamicin, Federspil et al. [9, 10] and Brummett et al. [7] found values of 12.0 and 9.5 hours, respectively. In each case, the half-life was longer in perilymph than in plasma.

The slower elimination of AAB from perilymph than from plasma has been considered responsible for their toxicity. The relationship between ototoxicity and perilymphatic clearance was emphasized as early as 1965 by Voldrich [22]. Comparing streptomycin, kanamycin, and neomycin, he noticed that neomycin, which is the most ototoxic of these AAB, had the slowest elimination rate from the perilymph. In his work, Stupp [19] developed the theory that the specific organ toxicity of the AAB is directly related to its specific accumulation in the inner ear fluids: the more ototoxic the aminoglycoside, the higher its concentration and the longer its retention in inner ear fluids. The accumulation phenomenon, which is of great therapeutic interest, has been investigated extensively after repeated intramuscular injections. Vrabec et al. [23] found accumulation of streptomycin in the perilymph of the cat after doses of 30 mg/kg given every 12 hours. The plateau values observed on the second day averaged 12 to 13 μg/ml, twice as high as those obtained after a single 30-mg/kg dose. This level was maintained regardless of the number of such doses subsequently given. Voldrich [22] also reported an accumulation after daily doses of 150 mg/kg of neomycin, yielding a concentration of 20 μg/ml after 4 days. Numerous studies performed subsequently on other AAB also showed accumulation [9, 20, 21]. Recently, Brummett et al. [7] demonstrated that, during administration of gentamicin or netilmicin, 150 mg/kg daily for 4 weeks, gentamicin accumulated in perilymph, whereas netilmicin did not. In contrast, the distribution kinetics after short-term administration was nearly identical for the two drugs. Brummett attributed this feature to "the gentamicin nephrotoxicity which could reduce its own elimination rate to a point yielding an accumulation whereas netilmicin would continue to be eliminated at the same rate." Thus, the differences between the perilymphatic concentrations of the two drugs reflect only the differences in plasma levels, with similar perilymph-to-plasma ratios for the two drugs: 12.5/98 = 0.13 for netilmicin and 32.7/402 = 0.08 for gentamicin. None of these experiments allows conclusions regarding any accumulation in perilymph, since they fail to take account of differences in nephrotoxicity and resulting accumulation in serum.

From a review of these studies, it is clear that "accumulation" does not have the same meaning for all investigators. Elimination of the AAB follows exponential (first-order) kinetics. This implies that a constant fraction of the drug is eliminated per unit time, and therefore that the elimination half-life is independent of drug concentration and dose. More than four half-lives are required for almost complete elimination from the perilymph. Thus, repeated administration of any aminoglycoside at intervals shorter than four half-lives must result in its accumulation in perilymph, which will continue until the amount eliminated (which increases as drug accumulation occurs) equals the amount administered per dose. In other words, the accumulation of AAB in perilymph reported by numerous investigators does not represent an abnormal phenomenon. Nor does apparent accumulation connote a continuous trapping of these drugs by their entry into the perilymph without clearance from this fluid, as described by Stupp [19]. Under the experimental conditions reported previously, accumulation resulted from the short dosage interval used by the authors for a given aminoglycoside, so that not enough time elapsed to permit the elimination of the previous dose from perilymph before the next dose was given.

A threshold for entry of the AAB into the inner ear has been reported by Stupp [19] and Wagner et al. [24]. Administering kanamycin in increasing doses of 15 to 250 mg/kg, Stupp observed an abrupt increase of the perilymph concentrations with doses above 40 mg/kg, and he designated this feature the toxic threshold of the inner ear. He therefore recommended avoiding high peak concentrations of AAB in blood. Such a critical level was also stated by Wagner et al. Using streptomycin in rabbits, they claimed that they were able to detect the drug in perilymph only when plasma concentrations exceeded 100 μg/ml, although our analysis of their data does not seem to sustain such a conclusion. At doses of streptomycin between 25 and 200 mg/kg, mean perilymph concentrations (y) were found to be directly related to the amount of the injected drug (x): $y = 0.178x - 0.174$; n = 8; r = 0.941.

In contrast, data on levels of AAB in the endolymph are scarce. Because of technical difficulties, very few studies have been conducted on this fluid, although its role in the hearing process is of primary importance. At 5 and 8 hours after a single subcutaneous injection of 250 mg/kg of kanamycin, Stupp [19] found endolymph concentrations of 18 and 11 μg/ml, respectively, approximately equal to the perilymph values at those times. From his report, however, it is not clear whether simultaneous determinations of perilymph and endolymph concentrations were performed on the same animal. After a single intramuscular injection of 400 mg/kg of kanamycin, Watanabe et al. [25] could not detect the drug in endolymph during the first 24 hours. Such negative results were observed even when the sample volume was increased to 7 μl to improve the sensitivity of the assay. With daily 400-mg/kg injections of kanamycin, the drug was present in endolymph at a concentration of 3 μg/g at

2 weeks and reached 10 μg/g at the end of 4 weeks. The endolymph-to-perilymph ratio of kanamycin concentrations increased from 0.13 to 0.83 during this period, but the surprising decrease of perilymph concentrations with time leads us to consider the six-fold increase of this ratio with caution. Moreover, the absolute increase of the endolymph concentration is likely to be related to a decrease in kidney function and a rise in plasma concentration, which can be expected after 10-day administration of 400 mg/kg of kanamycin per day. Nevertheless, the correlation made by the author between the decrease of the cochlear microphonic potentials and the increase of the drug concentration in endolymph is of great interest. Using the semiquantitative technique of autoradiography, Balogh et al. [2] injected ^{3}H-dihydrostreptomycin intraperitoneally in guinea pigs. They found greater quantities of the drug in perilymph than in endolymph. They proposed the hypothesis that the antibiotic entered into the perilymphatic space from the spiral ligament, and into the endolymphatic space from the stria vascularis and/or from the perilymphatic space.

Comments on Methodology

When the whole set of data is considered, it may be possible to explain the observed discrepancies among authors by differences in protocol. The methods used deserve some comments concerning the doses administered, routes of administration, fluid sampling, and the assays for AAB.

The doses administered were usually very large, producing levels in serum far higher than those customarily achieved in man. This experimental design could be explained by the relatively low sensitivity level of the antibiotic assays available at the time and the necessity to obtain, in some cases, a clear histologic pattern of drug toxicity. Such excessive dosage leads to the following problems: First, these high doses may induce disorders leading to experimental artifacts. Renal failure resulting from nephrotoxicity may increase the plasma levels and thus enhance the probability of ototoxic injury. Neuromuscular blockade by calcium depletion at the end-plate may result both in hypoxia caused by respiratory muscle paresis and in consequent acidosis. Under such conditions, any kinetics study conducted with high doses becomes questionable if renal function is not monitored at the same time. Second, the same dose of two AAB may yield slightly different peak plasma levels. Any comparative study should therefore emphasize plasma levels more than administered doses.

Usually, the AAB have been administered by single intramuscular or subcutaneous injections. Only Ohtani et al. [14] used the intraperitoneal route. Because half-lives of AAB differ in perilymph and plasma, the ratio of concentrations in these fluids determined after a single injection is a time-dependent variable and therefore has limited significance. Several investigators have used repeated intramuscular injections [7, 8, 9, 20, 21, 22, 23, 25], but in our experience such a technique does not yield reproducible peak plasma levels, probably because of local variations in absorption. Furthermore, investigators have rarely employed dosage intervals comparable to schedules that are standard in clinical practice. Extrapolation of results obtained in animals to the situation in man would require following dose regimens comparable to those used in man. The dose interval could be determined from the elimination half-life of the aminoglycoside from plasma, which is directly related to the glomerular filtration rate. In many rodent species, this consideration would lead to an increase in the frequency of drug administration. To obtain sustained plasma levels, some authors have ligated renal arteries [11, 15, 18]. This technique represents a remarkable attempt to achieve a steady state, but, for obvious reasons, it cannot be sustained for more than a few hours and therefore cannot be used in a chronic experiment. We would also like to emphasize that such a model does not, by any means, represent the conditions met in chronic renal failure observed in man, but only a model of acute anuria.

In most of the studies, perilymph rather than endolymph has been sampled. From the perilymph curves found in the literature, it appears that the number of determinations is often very small. This is especially noticeable in decay studies, in which half-lives were determined by the authors from only three or four values. A precise evaluation of kinetics would require more experimental points.

The numerous technical difficulties in the sampling of endolymph make the control of purity absolutely necessary, since, even with good technique, contamination of the specimen by blood or perilymph may readily occur. Measurement of sodium and potassium concentrations, demonstrating that the composition of this fluid resembles the intracellular milieu, is the best method of ensuring that the sample assayed for AAB is indeed endolymph. Normal values for sodium and potassium content reported by Bosher and Warren [5], who used emission spectrophotometry, averaged 0.91 and 154.0 millimoles/liter, respectively. Neither Stupp [19] nor Watanabe et al. [25], however, checked the purity of the samples used in their studies. Contamination, therefore, cannot be ruled out.

Regarding the assay for AAB in inner ear fluids, most of the reports describe microbiologic techniques that generally use *Bacillus subtilis* as a testing organism, either with a cup plate method or with a disk technique. When mentioned, the sensitivity limit averages 0.5 μg/ml for a 5-μl sample. Some authors, however, increased the sensitivity, detecting 0.625 μg/ml for a 1-μl sample [15, 18], 0.01 μg/ml for an unspecified sample volume [20], 0.015 μg/ml [23], and 0.003 μg by disk for a 1- to 2-μl sample [25]. The method of reverse vertical diffusion in capillary tubes, which is considered the most sensitive microbiologic technique, was not described in any of the cases. Radioenzymatic assays have been described by Russell, Fox, and Brummett [17]. When either acetylation of adenylylation is used, it seems difficult to lower the sensitivity limit to less than 0.5 μg/ml in a 5-μl sample. Radioactive ^{14}C-gentamicin has been used as a tracer by Federspil et al. [10], but the specific activity of this labeled compound is usually low, averaging 5 to 6 nCi/μg. ^{3}H-Gentamicin, with a specific activity of 1 to 2 μCi/μg, would be suitable for perilymph, but not for endolymph assays. Moreover, the high cost of such a technique makes it difficult to apply to a large-scale experiment.

Experimental Study with Gentamicin

This review of the studies published thus far showed that initial defects in methodology had prevented the elucidation of the kinetics of AAB in inner ear fluids. We therefore conducted a pharmacokinetic study of an aminoglycoside in endolymph and perilymph under controlled conditions, using a modified radioimmunoassay that allows precise determination of drug concentrations during the administration of doses producing serum levels comparable to those achieved in patients treated with AAB.

Gentamicin was chosen as the aminoglycoside for this study because it has undergone the most extensive investigation of ototoxicity in animals and in man. The drug was administered either by a single intramuscular injection of 4 mg/kg or by constant infusion of doses ranging from 7 to 150 μg per minute. The experiment involving a single intramuscular injection was conducted only to allow a comparison of our study with those previously reported. The constant-infusion technique was used as the primary method of administration since it proved to be the easiest means of obtaining the equilibrium necessary for measurement of the ratio of concentrations in the inner ear fluid and plasma in a steady state. In experiments lasting less than 15 hours, gentamicin in saline was infused via a jugular catheter at a rate of 30 μl per minute. We obtained a wide range of plasma gentamicin concentrations by varying the concentration in the infusate. A reproducible plasma level plateau was achieved after 45 minutes of infusion.

In continuous infusion experiments lasting for 6 days, gentamicin was administered via two implantable osmotic minipumps (Alzet, Alza Corp., Palo Alto, Calif.), which delivered 1 μl per hour of a 450-mg/ml solution of gentamicin at a constant rate, yielding a gentamicin infusion rate of 15 μg per minute. The rate of delivery of gentamicin was checked on the second day by assaying of gentamicin plasma concentrations in the first two aminals. Blood was sampled by puncture of the angular vein under brief anesthesia. The results were in agreement with those expected from the pumping rate according to the manufacturer's specifications. To avoid the need for anesthesia, we did not repeat this procedure on the other animals. We gave no priming dose, in order to avoid the consequences of the possible suprathreshold effect described by Stupp [19] and Wagner et al. [24].

Continuous infusion under anesthesia required a laboratory animal that would provide stable physiologic conditions. The rat appeared to be the most convenient animal, since it can be maintained under anesthesia for 15 hours without significant variations in blood pressure. Any experimental animal whose mean blood pressure fell below 100 mm Hg was discarded so that error related to the effect of a diminished glomerular filtration rate on gentamicin clearance was excluded. The glomerular filtration rate was measured by determination of the clearance of tritiated inulin in three animals.

Perilymph was collected by means of an external approach to the first coil of the scala vestibuli, with a beveled micropipette having a 10-μm (O.D.) tip. Suction was applied slowly over an average of 5 minutes to avoid rupture of the membranous labyrinth and subsequent contamination by endolymph. Any sample contaminated with blood was discarded. For the first 55 animals, the sample volume was adjusted to 10 μl with a calibrated glass capillary tube, but the volume of the sample collected was then reduced to 5 μl for the following 172 animals, in order to avoid contamination by cerebrospinal fluid via the cochlear aqueduct. The sample was diluted in 100 μl of distilled water and stored at −30°C.

An endolymph sample of about 100 nl was collected by an external approach to the second coil, with a beveled micropipette having a 5-μm (O.D.) tip. The sample was placed under water-saturated oil to avoid evaporation, and its purity was immediately assessed according to determination of the Na^+ and K^+ concentrations by ultramicrospectrophotometry of 1-nl samples. The mean sodium concentration was 1.58 ± 0.3 millimoles/liter (mean ± SEM), and the mean potassium concentration was 146 ± 2.3 millimoles/liter. Twenty percent of our samples had to be discarded because of electrolyte abnormalities. In each of these cases, the sodium concentration was far above the upper limit of the spectrophotometer sodium channel, which was adjusted for measurements in the range 0.2 to 6 millimoles/liter.

In our study, we required sensitivity for detection of gentamicin concentrations as low as 100 pg in 1 μl of perilymph and 10 to 20 pg in 100 nl of endolymph. Thus, radioimmunoassay was the method of choice, since it can detect 10 pg of gentamicin.

With this method, our results were the following: After a single intramuscular injection of 4 mg/kg, a peak occurs in plasma at 15 minutes and in perilymph at about 3 hours (Fig. 5-1). At the perilymphatic peak, the perilymph-to-plasma ratio of gentamicin concentrations averages 0.20. The slow perilymphatic uptake is also clearly demonstrated during the continuous infusion experiment, the results of which are presented in Table 5-2. With a 15-μg per minute gentamicin infusion rate yielding a plasma plateau after 45 minutes of infusion, the perilymphatic concentration slowly increased from 0.06 μg/ml at 45 minutes to 2 μg/ml at 12 hours. The rate of increase of the gentamicin concentration in perilymph, however, was extremely slow after the twelfth hour and reached a value of 2.4 μg/ml at 2 days, suggesting that a plateau was being achieved. At 6 days, the further rise in plasma levels suggested the development of renal failure. Such a possibility was demonstrated by the dramatic decrease of the glomerular filtration rate as determined in three animals. Throughout the 6-day experiment, however, the perilymph-to-plasma ratio of gentamicin concentrations remained in a narrow range, regardless of the plasma levels. The fact that the perilymphatic concentration reached a value of 5 μg/ml at 6 days, when the plasma concentration was 25.8 μg/ml, is evidence against any substantial accumulation of the drug in the perilymph.

We explored the hypothesis of a "toxic threshold" by varying the gentamicin

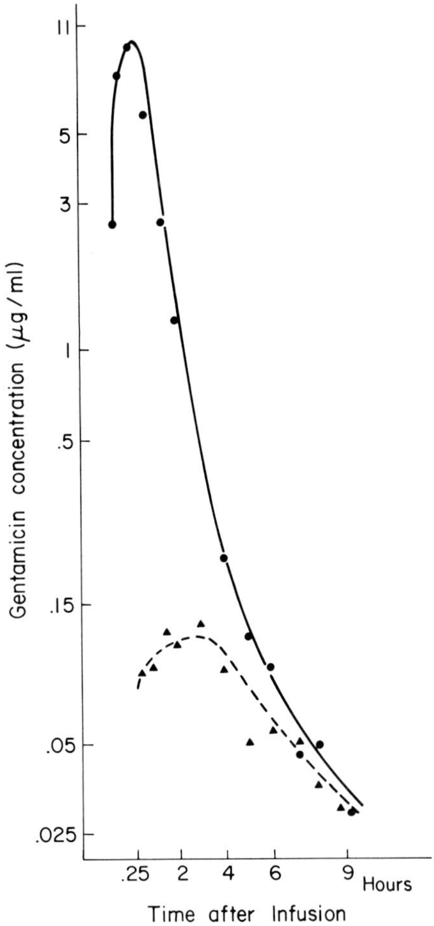

Figure 5-1. Kinetics of gentamicin in plasma (●) and perilymph (▲) after a single intramuscular injection of 4 mg/kg. Each perilymph point represents the mean of assays of two samples.

infusion rate from 7 to 150 μg per minute. A linear relationship was found between the perilymph concentration and the plasma level, suggesting that there was no threshold for entry of gentamicin into perilymph, at least within the limits of our experiment.

The decay curve of gentamicin in perilymph was studied with two distinct methods: following a single intramuscular injection, and after cessation of a 4-hour constant infusion of 15 μg per minute. A half-life of 3 hours and 12 minutes was calculated from 14 experimental points during the decay period in the single-injection experiments (Fig. 5-1) and a half-life of 2 hours and 57 minutes from 27 experimental points obtained in the intravenous infusion experiments (Fig. 5-2). Although early points following the cessation of a 4-

Table 5-2. Kinetics of Gentamicin during Continuous Infusion

Rate of Infusion	Time of Sampling	Concentration in Plasma (μg/ml)	Concentration in Perilymph (μg/ml)	Concentration in Endolymph (μg/ml)	Ratio of Concentrations—Endolymph/Perilymph
15 μg/min	45 min	11.47 ± 1.8	0.06	<0.05	
	2 hr	11.47 ± 1.8	0.4 ± 0.15	<0.05	
	7 hr	11.47 ± 1.8	0.81	<0.05	
	9 hr	11.47 ± 1.8	1.04 ± 0.5	<0.05	
	10 hr	11.47 ± 1.8	1.84 ± 0.14	1.03 ± 0.3	0.56
	12 hr	11.47 ± 1.8	2 ± 0.19	1.03 ± 0.3	0.56
	2 days	12.6 ± 1.3	2.4 ± 0.1	1 ± 0.5	0.42
	6 days	25.8 ± 2.5	5.1 ± 0.5	1.2 ± 0.4	0.23
150 μg/min	3 hr	164 ± 8	3.18 ± 0.6	<0.05	
	8 hr	171 ± 9	3.7 ± 0.2	1.6 ± 0.5	0.43

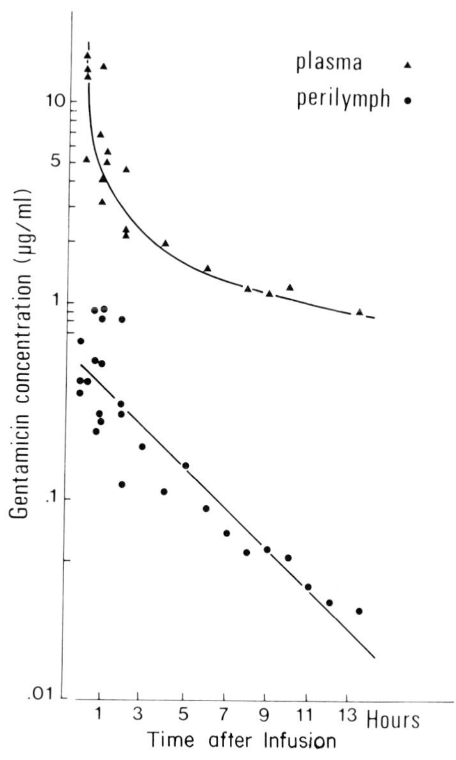

Figure 5-2. Disappearance of gentamicin from plasma and perilymph after the end of a 4-hour infusion at a constant rate of 15 μg/minute.

hour constant-rate infusion of gentamicin may suggest an initial rapid decline of the concentration in perilymph, the rest of the curve appears to be monoexponential. If the decay curve were truly monoexponential, it would suggest that gentamicin in perilymph has no exchange with any deeper compartment, i.e., tissues of the inner ear. On the other hand, since ototoxicity undoubtedly involves binding of the aminoglycoside to tissue receptors, such exchange of gentamicin in perilymph with inner ear tissue must occur. The sensitivity limit of our radioimmunoassay did not allow us to detect such an exchange, however. A study with a more sensitive assay of gentamicin in inner ear tissues as well as in fluids could detect the influence of gentamicin uptake and release from inner ear tissues on clearance from the perilymph.

Under our experimental conditions, the main factor influencing disappearance of gentamicin from the perilymph seems to be the turnover of perilymph itself. Unfortunately, the exact physiology of the labyrinthine fluids is still not clear. The slow disappearance from perilymph of gentamicin, and presumably of other AAB as well, is not entirely responsible for their toxicity, however. The high affinity that exists between AAB and some compounds of the cell membrane (see Chap. 7) most probably plays the major role in the mechanism of ototoxicity. It must be emphasized that, if the low clearance indeed facilitates the uptake of the drug by the tissues of the inner ear, this does not argue for or against a special affinity of these drugs for these tissues.

The endolymph data reported in Table 5-2 show that gentamicin was undetectable (<0.05 μg/ml) for 9 hours with a 15 μg per minute infusion rate. By 10 hours, the concentration in endolymph had risen to about 1 μg/ml, and it remained at about the same level throughout the 6-day infusion. The ratio of gentamicin in endolymph and perilymph declined from 0.56 to 0.23. The ratio in endolymph and plasma ranged from 0.09 to 0.05 throughout the 6-day infusion. When the rate of infusion was increased to 150 μg per minute, gentamicin was still undetectable in endolymph at 3 hours. At 8 hours, the concentration was 1.58 ± 0.48 μg/ml, and the ratio of concentrations in endolymph and perilymph was about 0.43. Such data do not permit any conclusions as to whether gentamicin is actively transported into endolymph, nor do they allow one to assess the role of endolymph in the transport of the drug to the organ of Corti, but the delayed detection of gentamicin in endolymph, as compared to perilymph, must be emphasized, whatever its significance.

The results of a recent unpublished experiment provide new information regarding the route by which gentamicin reaches the hair cells of the cochlea. For many years, this route has been presumed to be the perilymph, probably because the numerous technical difficulties encountered in the collection of endolymph restricted measurements on this fluid. In studying the effect on gentamicin kinetics when ethacrynic acid was administered at low doses (8 mg per hour), thus producing no diuretic effects, we found that penetration of gentamicin into endolymph was increased, whereas gentamicin penetration into perilymph was not affected. Since ethacrynic acid seems to increase the ototoxicity of AAB in animals (see Chap. 4) and man (see Chap. 26), our results would suggest that the concentration of gentamicin in endolymph is probably a critical factor in toxicity that has been insufficiently evaluated in the past. Konishi recently demonstrated [12] that the concentration of AAB necessary to suppress the cochlear microphonic potentials was always lower when the drug was administered into the endolymph rather than into the perilymphatic space. Thus, for potentiation between diuretics and AAB, endolymph may provide the main route of access of AAB to the sensory structures.

To approach the basic question regarding the influence of the mode of administration upon drug kinetics, we are in the process of comparing gentamicin concentrations in inner ear fluids after administering equal doses either by continuous infusion or by sequential intravenous injections. Preliminary results show that continuous infusion yields higher concentrations in endolymph and perilymph than are seen with the intermittent-dose regimen.

Therapeutic Considerations

One of the aims of experimental pharmacokinetic studies is to provide clinicians with guidelines for administration of AAB with the lowest toxic risk for both the kidney and the inner ear. The conditions favoring development of minimal renal toxicity have been explored in a variety of experimental studies. Bennett et al. [4] showed in rats that the frequency of doses of gentamicin was a more important factor in the development of nephrotoxicity than the peak serum concentration, i.e., increase of plasma creatinine (an index of nephrotoxicity) was directly related to the number of daily doses for a given total daily dose. Reiner et al. [16] also showed in dogs that the same total dose of gentamicin was significantly less nephrotoxic when given by one daily intravenous injection than when administered by continuous infusion. If nephrotoxicity is mainly related quantitatively to the uptake of AAB by the kidney, one should observe different amounts of AAB bound to the renal tissue following different modes of administration; however, such a direct causal relationship between toxicity and renal tissue concentration of AAB has not been observed. According to Bennett et al. [4], the more frequent the doses, the higher the cortical gentamicin concentration, whereas, according to Reiner et al. [16], the mass of gentamicin found in the renal cortex is paradoxically the same, regardless of the frequency of administration. Moreover, Bowman et al. [6] showed in rats that the difference in nephrotoxicity between gentamicin and netilmicin cannot be accounted for by a difference in drug concentration in the renal cortex. This fact leads us to consider the possibility of intrinsic toxicity of the AAB, independent of their pharmacokinetic properties.

The intrinsic toxicity of various AAB has been studied in vitro. By using either lysosome preparations extracted from renal tubular cells [13] or mitochondrial suspensions prepared with hepatocytes [3], some authors have developed a scale of relative toxicity for various AAB that generally agrees with the conclusions established in human beings, as reported by Appel and Neu [1].

As far as ototoxicity is concerned, what is known about gentamicin kinetics in inner ear fluids—and this can probably be extrapolated to most of the other AAB—yields the following conclusions:

1. Ototoxicity seems to depend on two factors: the affinity of the drug for some compounds (these could be polyphosphoinositides; see Chap. 7) located in the membranes of cochleovestibular sensory cells, and a complex factor implicating both plasma concentration of the drug and time.
2. The strong correlation observed among plasma, perilymph, and endolymph concentrations of gentamicin under equilibrium conditions shows that sustained high plasma levels, as encountered in chronic renal failure, may give rise to cochleovestibular disorders by leading to high and sustained inner ear fluid levels of the drug that facilitate its uptake by the susceptible inner ear tissues.
3. From our experiments, it can be seen that high, but brief, peak plasma levels might not yield the same risk as more sustained elevated levels, because perilymph and especially endolymph are in deep compartments that require time for the drug to reach significant concentrations. When AAB are administered clinically, intermittent injections, which yield lower inner ear fluid concentrations than does continuous infusion, would be expected to produce less ototoxicity.
4. In determining the dosage interval of an aminoglycoside, we should consider the elimination half-life of the drug from the inner ear fluids. Since the half-life in endolymph is difficult to assess at present, four perilymphatic half-lives should be allowed between successive injections for elimination from the perilymph. For gentamicin, such considerations would lead to a theoretical dose interval of 12 hours, although in fact an interval of 8 hours is generally used because of therapeutic considerations.
5. Since the concentration of AAB in endolymph is probably a prominent factor in the mechanism of ototoxicity, drugs such as diuretics, which may modify penetration into the membranous labyrinth, would be expected to increase the risk of toxicity.
6. If all pharmacokinetic and bacteriologic parameters are equal, the clinician should select the aminoglycoside that shows the least affinity for the sensory structures of the inner ear. In the future, this affinity has to be studied comparatively for the various AAB used therapeutically, and studies on kinetics must be conducted concomitantly in endolymph and tissues of the inner ear, such as the organ of Corti and stria vascularis.

References

1. Appel, G. B., and Neu, H. C. The nephrotoxicity of antimicrobial agents. *N. Engl. J. Med.* 296:722, 1977.
2. Balogh, K., Jr., Hiraide, F., and Ishii, D. Distribution of radioactive dihydrostreptomycin in the cochlea. An autoradiographic study. *Ann. Otol. Rhinol. Laryngol.* 79:641, 1970.
3. Bendirdjian, J-P., Foucher, B., and Fillastre, J-P. Influence des aminoglycosides sur le métabolisme respiratoire des mitochondries isolées de foie et de rein de rat. In J-P. Fillastre (Ed.), *Nephrotoxicity, Interaction of Drugs with Membrane Systems: Mitochondria-Lysosomes.* New York: Masson, 1978. P. 315.
4. Bennett, W. M., Plamp, C. E., Gilbert, D. N., Parker, R. A., and Porter, G. A. The influence of dosage regimen on experimental gentamicin nephrotoxicity: Dissociation of peak serum levels from renal failure. *J. Infect. Dis.* 140:576, 1979.

5. Bosher, S. K., and Warren, R. L. Observations on the electrochemistry of the cochlear endolymph of the rat: a quantitative study of its electrical potential and ionic composition as determined by means of flame spectrophotometry. *Proc. R. Soc. Lond. [Biol.]* 171:227, 1968.
6. Bowman, R. L., Silverblatt, F. J., and Kaloyanides, G. J. Comparison of the nephrotoxicity of netilmicin and gentamicin in rats. *Antimicrob. Agents Chemother.* 12:474, 1977.
7. Brummett, R. E., Fox, K. E., Brown, R. T., and Himes, D. L. Comparative ototoxic liability of netilmicin and gentamicin. *Arch. Otolaryngol.* 104:579, 1978.
8. Christensen, E. F., Reiffenstein, J. C., and Madissoo, H. Comparative ototoxicity of amikacin and gentamicin in cats. *Antimicrob. Agents Chemother.* 12:178, 1977.
9. Federspil, P. Zur Ototoxizität der Aminglykosid-Antibiotika. *Infection* 4:239, 1976.
10. Federspil P., Schätzle, W., and Tiesler, E. Pharmacokinetics and ototoxicity of gentamicin, tobramycin, and amikacin. *J. Infect. Dis.* 134 [Suppl]:S200, 1976.
11. Von Ilberg, C., Arnold, W., and Ritter R. Ursachen und Beeinflussung der Ototoxizität des Streptomycins und verwandter Antibiotika. *Z. Laryngol. Rhinol. Otol.* 53:112, 1974.
12. Konishi, T. Effects of local application of ototoxic antibiotics on cochlear potentials in guinea pigs. *Acta Otolaryngol.* 88:41, 1979.
13. Morin, J. P., Fresel, J., Fillastre, J-P., and Vaillant, R. Aminoglycoside Actions on Rat Kidney Lysosomes in vivo and in vitro. In J-P. Fillastre (Ed.), *Nephrotoxicity, Interaction of Drugs with Membrane Systems: Mitochondria-Lysosomes.* New York: Masson, 1978. P. 253.
14. Ohtani, I., Ohtsuki, K., Omata, T., Ouchi, J., and Saito, T. Potentiation and its mechanism of cochlear damage resulting from furosemide and aminoglycoside antibiotics. *ORL* 40:53, 1978.
15. Quante, M., Strauss, P., and Rosin, H. Gentamicin level in the guinea-pig's perilymph and liquor subject to the dosis distribution. *Arch. Otorhinolaryngol.* 208:295, 1974.
16. Reiner, N. E., Bloxham, D. D., and Thompson, W. L. Nephrotoxicity of gentamicin and tobramycin given once daily or continuously in dogs. *J. Antimicrob. Chemother.* 4[Suppl. A]:85, 1978.
17. Russell, N. J., Fox, K. E., and Brummett, R. E. Ototoxic effects of the interaction between kanamycin and ethacrynic acid. *Acta Otolaryngol.* 88:369, 1979.
18. Strauss, P., Rosin, H., Quante, M., Harari, G., Winter, V., and Löbner, S. Gentamicin im Verteilungsgleichgewicht zwischen Serum, Perilymphe und Liquor beim Meerschweinchen nach Dosierung im therapeutischen Bereich. *Arch. Otorhinolaryngol.* 218:79, 1977.
19. Stupp, H-F. Untersuchung der Antibiotikaspiegel in den Innenohrflüssigkeiten und ihre Bedeutung für die spezifische Ototoxizität der Aminoglykosidantibiotika. *Acta Otolaryngol. (Stockh.)* [Suppl. 262], 1970.
20. Tachibana, M., Mizukoshi, O., and Kuriyama, K. Inhibitory effects of kanamycin on glycolysis in cochlea and kidney—possible involvement in the formation of oto- and nephrotoxicities. *Biochem. Pharmacol.* 25:2297, 1976.
21. Toyoda, Y., and Tachibana, M. Tissue levels of kanamycin in correlation with oto- and nephrotoxicity. *Acta Otolaryngol.* 86:9, 1978.
22. Voldrich, L. The kinetics of streptomycin, kanamycin and neomycin in the inner ear. *Acta Otolaryngol.* 60:243, 1965.
23. Vrabec. D. P., Cody, D. T., and Ulrich, J. A. A study of the relative concentrations of antibiotics in the blood, spinal fluid and perilymph in animals. *Ann. Otol. Rhinol. Laryngol.* 74:688, 1965.
24. Wagner, W. H., Chou, J. T., von Ilberg, C., et al. Untersuchungen zur Pharmakokinetik von Streptomycin. *Arzneim. Forsch.* 21:2006, 1971.
25. Watanabe, Y., Nakajima, R. Oda, R., et al. Experimental study on the transfer of kanamycin to the inner ear fluids. *Med. J. Osaka Univ.* 21:257, 1971.

6. Pharmacokinetics of Aminoglycoside Antibiotics in the Perilymph

Pierre Federspil

The specific toxic effect of aminoglycoside antibiotics on the inner ear may be explained in part by the fact that these antibiotics are eliminated more slowly from the inner ear fluids than from serum. This retention was described initially for streptomycin [15, 23], dihydrostreptomycin [15, 18], neomycin [15, 21, 23], and kanamycin [19, 23]. The first studies on the pharmacokinetics of gentamicin in the inner ear fluids were published in 1973 [4, 10], and comparable studies on tobramycin and amikacin first appeared in 1975 [6]. All of these experiments were performed on guinea pigs.

In this review, we will provide some additional data on the inner ear pharmacokinetics of gentamicin, tobramycin, amikacin, and neomycin, as well as of a newer aminoglycoside, netilmicin. Comparative studies with almost similar results will be reported for mezlocillin, a new penicillin. In addition, we shall discuss the application of experimental pharmacokinetic studies in animals to questions of clinical ototoxicity of aminoglycosides in patients.

Figure 6-1A depicts the pharmacokinetics of ^{14}C-labeled gentamicin in the serum, perilymph, aqueous and vitreous humors, and brain of guinea pigs after a subcutaneous injection of 100 mg/kg. The concentration of gentamicin in the serum of the guinea pig is maximal soon after the injection, and elimination of the drug is rapid, with a half-life of about 60 minutes. The rapid rise to a maximal serum concentration and the subsequent rapid decline are seen with all aminoglycoside antibiotics and in all mammalian species studied [2]. If, however, a given dose of an aminoglycoside, expressed as mg/kg body weight, is administered to animals of different species, the maximal serum concentrations observed in the guinea pig or mouse are much lower than those observed, for example, in the dog or in man. This finding is related to the ratio of body surface area and relative blood volume to total body weight. Such considerations are important in comparisons of pharmacokinetics and toxicity of aminoglycosides in different mammalian species. This principle probably explains the observation by Waitz [26] that several authors evaluating the

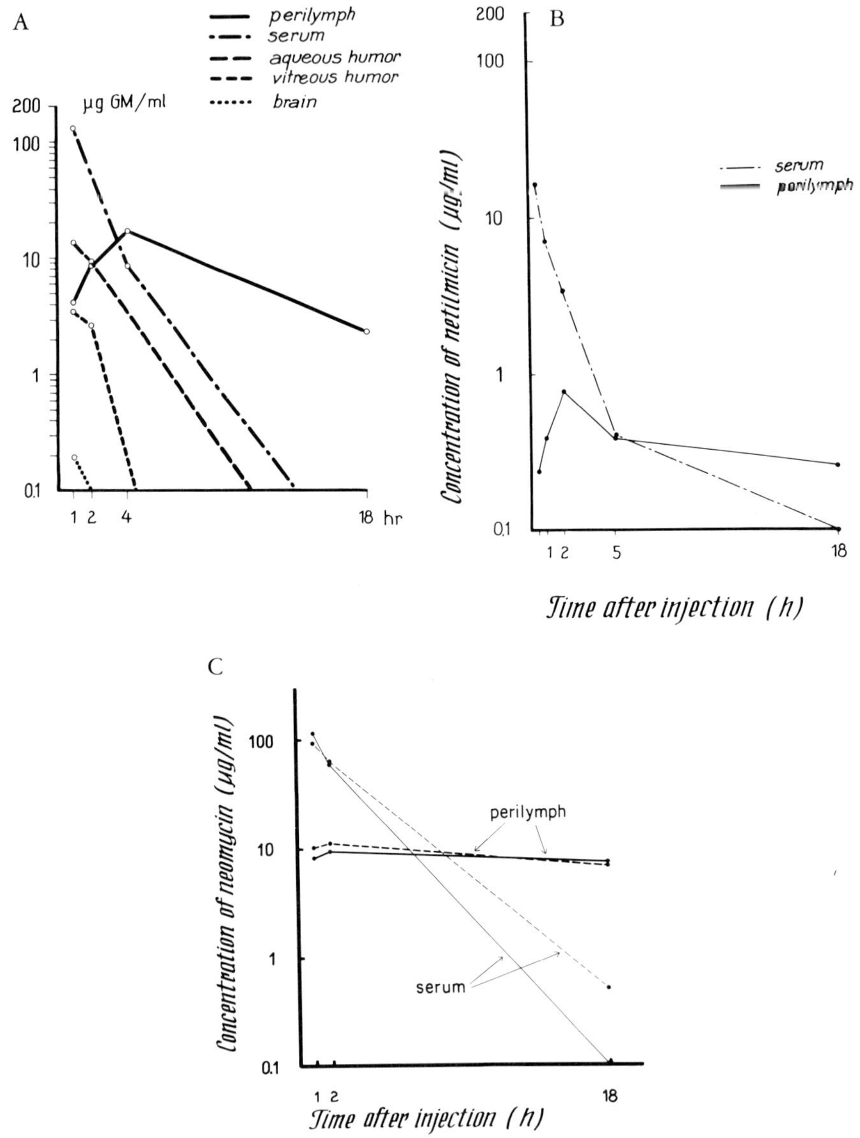

Figure 6-1. A. Pharmacokinetics after subcutaneous injection of 100 mg/kg of ^{14}C-labeled gentamicin in the guinea pig. Each point gives the average of the results determined in two or four samples obtained from one or two guinea pigs. B. Pharmacokinetics after subcutaneous injection of 8 mg/kg of ^{14}C-labeled netilmicin in the guinea pig. Each point is the average of the results determined in two or four samples from one or two guinea pigs. C. Neomycin pharmacokinetics in serum and perilymph after intraperitoneal (continuous curves) and subcutaneous (interrupted curves) injection of 100 mg/kg. Each point is the average of the results for six different animals.

aminoglycoside antibiotics used a "human-size dose" in mice and wondered why the efficacy was less than expected. One solution is to adjust the dosage for different species to obtain comparable serum levels.

The concentration of gentamicin in the perilymph increases more slowly than that in serum. The maximal concentration in the perilymph, about 6 percent of that in serum, is reached 2 hours after the subcutaneous injection and persists up to 5 hours, by which time the concentration in serum has become lower than that in perilymph (Fig. 6-1A). After 18 and 25 hours, the level of gentamicin in perilymph has fallen slowly, long after gentamicin is no longer detectable in serum. Thus, there is retention of gentamicin in the perilymph compared with serum, as shown in Fig. 6-1A and confirmed by similar data in Fig. 6-5. The half-lives of gentamicin and other new aminoglycosides in the perilymph of the guinea pig are all about 10 hours [4, 13]. Figure 6-1A also shows the maximal concentrations of gentamicin in eye humors and brain of guinea pigs compared to the maximal serum concentration after a subcutaneous injection. The maximal aqueous humor concentration of gentamicin is 20 percent, and the maximal cerebrospinal fluid concentration about 3 percent, of the maximal serum concentration, whereas the vitreous humor concentration is 10 to 15 percent of the aqueous humor concentration [4, 13].

The pharmacokinetics of aminoglycosides in endolymph appears to be similar to that in perilymph. Two to five hours after the subcutaneous injection of 50 mg of gentamicin per kg into guinea pigs, the endolymph concentration of gentamicin is 80 to 90 percent of the perilymph level [4, 13]. Stupp [17] found that concentrations of kanamycin in the endolymph and perilymph of the guinea pig were similar, i.e., 18.0 and 23.5 μg/ml at 5 hours and 11 and 13 μg/ml at 18 hours, respectively, after the subcutaneous injection of kanamycin, 250 mg/kg body weight. Watanabe et al. [27] did not detect any kanamycin in the endolymph of the guinea pig 24 hours after a single intramuscular injection of 400 mg/kg, or after the last of eight daily injections of the same dose, whereas the perilymph concentrations were about 5 and 20 μg/ml, respectively. Twenty-four hours after the last of 15 daily injections of 400 mg/kg, however, a small quantity of kanamycin (3 μg/ml) was observed in the endolymph. The endolymph concentrations increased in the third and fourth weeks of treatment, reaching the values of the decreasing perilymph concentrations (11 μg/ml).

Netilmicin is a new semisynthetic aminoglycoside antibiotic that exhibits cochlear and vestibular toxicity less than one-fifth that of gentamicin in the guinea pig [3]. Figure 6-1B shows the pharmacokinetics of netilmicin in the serum and perilymph of guinea pigs after a single subcutaneous injection of 8 mg/kg of radioactively labeled drug. The curves indicate that, while netilmicin rapidly disappears from serum, as expected, its concentration in perilymph reaches a peak (at about 5 percent of that of the maximal serum concentration) after 2 hours and then declines slowly. If one compares the pharmacokinetics of netilmicin in the perilymph of the guinea pig (Fig. 6-1B) with that of gentamicin (Fig. 6-1A), one cannot see any significant difference after adjustment for dosage on the basis of mg/kg body weight. Thus, for the guinea pig, differences in ototoxicity of netilmicin and gentamicin cannot be explained by pharmacokinetic variations.

Neomycin has long been known to be exceedingly ototoxic. In fact, its ototoxicity in man is so great that its parenteral use was abandoned [11]. In order to see whether the perilymph pharmacokinetics of this aminoglycoside differs from that of gentamicin and the other newer aminoglycosides, we carried out pharmacokinetic studies in guinea pigs after injection of neomycin. Figure 6-1C illustrates the pharmacokinetics of neomycin in perilymph and serum after a single subcutaneous or intraperitoneal injection of 100 mg/kg [11]. Results with the two routes of administration are comparable. The peak concentration of neomycin in perilymph is similar to that of gentamicin (Fig. 6-1A) and to that of netilmicin (Fig. 6-1B), after adjustment for dosage. Neomycin, like the other aminoglycosides, is retained in perilymph; the decline of neomycin seems to be even slower. Our results consistently differ from those obtained by Stupp [17], who measured neomycin concentrations of 60 to 100 μg/ml in perilymph after injecting 100 mg/kg, whereas we found about 10 μg/ml after injecting the same dose. Our results are comparable to those of Vrabec et al. [23]. Thus, it seems unlikely that the greater ototoxic potential of neomycin can be accounted for by markedly elevated levels in the perilymph, although the apparently slower exit from the perilymph may thus be important for ototoxicity.

Such a delayed exit from perilymph is also seen, however, in the case of non-ototoxic antibiotics such as the acylureidopenicillin mezlocillin. As shown in Fig. 6-2, the concentration of mezlocillin in perilymph fell at a slower rate (half-life of 3.7 hours) than in serum (half-life of 24 minutes). Therefore, retention of aminoglycoside antibiotics in inner ear fluids cannot account completely for their ototoxicity.

Perilymph levels themselves do not give us any information on aminoglycoside binding within tissues of the inner ear, which may be more relevant. Von Ilberg et al. [22] noted a specific affinity of radioactively labeled dihydrostreptomycin for the cytoplasm of the inner and outer hair cells after local application of the drug. In contrast, Balogh et al. [1] and Kraus et al. [14] observed a nonspecific pattern of distribution of radioactively labeled dihydrostreptomycin in the inner ear after parenteral administration of the drug.

Many clinically important facts have been revealed by our study of the pharmacokinetics of the new aminoglycoside antibiotics in the inner ear. Figure 6-3 shows the perilymph levels of gentamicin in guinea pigs 2, 5, and 18 hours after subcutaneous injection of single doses ranging from 5 to 100 mg of gentamicin per kg. The perilymph concentration at each time increases linearly with the injected dose. Our finding [4, 10] was later confirmed by Quante et al. [16] in experimental studies with a different method. Figure 6-3 does not show a tenfold increase in perilymph levels analogous to that observed by Stupp [17] when he increased the dose of kanamycin from 25 to 50 mg/kg. We did not find a critical serum level for the penetration of gentamicin or tobramycin into the inner ear of the guinea pig. The linear increase of the concentration in

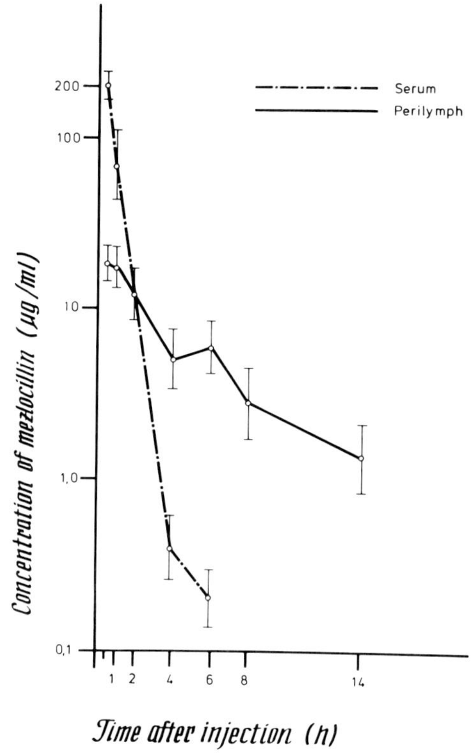

Figure 6-2. Mezlocillin pharmacokinetics in serum and perilymph of the guinea pig after a single intramuscular injection of 200 mg/kg. Each point is the average of the results for six different animals.

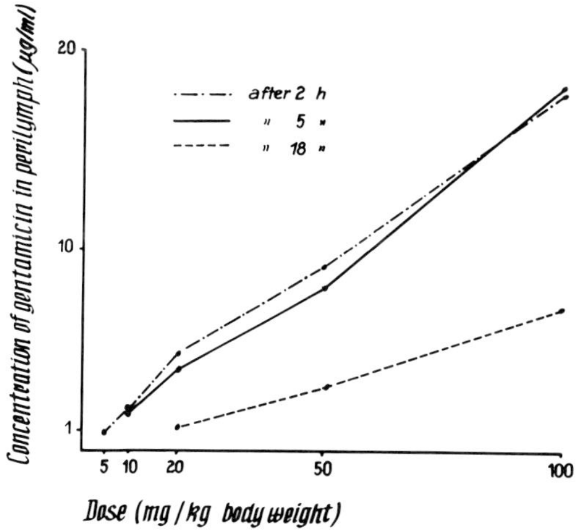

Figure 6-3. Relationship between the dose administered subcutaneously and the concentration of gentamicin in the perilymph of guinea pigs. Each point is the average of the results for at least six different animals.

perilymph with increasing doses of the drug argued against the critical serum level or threshold level that Wagner et al. [25] had reported for streptomycin in the rabbit. These results help to explain in part the observation that, although the risk of ototoxicity for a patient probably increases with the daily dose, there is no absolute threshold daily dose for the development of ototoxicity. Together with histologic investigation in the guinea pig showing an increase of ototoxicity of the aminoglycosides when the daily dose is divided [2], these results are the best argument for the fact that an occasional transient high aminoglycoside serum level does not lead to excessively high inner ear concentrations or to any damage. Our functional and histologic studies on ototoxicity in guinea pigs [5, 12] have suggested that the threshold for ototoxicity of the aminoglycosides is determined by the total dose, and that renal function is the major factor influencing this threshold. Diminution of high peak concentrations of aminoglycosides in serum by means of depot preparations or by continuous infusion to achieve sustained serum levels is not likely to decrease the ototoxic risk; in fact, it may even allow the aminoglycoside concentrations in perilymph to reach the serum level and, in this way, actually increase the ototoxic risk.

The concentrations of gentamicin, tobramycin, amikacin, and netilmicin in both inner ears are similar, i.e., they do not vary by more than 20 percent in both inner ears of 90 percent of the guinea pigs tested; this provides pharmacokinetic confirmation of the clinical observation that ototoxic damage is generally symmetric [7], although it is sometimes unilateral. In our histologic and functional investigations with the new aminoglycosides, major asymmetric cochlear damage was observed in about 15 percent of the guinea pigs tested. Early ototoxic damage is probably more often asymmetric than is severe ototoxicity. Pharmacokinetic studies with streptomycin in the rabbit have shown a high percentage of asymmetric perilymph concentrations [24]. The reasons for this discrepancy are not clear.

The ototoxicity of the new aminoglycoside antibiotics in patients without renal impairment occurs mainly during long-term treatment [5]. In order to explore the consequences of chronic treatment with an aminoglycoside for perilymph pharmacokinetics, we treated guinea pigs over longer periods of time, i.e., 10 days of treatment with single daily subcutaneous doses of 50 mg gentamicin per kg, 28 single daily subcutaneous doses of 80 mg tobramycin per kg, or 28 days of 100 mg amikacin per kg given subcutaneously twice daily. After the last dose of each of these courses, the pharmacokinetics of the aminoglycoside was similar to that in control animals treated with only a single dose (gentamicin is shown in Fig. 6-4). This result is in apparent contradiction to the experimental studies with other aminoglycosides [17, 21, 23, 27]. The aminoglycoside dosage chosen in those experiments may have produced renal functional disturbances that were not registered by serum determinations. The lack of accumulation in the perilymph during chronic aminoglycoside administration may suggest that, in patients with normal renal function, the risk of ototoxicity remains linear with time during long-term therapy until the total dose threshold is reached (see above).

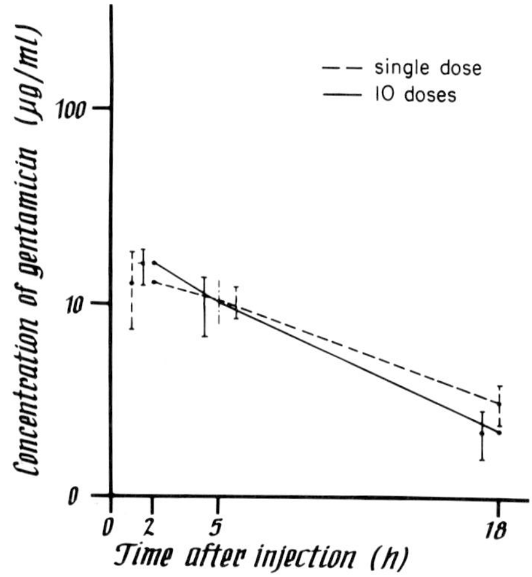

Figure 6-4. Gentamicin concentrations in the perilymph after a single subcutaneous injection (interrupted curve) and the last of 10 daily subcutaneous injections (continuous curve) of 50 mg gentamicin per kg in the guinea pig (36 samples).

There is an increased risk of aminoglycoside ototoxicity in patients with renal failure [2]. This may be due in part to accumulation of excessively high levels in serum as a result of decreased renal excretion, presumably leading to higher levels in the perilymph. In order to study the perilymph pharmacokinetics of a representative aminoglycoside under conditions of decreased renal excretion, we administered 50 mg gentamicin per kg subcutaneously to nephrectomized and normal control guinea pigs. As shown in Fig. 6-5A and 6-5B, the serum level fell off rapidly in the normal animals, as expected, but in the anuric animals there was prolonged persistence of a high level in the serum. As shown in Fig. 6-5, the gentamicin level in the perilymph of nephrectomized animals rose over several hours to a maximum at about 50 percent of that in serum. As the serum level declined slowly over 18 hours, the perilymph level remained nearly constant. Thus, whereas the perilymph level in normal animals remained at a low value (10 μg/ml) as the concentration in serum rose sharply and fell quickly, the perilymph level in nephrectomized animals rose to a higher range (around 50–70 μg/ml) and persisted while the serum level remained elevated. The persistent serum levels of gentamicin in anuric guinea pigs may be considered a short-term experimental model for continuous intravenous infusion of aminoglycosides. Such continuous administration to patients may result in constant serum levels in the therapeutic range. One might expect, however, that perilymph levels would also rise toward this range and persist as the aminoglycoside equilibrates in the serum and perilymph. Thus, although aminoglycosides appear to have increased efficacy in neutropenic patients when they are administered by continuous infusion

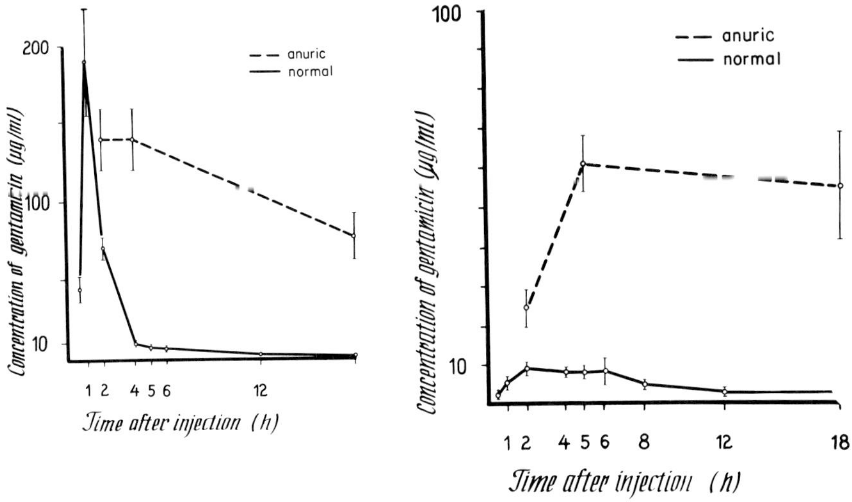

Figure 6-5. Pharmacokinetics of gentamicin in serum (A) and perilymph (B) of normal (continuous curve) and anuric (interrupted curve) guinea pigs after subcutaneous injection of 50 mg/kg. Gentamicin concentrations were determined by microbiologic assays. Each point is the average of the gentamicin determinations in six guinea pigs. To produce anuria, a bilateral nephrectomy was performed 2 to 3 hours before the administration of gentamicin.

[20], such a regimen might be expected to incur an increased risk of ototoxicity and nephrotoxicity [2, 5, 13, 19].

Furthermore, Fig. 6-5 indicates that treatment of ototoxicity with hemodialysis is not indicated in a patient with normal renal function, since the serum level of gentamicin falls rapidly even without dialysis. On the other hand, prolonged high serum levels in nephrectomized animals may lead to higher perilymph levels. Therefore, hemodialysis in patients with severe renal impairment may be helpful in reducing ototoxicity by decreasing the serum level and thus promoting exit from the perilymph. In assessing the effectiveness of other types of treatment for ototoxic damage caused by aminoglycoside antibiotics, we assumed initially that the concentration of aminoglycoside antibiotics in the inner ear fluids is an indicator of ototoxicity; thus, we would expect that a reduction of antibiotic concentration in the perilymph would lead to a reduction in ototoxicity. In 16 experimental series of about 8 guinea pigs each, however, no significant effect on gentamicin perilymph levels could be demonstrated by suboccipital puncture or by hydro-, osmo-, or salidiuresis [2, 4].

Patients with inner ear infections have long been known to have an increased risk of ototoxicity with aminoglycoside therapy [6]. Such an increase has not been so well established in patients with otitis media [2]. In pharmacokinetic studies, we were able to demonstrate a rise in perilymph levels of gentamicin and amikacin in otitis media during the first hours after subcutaneous injection, but not in all of the animals tested. We also found a diminution of the aminoglycoside antibiotic concentrations in the perilymph in otitis media a long time after the injection in some cases [2, 4]. Our pharmacokinetic studies confirm those of Voldrich and Petrcelkova [21] and of Wagner et al. [25] only inasmuch as these authors found a rise in streptomycin perilymph levels in all cases of otitis media. In our functional and histologic studies on the effect of otitis media on the ototoxicity of gentamicin, tobramycin, and amikacin, we were able to demonstrate an increase in ototoxicity [8].

Comparative pharmacokinetic studies of the aminoglycoside antibiotics in the inner ear make it possible to give an estimate of their ototoxic potential [11]. As already mentioned, the pharmacokinetics of netilmicin and gentamicin in the perilymph of the guinea pig is similar (Figs. 6-1B, 6-1A). Thus, we may assume that the ototoxic potential of netilmicin is much lower than that of gentamicin, because the semichronic toxicity of netilmicin is much lower than that of gentamicin. This evaluation is not as secure, however, as that based on well-conducted functional and histologic comparative studies.

Finally, it is important that some of the experimental results on the pharmacokinetics of the newer aminoglycoside antibiotics in the inner ear of animals could be confirmed in man for gentamicin by Federspil [2, 4] and in the more extended pharmacokinetic studies by Lerner et al. (see Chap. 25).

References

1. Balogh, K., Jr., Hiraide, F., and Ishii, D. Distribution of radioactive dihydrostreptomycin in the cochlea. An autoradiographic study. *Ann. Otol. Rhinol. Laryngol.* 79:641, 1970.
2. Federspil, P. *Antibiotikaschäden des Ohres.* Leipzig: Barth, 1979.
3. Federspil, P. Evaluation of the ototoxicity of netilmicin. *Current Chemotherapy,* Washington: Amer. Soc. for Microbiology. (Proceedings of 10th Internat. Congress of Chemotherapy, Zürich, 18–23 Sept. 1977.) P. 975, 1978.
4. Federspil, P. Experimentelle Untersuchungen zur Ototoxizität des Gentamycins. Habilitationsschrift, Medizinische Fakultät, University of the Saar, Homburg, W. Germany, 1973.
5. Federspil, P. Die klinische Ototoxizität und ihre Prophylaxe. In K. Hierholzer and N. Rietbrock (Eds.), *Physiologische und pharmakologische Grundlagen der Therapie.* Berliner Seminar 2. Braunschweig: Vieweg Verlag, 1979. P. 51.
6. Federspil, P. Oto-Rhino-Laryngologie. In H. P. Kuemmerle, E. R. Garrett, and K. H. Spitzy (Eds.), *Klinische Pharmakologie und Pharmakotherapie.* Munich/Berlin/Vienna: Urban & Schwarzenberg, 1976. P. 521.
7. Federspil, P. Ototoxicity. In Robert G. Richardson (Ed.) *Round Table Discussion on Gentamicin and Tobramycin.* The Royal Society of Medicine. London: Academic; New York: Grune & Stratton, 1978. P. 15.
8. Federspil, P. Ototoxizität der Aminoglykosid-Antibiotica und Otitis media. *Arch. Ohr.-, Nas.- u. Kehlk.-Heilk.* 207:487, 1974.
9. Federspil, P. Pharmakokinetik der neuen Aminoglykosid-Antibiotica im Innenohr und Ototoxizität. *Arch. Ohr.-, Nas.- u. Kehlk.-Heilk.* 210:363, 1975.
10. Federspil, P. Pharmakokinetik des Gentamycins in Serum und Innenohrflüssigkeiten. *Aktuel. Med.* in *Münch. Med. Wschr.* 115:8, 1973.
11. Fedespil, P. Zur Neomycin-Resorption aus dem gesunden und entzündlich veränderten Peritoneum. *Fortschr. Med.* 97:1517, 1979.
12. Federspil, P., Schätzle, W., Kayser, M., Sack, K., and Schentag, J. Influence of Total Dose, Division of Daily Dose, Age, and Pregnancy on Aminoglycoside

Ototoxicity. In J. D. Nelson and C. Grassi (Eds.), *Current Chemotherapy and Infectious Disease.* Washington, D.C.: American Society for Microbiology, 1980. Vol. 1, p. 607.

13. Federspil, P., Schätzle, W., and Tiesler, E. Pharmacokinetics and ototoxicity of gentamicin, tobramycin, and amikacin. *J. Infect. Dis.* 134[Suppl.]:200, 1976.
14. Kraus, H., Richrath, W., Borchard, K., Hägele, W., and Reinhold, B. Historadiographische Versuche zum Nachweis von 3H-Dihydrostreptomycin in der Cochlea des Meerschweinchens. In H. Jakobi and A. Herrmann (Eds.), *Hals-Nasen-Ohrenheilkunde.* Leipzig: Barth, 1973. P. 307.
15. Muraveiskaya, V. S. Determination of streptomycin, dihydrostreptomycin, colimycin, and monomycin concentrations in labyrinth fluid of guinea pigs. *Antibiotiki* 10:245, 1965.
16. Quante, M., Strauss, P., Harai, G., Winter, V., and Rosin, H. Die Abhängigkeit der Gentamicinkonzentration in der Perilymphe des Meerschweinchens von der Serumkonzentration. *Arch. Otorhinolaryngol.* 210:267, 1975.
17. Stupp, H-F. Untersuchung der Antibiotikaspiegel in den Innenohrflüssigkeiten und ihre Bedeutung für die spezifische Ototoxizität der Aminoglykosidantibiotika. *Acta Otolaryngol. (Stockh.)* [Suppl. 262], 1970.
18. Stupp, H., Rauch, S., Sous, H., Lagler, F., and Brun, J-P. Die Ursache der spezifischen Ototoxizität der basischen Streptomyces-Antibiotica—ein Permeabilitätsproblem. *Méd. Hyg.* 23:988, 1965.
19. Thompson, W. L. Néphrotoxicité de la gentamicine et de la tobramycine chez le chien. Comparaison après perfusion continue ou injection intraveineuse unique. *Nouv. Presse Méd.* 43:380, 1978.
20. Valdivieso, M., Feld, R., Rodriguez, V., and Bodey, G. P. Amikacin therapy of infections in neutropenic patients. *Am. J. Med. Sci.* 270:453, 1975.
21. Voldrich, L., and Petrcelkova, D. Neomycin levels in the inner ear fluids of guinea pigs. *Cesk. Otolaryngol.* 14:277, 1965.
22. Von Ilberg, C., Arnold, W., and Ritter, R. Ursachen und Beinflussung der Ototoxizität des Streptomycins und verwandter Antibiotika. *Laryngol. Rhinol. Otol.* 53:112, 1974.
23. Vrabec, D. P., Cody, D. T., and Ulrich, J. A. A study of the relative concentrations of antibiotics in the blood, spinal fluid, and perilymph in animals. *Ann. Otol. Rhinol. Laryngol.* 74:689, 1965.
24. Wagner, W. H. Spezifische Ototoxizität von Aminoglykosid-Antibiotika. *Immun. Infekt.* 3:241, 1975.
25. Wagner, W. H., Chou, J. T., von Ilberg, C., Ritter, R., and Vosteen, K. H. Untersuchungen zur Pharmakokinetik von Streptomycin. *Arzneim. Forsch.* 21:2006, 1971.
26. Waitz, J. A. Laboratory Evaluation of Aminoglycoside Antibiotics. In *Development in Industrial Microbiology.* Washington, D.C.: American Institute of Biological Sciences, 1975. Vol. 16, P. 161.
27. Watanabe, Y., Nakajima, R., Oda, R., Uno, M., and Naito, T. Experimental study on the transfer of kanamycin to the inner ear fluids. *Med. J. Osaka Univ.* 21:257, 1971.

Discussion of Chapters 5 and 6

Dr. Honrubia: I would like to report on an observation by Himmelfarb and Strelioff. They concluded from measurements of the cochlear potentials after administration of ethacrynic acid that the impedance of the cochlear partitions was affected by the action of this drug. This impedance change took place after the decline in the cochlear potentials and microphonics. Thus, it appears that there was a delayed effect on the cochlear potentials, due to a change in the impedance of the walls of the scala media. If that is the case, I think it is very important; we suggest that the effect of ototoxic drugs may be enhanced by ethacrynic acid because of the increased permeability of the membranes for the passage of drugs into the endolymphatic space. I would like to ask our speakers whether they could agree that the cochlear hair cells are most sensitive to kanamycin, due to the fact that kanamycin doesn't enter the endolymphatic spaces of the vestibular labyrinth because there is no change in the permeability of the endolymphatic membranes in the vestibule. I presume that the change in permeability of the scala media is due to the edema that ethacrynic acid produces around the stria vascularis, a structure unique to the cochlear labyrinth.

Dr. Federspil: Phase contrast microscopy shows that hair cells are characteristically altered by diuretics. Potentiation of ototoxicity occurs with aminoglycosides and ethacrynic acid; however, in my opinion, ethacrynic acid and not the aminoglycosides plays the important role. For instance, after having treated a guinea pig for 8 days with 100 mg of gentamicin per kg, and giving a dose of ethacrynic acid that is not ototoxic in itself, we could not find any potentiation of the ototoxicity. I think the main part of this toxicity is due to the ethacrynic acid or furosemide.

Dr. Honrubia: What causes the potentiation is the question—whether it is a direct action of the drug on the membranes or on the physiology of the hair cell; or it may be that it changes the passage of fluids through the cochlear partition, which allows the kanamycin to enter the scala media.

Dr. Federspil: Yes, that could also be a good explanation.

Dr. Wersäll: This leads to an important question dealing with pharmacology—that of the actual relationship between perilymph and endolymph concentrations under various conditions. There are rather few data on endolymph concentrations. Stupp, of course, put very much stress on endolymph concentrations. I think we will have to wait for future pharmacokinetic studies to find out what happens in the endolymph after the injection of ethacrynic acid.

I also think some of this material has to be studied in vitro with regard to the direct action of the two drugs on the cells. The direct effect on the membrane is important. What does the interaction of ethacrynic acid with neomycin or any other antibiotic mean? I think this has to be resolved by a combination of morphologic, histochemical, and physiologic methods.

Dr. Lerner: Dr. Tran Ba Huy, are you able with your methodology to distinguish among gentamicins C_1, C_{1a}, and C_2, and if so, was there any difference in the pharmacokinetics?

Dr. Tran Ba Huy: No.

Dr. Schacht: It seems to me we are trying to solve a problem with inadequate background. The action of the drugs obviously is in the tissues, and we are talking about extracellular levels of these drugs. I don't want to detract from the value of these studies; they do give us useful information. However, they only give us indirect information on what is happening in the tissues. I would like to see studies of drug concentrations in the tissues.

Dr. Manuel: Dr. Schacht, it seems to me that you don't agree with Dr. Tran Ba Huy's postinfusion decay curve for perilymph. It seems to be monoexponential. I agree with the thoughts you have about that, but it isn't fair to say that the curve may have two or more components, because you know the change in the precision of the model when the precision of the data decreases just a little. Since the dispersion of the points is very high, I think we cannot treat the curve mathematically at present.

Biochemistry of Aminoglycoside Effects on the Cochlea

Chapter 7, which is concerned with the effect of aminoglycosides on phospholipid metabolism in the hair cells, constitutes a novel approach to explaining the toxicity of aminoglycosides at the cellular level. Evidence provided by Norman Weiner and Jochen Schacht suggests that the initial step in the ototoxic action of these drugs may involve their binding to polyphosphoinositides in the cell membranes of inner ear tissues. After reviewing this evidence, they describe an artificial membrane system in which they study the effects of aminoglycosides at the molecular level. If the critical action of these agents can be elucidated, we might be able to reduce their ototoxic potential by chemical or pharmacologic manipulation.

7. Biochemical Model of Aminoglycoside-Induced Hearing Loss

Norman D. Weiner and Jochen Schacht

Most of the efficacious therapeutic agents in use today possess various degrees of toxic side effects that limit their clinical usefulness. In a number of instances, both the therapeutic and toxic actions of drugs at the cellular level are believed to be similar (e.g., the cytotoxic effects of alkylating agents). In other cases, the therapeutic and toxic actions at the cellular level are different (e.g., anticholinergic side effects of antihistamines). For many drugs, however, the biochemical events at the cellular level have not been clearly defined for either the therapeutic activity or the toxic side effects.

Although the site and mechanism of antibacterial action of aminoglycoside antibiotics are fairly well known at the biochemical level, a clear picture of their toxic action at the cellular level in the kidney and inner ear is still elusive. Their capacity to kill bacteria has been related to their affinity for the 30 S ribosomal subunit, resulting in interference with protein synthesis [22]. Ribosomes in the cytoplasm of eukaryotic (e.g., mammalian) cells are composed of subunits different from those of bacterial ribosomes. Although aminoglycosides may have some effect on mammalian protein synthesis, there are significant differences from the bacterial system [2].

Our work has been directed toward elucidation of the molecular mechanisms of antibiotic-induced hearing loss. If the molecular mechanism of ototoxicity is known, we can determine those sites on the antibiotic that are responsible for this toxicity. Such knowledge would provide a rational basis for future attempts at chemical modification of existing antibiotics to render them less ototoxic while they retain their antibacterial properties.

It is well established that the first step in the action of many hormones and drugs is their binding to receptor sites in the cell membrane. Receptor sites have been characterized as proteins in the case of many neurotransmitters and

The authors wish to acknowledge the collaboration of Dr. Shahid Lodhi and Iris Mechigian in the experimental work underlying this article. The research was supported by Grant NS 13792 and Program Project Grant NS 05785 from the National Institutes of Health.

hormones, as glycoproteins in the case of lectins, and as glycolipids in the case of glycoprotein hormones and bacterial toxins [3, 10]. Based on the experimental evidence discussed below, we suggest the polyphosphoinositides as receptors for aminoglycoside antibiotics.

Experimental Background

The strongly basic aminoglycosides do not readily penetrate cells [23], and it has been shown that these antibiotics accumulate in membrane structures [1, 30]. The initial action of these drugs may therefore occur at the cell membrane. This is also suggested by the rapid but reversible suppression by streptomycin of the microphonic output from the lateral line organ [37]. A number of drugs acting on the nervous system, as well as neurohumors modulating membrane permeability, alter the metabolism of membrane phospholipids, particularly the phosphoinositides [16]. We have previously provided evidence for involvement of polyphosphoinositides in the toxic actions of aminoglycoside antibiotics:

1. After chronic treatment of guinea pigs with neomycin, labeling of phosphatidylinositol diphosphate by [^{32}P]-orthophosphate was reduced in inner ear tissues [19].
2. After 6 days of treatment with neomycin, the incorporation of ^{32}P into polyphosphoinositides, but not into other lipids, was reduced in the kidney, and the amount of phosphatidylinositol diphosphate present was decreased [28].
3. In short-term experiments in which cochlear perilymphatic spaces were perfused with artificial perilymph containing neomycin at various concentrations, concentration-dependent decreases of cochlear microphonic potentials were paralleled by decreased labeling of cochlear [^{32}P]-phosphatidylinositol diphosphate [18, 31].
4. Neomycin inhibited the labeling of phosphatidylinositol diphosphate from [γ-^{32}P]-ATP in subcellular fractions of guinea pig brain, and it blocked the hydrolysis of previously labeled polyphosphoinositides. The actions of neomycin were shared by related ototoxic antibiotics, but not by chemically related non-ototoxic substances [26].
5. Low concentrations of neomycin competitively displaced Ca^{++} from polyphosphoinositides and synaptosomal membranes, whereas higher drug concentrations acted noncompetitively [12].

Furthermore, we have identified polyphosphoinositides as potential aminoglycoside receptors by using affinity chromatography. Neomycin was immobilized on glass beads and served as the stationary phase in column chromatography. Fractionation of an organic tissue extract of inner ear tissue or kidney demonstrated two components with high affinity for neomycin: phosphatidylinositol phosphate and phosphatidylinositol diphosphate [27].

The lipid specificity of the neomycin action was then investigated in monomolecular lipid films. Neomycin did not interact significantly, or it exerted a calciumlike effect (i.e., decrease of surface pressure) on films of phosphatidylcholine, -ethanolamine, -serine, and -inositol, and of cardiolipin, phosphatidic acid, and cerebroside. Films of polyphosphoinositides showed a unique reaction with the drug: a large increase in surface pressure that was already apparent at low drug concentrations [13]. From these experiments, an approximate dissociation constant for neomycin/polyphosphoinositide was calculated, $K_d = 3 \times 10^5$M, indicative of a rather stable complex.

Hypothesis

The formation of such an aminoglycoside-polyphosphoinositide complex should have a strong influence on the integrity of the plasma membrane. The polyphosphoinositides are believed to be involved in the control of membrane permeability [6, 9], so that complex formation would interfere not only with the structure, but also with the function of the membrane, e.g., excitability. Such a disturbance of membrane structure and function may be sufficient to explain most of the toxic actions of the drugs. It seems attractive, however, to speculate that this effect on membrane permeability is the first prerequisite for the drug to enter the cell. Inside the cell, the drug then may exert further toxic actions at different locations.

There is no shortage of other suggested mechanisms of aminoglycoside toxicity. Early hypotheses, primarily based on semi-quantitative techniques such as radioautography or histochemistry, have not provided rational explanations and need not be reviewed here. In the past few years, possible ototoxic mechanisms have been suggested involving mucopolysaccharides [4], nucleic acids [8], glycolysis [33], and glucose transport [5].

The polyphosphoinositides are not uniformly distributed among body tissues. Besides the brain, which has a high polyphosphoinositide content, but is protected from the aminoglycosides by the blood-brain barrier, the only organ known to have a high content of these lipids is the kidney [7]. This correlates well with the susceptibility of the kidney as a major target organ for toxic injury by aminoglycosides. The amounts of these lipids in the inner ear are presently being measured, and our labeling studies with ^{32}P already indicate that the polyphosphoinositides are highly active constituents of cochlear tissues, which are the other major target of aminoglycoside toxicity. It therefore seems appropriate to assume that the presence of these lipids makes a tissue susceptible to attack by aminoglycoside antibiotics. Although the studies cited above indicate that cochlear carbohydrate metabolism and energy utilization are affected by aminoglycosides,* there is no evidence that enzymes of glycolysis (or, for that matter, nucleic acids) in the cochlea differ from those in other tissues. Selective effects on various tissues are best explained by selec-

For a recent review of antibiotic toxicity, see ref. 25.

tive effects on their permeability. Thus, if the interaction of aminoglycoside antibiotics with polyphosphoinositides at the cell membrane is considered to be the initial causative action, a variety of intracellular effects may follow. Subsequent involvement of glycolysis and nucleic acids following antibiotic challenge is therefore not mutually exclusive with our hypothesis.

As another hypothesis, glucose transport has been suggested as a site of aminoglycoside action [5] on the basis of experiments showing that hyperglycemia (alloxan "diabetes") protects animals against kanamycin ototoxicity. These results still seem to be preliminary and, by the authors' own admission, are open to alternative explanations. For instance, drug excretion is considerably more rapid in hyperglycemic animals, and this might cause perilymph levels of kanamycin to be lower than in normal controls. Drug levels in serum and perilymph were not measured in the study cited.

An earlier study implying interference with glucose transport as a mechanism of antibiotic toxicity is in apparent contrast to recent preliminary results from our laboratory. Owada [20] reported that 3-aminoglucose, a fragmentation product of kanamycin, is more toxic than kanamycin itself. As far as we know, this is the only report ascribing ototoxic properties to aminosugars. We have used 3-aminoglucose in cochlear perfusions and found no indication of an effect on cochlear microphonics [34], whereas kanamycin showed a significant action under identical conditions. More data are needed for evaluation of glucose transport as a site of aminoglycoside toxicity.

Binding of aminoglycosides to mucopolysaccharides [4, 14, 24, 32] appears to be incompatible with our hypothesis, since it implies a different mechanism at the cell membrane. Although aminoglycosides might have more than one site of membrane action, it appears that binding to mucopolysaccharides is not sufficient to cause cellular toxicity. Tissues high in mucopolysaccharide content, such as liver, remain largely unaffected by the aminoglycosides. Complexes between these drugs and mucopolysaccharides have been demonstrated in vitro, but it is difficult to evaluate their significance. Mucopolysaccharides have a high affinity for calcium, which should be their physiologic counter-ion, but the above studies have been limited to Na^+ and K^+ as cations.

On the other hand, polyphosphoinositides appear to meet major criteria as a receptor site for aminoglycoside antibiotics; the polyphosphoinositides are preferentially distributed in tissues that are sensitive to aminoglycosides, and they bind the antibiotics at high ionic strength and in competition with calcium ion.

Models of Ototoxicity

The determination of the mechanism of toxic action at the cellular level of a systemically administered drug is extremely complex. Pharmacokinetic parameters, such as distribution, metabolism, and elimination, often critically influence the tissue levels and activity of the drug and prevent reliable determination of toxicity.

We have attempted to eliminate these uncertainties by administering drugs

Table 7-1. Effect of Drugs on Cochlear Microphonics

Drug	Rate of Loss ($-\mu V/min$)	Percent Loss	Significance (p value)
None	0.10 ± 0.26	7 ± 1	
Methylneobiosamine	0.23 ± 0.31	6 ± 5	>0.5
Neamine	0.36 ± 0.29	10 ± 7	>0.3
Kanamycin A	1.06 ± 0.30	29 ± 6	0.025
G-418	1.09 ± 0.21	24 ± 7	0.02
Ribostamycin	1.72 ± 0.24	51 ± 6	<0.01
Gentamicin C_{1_a}	1.77 ± 0.34	47 ± 4	<0.01
Neomycin B	3.34 ± 0.63	79 ± 7	<0.01
Kanamycin B	4.15 ± 0.75	76 ± 10	<0.01

Perilymphatic spaces of the guinea pig cochlea were perfused for 30 minutes with artificial perilymph, followed by 60 minutes with artificial perilymph containing the respective drug (10 mM). Loss of cochlear microphonics was determined 30 minutes after introduction of the drug. Numbers are means ± s.e.m. of five experiments. For experimental details, see S. Lodhi et al., Ototoxicity of aminoglycosides correlates with their action on monomolecular films of polyphosphoinositides. *Biochem. Pharmacol.* 29:597, 1980. G-418 (Schering) is an aminoglycoside produced by micromonospora.

directly into the cochlea [11, 31] (see also Chap. 3). Such experiments in situ allow direct control of drug concentrations and duration of treatment, and they provide an assessment of the intrinsic ototoxicity of a drug. The ototoxic potency of six aminoglycoside antibiotics and two fragments of aminoglycosides was measured in this way by cochlear perfusion in the guinea pig. Perilymphatic spaces were perfused with "artificial perilymph" containing 10 mM drug for 1 hour, during which time continuous measurements of cochlear microphonic potentials were made. Kanamycin B and neomycin B caused the most rapid decline of cochlear microphonic potentials, followed by gentamicin C_{1_a} = ribostamycin > kanamycin A = G-418. Neamine and methylneobiosamine, the aminoglycoside fragments, did not show any significant effect (Table 7-1).

Studies performed in situ provide a necessary link between experiments in vivo and attempts to investigate molecular mechanisms in vitro. Being less complex than in vivo studies, they provide more easily quantitated information about the physiologic action of the drug. Such assessment of physiologic effects cannot be gained from in vitro systems because of their greater simplicity.

Physicochemical in vitro models have been used in studies on mechanisms of drug action since Meyer's classical experiments on the mechanism of anesthetic action [15]. Although volumes of incorrect or highly speculative hypotheses have been generated by the use of naive models and their incorrect interpretation, there are numerous examples of physicochemical models that have given us insight into the molecular action of drugs.

These physicochemical models may range in complexity from simple studies of partition coefficients to systems allowing the investigator to separate such complex and interrelated factors as lipoidal membrane permeability, membrane pore permeability, unstirred-layer effects, enzyme activity, and specific protein binding [36].

The choice of the model system to be used in a given study must be considered with great care. Most drugs show more than one action on a tissue. Although secondary effects may contribute to the toxicity of a drug, it is most important to determine the initial reaction, for this is the reaction that must be prevented if an attempt to abolish toxicity is to be successful. Thus, the prime criterion for the selection of a model is its capacity to focus on the causative action at the molecular level. A second and possibly equally important criterion is its capacity to test and eliminate alternative hypotheses.

By far the most successful approaches to physicochemical modeling have been carried out with drugs that are believed to exert their action at the membrane. A number of pharmacologically active agents such as steroids [29], polyene antibiotics [35], local anesthetics [21], and phenothiazine derivatives [17] have been studied extensively by means of a variety of "model membrane" systems. The success of these model systems in elucidating molecular mechanisms, and even predicting structural requirements for activity, relies on the fact that the primary event is an interaction of the agent with one or more specific membrane components, which results in a measurable modification of a membrane property.

The choice of an appropriate model system is often a compromise. A complex system (e.g., cell culture) may better mimic the natural membrane, but does not easily allow one to vary membrane composition, surface charge, etc. A simpler system (e.g., monolayers) will allow control of these parameters, but the complexity of the natural membrane is lost.

Since polyphosphoinositides have been strongly indicated as membrane receptors for aminoglycoside antibiotics, we have chosen monolayers as the model system to study the interactions of various antibiotics with this class of lipids. Monolayers represent a relatively simple type of membrane model having a well-defined, organized structure. They provide a convenient and promising method of studying molecules in a fixed orientation, as well as in a single layer where the orientation of the molecules can be changed by compression or expansion. Thus, monolayers constitute an important model system for the study of many natural phenomena involving surfaces with an oriented array of molecules.

Studies with such a monolayer system showed that different aminoglycosides elicited different responses (Fig. 7-1). The magnitude of the response appeared to increase with the ototoxicity of the drug. All drugs that had previously been tested in cochlear perfusions (Table 7-1) were tested for their interaction with monomolecular films of polyphosphoinositides, and relative binding constants were determined. Neomycin B and kanamycin B had the highest affinity for the lipids, followed by the other drugs in the order seen for ototoxity. A comparison of the in situ and the in vitro results showed a remarkably high degree of correlation between these two actions (Fig. 7-2).*

*For experimental details, see refs. 11, 13.

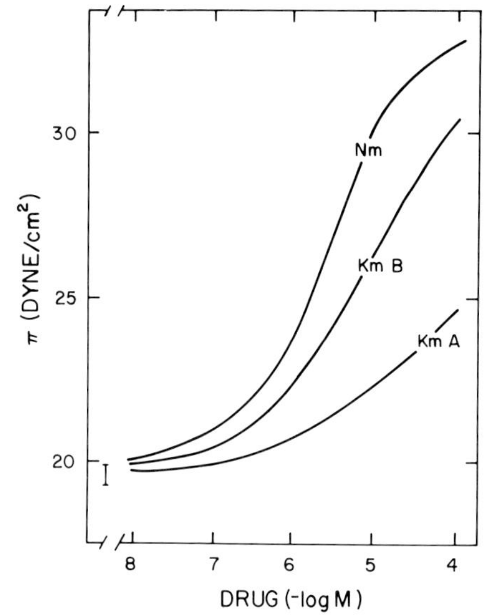

Figure 7-1. Effect of aminoglycoside concentration on surface pressure (π) of a polyphosphoinositide film. Increasing amounts of neomycin B (Nm), kanamycin B (Km B), or kanamycin A (Km A) were added to the subphase of a monomolecular film of polyphosphoinositides. (From S. Lodhi et al., Ototoxicity of aminoglycosides correlates with their action on monomolecular films of polyphosphoinositides. *Biochem Pharmacol.* 29:597, 1980. Reprinted by permission.)

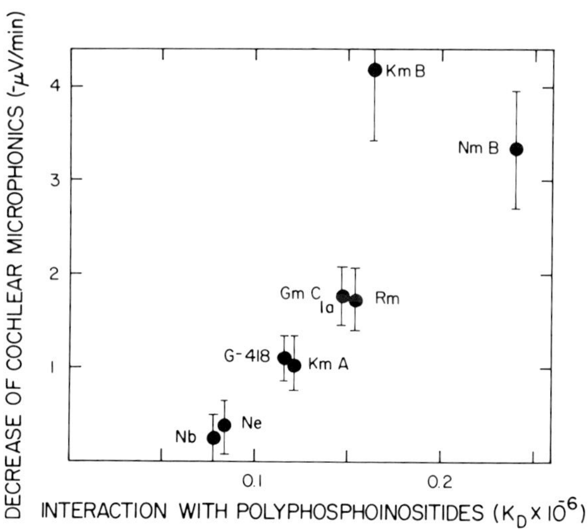

Figure 7-2. Correlation between drug effects on cochlear microphonics and on polyphosphoinositides. (Nb = Neobiosamine; Ne = neamine; G-418 = antibiotic G-418; Km A = kanamycin A; GmC_{1a} = gentamicin C_{1a}; Rm = ribostamycin; Km B = kanamycin B; Nm B = neomycin B.)

Comments

This study on the interactions between polyphosphoinositide monolayers and antibiotics with various structures and degrees of ototoxicity provides a critical test of the hypothesis of the polyphosphoinositides as cell receptors for ototoxicity. Furthermore, such studies should provide insight into the structural requirements for ototoxicity and lead to a more rational approach to chemical modification, which may in turn reduce toxicity. Such studies could also provide a basis for the screening of suspected ototoxic antibiotics and newly designed drugs.

References

1. André, T. Studies on the distribution of tritium-labeled dihydrostreptomycin and tetracycline in the body. *Acta Radiol (Stockh.)* [*Suppl.* 142]1, 1956.
2. Beard, N. S., Jr., Armentrout, S. A., and Weisberger, A. S. Inhibition of mammalian protein synthesis by antibiotics. *Pharmacol. Rev.* 21:213, 1969.
3. Cuatrecasas, P. Membrane receptors. *Annu. Rev. Biochem.* 43:169, 1974.
4. Deguchi, T., Ishii, A., and Tanaka, M. Binding of aminoglycoside antibiotics to acidic mucopolysaccharides. *J. Antibiot.* 31:150, 1978.
5. Garcia-Quiroga, J., Norris, C. H., Glade, L., Bryant, G. M., Tachibana, M., and Guth, P. The relationship between kanamycin ototoxicity and glucose transport. *Res. Commun. Chem. Pathol. Pharmacol.* 22:535, 1978.
6. Griffin, H. D., and Hawthorne, J. N. Calcium-activated hydrolysis of phosphatidyl-myo-inositol 4-phosphate and phosphatidyl-myo-inositol, 4,5 bisphosphate in guinea-pig synaptosomes. *Biochem. J.* 176:541, 1978.
7. Hauser, G., and Eichberg, J. Improved conditions for the preservation and extraction of polyphosphoinositides. *Biochim. Biophys. Acta* 326:201, 1973.
8. Jarlstedt, J., and Bagger-Sjöbäck, D. Gentamicin-induced changes in RNA content in sensory and ganglionic cells in the hearing organ of the lizard *Calotes versicolor. Acta Otolaryngol. (Stockh.)* 84:361, 1977.
9. Kai, M., and Hawthorne, J. N. Physiological significance of polyphosphoinositides in brain. *Ann. N.Y. Acad. Sci.* 165:761, 1969.
10. Kohn, L. D., Lee, G., Grollman, E. F., Ledley, F. D., Mullin, B. R., Friedman, R. M., Moldolesi, M. F., and Aloj, S. M. Membrane Glycolipids and Their Relationship to Structure and Function of Cell Surface Receptors for Glycoprotein Hormones, Bacterial Toxins, and Interferon. In R. E. Harmon (Ed.), *Cell Surface Carbohydrate Chemistry.* New York: Academic, 1978. Pp.103–134.
11. Lodhi, S., Weiner, N. D., Mechigian, I., and Schacht, J. Ototoxicity of aminoglycosides correlates with their action on monomolecular films of polyphosphoinositides. *Biochem. Pharmacol.* 29:597, 1980.
12. Lodhi, S., Weiner, N. D., and Schacht, J. Interactions of neomycin and calcium in synaptosomal membranes and polyphosphoinositide monolayers. *Biochim. Biophys. Acta* 426:781, 1976.
13. Lodhi, S., Weiner, N. D., and Schacht, J. Interactions of neomycin with monomolecular films of polyphosphoinositides and other lipids. *Biochim. Biophys. Acta* 557:1, 1979.
14. Lotz, P. Die Ursache der Ototoxizität basischer Zuckerantibiotika. *Wiss. Z. Univ. Halle* 26:87, 1977.
15. Meyer, H. Welche Eigenschaft der Anästhetica bedingt ihre narkotische Wirkung. *Arch. Exp. Pathol. Pharmakol.* 42:109, 1899.
16. Mitchell, R. H. Inositol phospholipids and cell surface receptor function. *Biochim. Biophys. Acta* 415:81, 1975.

17. Naoi, M., Suzuki, T., and Yagi, K. Effects of chlorpromazine and other phenothiazine derivatives on the permeability of liposomes. *Biochem. Pharmacol.* 28:295, 1979.
18. Nuttall, A. L., Marques, D. M., and Lawrence, M. Effects of perilymphatic perfusion with neomycin on the cochlear microphonic potential in the guinea pig. *Acta Otolaryngol.* 83:393, 1977.
19. Orsulakova, A., Stockhorst, E., and Schacht, J. Effect of neomycin on phosphoinositide labelling and calcium binding in guinea-pig inner ear tissues *in vivo* and *in vitro*. *J. Neurochem.* 26:285, 1976.
20. Owada, K. Experimental studies on the toxicity of kanamycin, its hydrolyzed products and neomycin. *Chemotherapia* 5:277, 1962.
21. Papahadjopoulos, D. Phospholipid model membranes. III. Antagonistic effects of Ca^{2+} and local anesthetics on the permeability of phosphatidylserine vesicles. *Biochim. Biophys. Acta* 211:467, 1970.
22. Pestka, S. Inhibitors of ribosome functions. *Annu. Rev. Biochem.* 40:697, 1971.
23. Robson, J. M., and Sullivan, F. M. Antituberculosis drugs. *Pharmacol. Rev.* 15:169, 1963.
24. Saito, H., and Daly, J. F. Quantitative analysis of acid mucopolysaccharides in the normal and kanamycin intoxicated cochlea. *Acta Otolaryngol.* 71:22, 1971.
25. Sanders, W. E., Jr., and Sanders, C. C. Toxicity of antibacterial agents: Mechanism of action on mammalian cells. *Annu. Rev. Pharmacol. Toxicol.* 19:53, 1979.
26. Schacht, J. Inhibition by neomycin of polyphosphoinositide turnover in subcellular fractions of guinea-pig cerebral cortex *in vitro*. *J. Neurochem.* 27:1119, 1976.
27. Schacht, J. Isolation of an aminoglycoside receptor from guinea pig inner ear tissues and kidney. *Arch. Otorhinolaryngol.* 224:129, 1979.
28. Schibeci, A., and Schacht, J. Action of neomycin on the metabolism of polyphosphoinositides in the guinea pig kidney. *Biochem. Pharmacol.* 26:1769, 1977.
29. Sessa, G., and Weissmann, G. Differential effects of etiocholanolone on phospholipid/cholesterol structures containing either testosterone or estradiol. *Biochim. Biophys. Acta* 150:173, 1968.
30. Staemmler, M., and Dudkowiak, V. Über die Wirkung des Kanamycins auf die Nieren. *Med. Welt* 24:1296, 1961.
31. Stockhorst, E., and Schacht, J. Radioactive labeling of phospholipids and proteins by cochlear perfusion in the guinea pig and the effect of neomycin. *Acta Otolaryngol.* 83:401, 1977.
32. Tachibana, M., Mizukoshi, O., and Kuriyama, K. Inhibitory effects of kanamycin on glycolysis in cochlea and kidney—possible involvement in the formation of oto- and nephrotoxicities. *Biochem. Pharmacol.* 25:2297, 1976.
33. Tachibana, M., Saito, H., Yamamichi, I., and Morioka, H. A possible involvement of acidic glycosaminoglycans in kanamycin ototoxicity. *Acta Otolaryngol.* 86:15, 1978.
34. Tachibana, M., and Schacht, J. Unpublished.
35. Tillack, T. W., and Kinsky, S. C. A freeze-etch study of the effects of filipin on liposomes and human erythrocyte membranes. *Biochim. Biophys. Acta* 323:43, 1973.
36. Turi, J. S., Ho, N. F., Higuchi, W. I., and Shipman, C., Jr. Systems approach to study of solute transport across membranes using suspension cultures of mammalian cells. *J. Pharm. Sci.* 64:631, 1975.
37. Wersäll, J., and Flock, A. Suppression and restoration of the microphonic output from the lateral line organ after local application of streptomycin. *Life Sci.* 3:1151, 1964.

Discussion of Chapter 7

Dr. Brummett: Dr. Schacht, did you perform a cochlear perfusion with the aminoglycosides and then look at the binding capacity of the cochlear tissues?

Dr. Schacht: These binding experiments were not correlated with perfusion. These were dissected cochlear tissues, radioactively labeled for convenience, and we tried to isolate anything that would bind to neomycin.

Dr. Brummett: What kind of cochlear tissues did you use?

Dr. Schacht: We used combinations of stria vascularis, spiral ligament, and organ of Corti. We also separated the tissues and found that the highest concentration of polyphosphoinositides is probably in the stria vascularis; the next-highest concentration is found in the organ of Corti.

Dr. Brummett: One of the things we need to explain is the mechanism by which the hair cells are selectively affected by aminoglycosides. I think your experimental model is excellent, but I still don't see any answer to this question. I thought perhaps you had isolated phosphoinositides from the hair cells.

Dr. Schacht: Let's make a deal. You give me 1 mg of isolated hair cells, and I will analyze them for polyphosphoinositides. The question of selectivity is a good one, but without knowledge of the lipid distribution, we cannot answer it.

It is not only the hair cells that are defective after aminoglycoside treatment; the supporting cells are also affected.

Dr. Lerner: Have you looked at any nonaminoglycosidic aminocyclitols like spectinomycin, either in situ or in your artificial membrane system?

Dr. Schacht: We have looked at more drugs in the in vitro system of the monolayers, but not in perfusion experiments. Spectinomycin interacted with monolayers even less than neamine and neobiosamine.

Dr. Lietman: Although I am one of those who is wedded to another system, that is, sodium-potassium-ATPase as a site of effect, I have been an admirer of your work for a long time. I think it might, however, have greater applicability to the transport of the aminoglycoside than to the ultimate biochemical toxicity. What I am suggesting is that the autoradiographic evidence, at least in the kidney, is that the drug doesn't stay bound at the luminal side of the proximal tubule, but instead is "gobbled up" by a lysosome, in which case it wouldn't then be responsible for destroying the integrity of the outer cellular membrane.

I wonder if you would comment on the evidence you have that the interaction with the polyphosphoinositide, instead of the transport mechanism, has anything to do with the ultimate toxicity of the cell.

Dr. Schacht: I think we are in agreement. We say that the interaction with the polyphosphoinositides is a necessary prerequisite for toxicity, and that aminoglycosides then act intracellularly. This intracellular activity is, for instance, not found in the liver, which has a low concentration of polyphosphoinositides.

Dr. N. G. Toremalm (Malmö General Hospital, Malmö, Sweden): It is well known that penicillins can be divided into two groups according to their different neurotoxicity. This is due to their different hydrophobic character. Have you found any similarity in this respect among different aminoglycosides?

Dr. Weiner: Not in that respect, because all of the aminoglycosides are extremely hydrophilic, and really there can't be any hydrophobic interaction that could result in any change of permeability. For example, if the interaction does result in a displacement of calcium, then we would see an even greater differential in the calcium gradient, at least initially, on the outside and inside of the cell membrane. This early change in the calcium gradient occurs before the aminoglycoside can get through the membrane. This gradient can cause tremendous variation in the effects on the membrane, such as an even further aggregation of the negatively charged lipids and small changes in permeability.

Try to picture this interaction as taking place in a balloon. There is only a small percentage of polyphosphoinositides in the membrane, but if they are aggregated in the presence of neomycin or calcium, then all you need is one little hole in the balloon to cause drastic changes in permeability.

Dr. Wersäll: We have had a lot of discussions about whether the reversibility with potassium ions or low-concentration aminoglycosides on the surface actually means that there is one reaction which is reversed with potassium and another reaction which acts on the calcium site. This agrees well with the fact that, at low concentrations of aminoglycosides after short exposure, you have complete reversibility of the action on the microphonics, whereas the secondary effects, with complete incorporation and no reversibility, could be correlated to your finding that binding occurs on the calcium sites.

Dr. Weiner: We still don't know whether the polyphosphoinositides in the membrane are uniformly dispersed laterally, or even uniformly dispersed between the outside and the inside parts of the membrane.

Vestibular Function

It is well known that the aminoglycosides can be vestibulotoxic as well as cochleotoxic. However, in animals as in man, assessment of vestibular toxicity has been compromised by considerable test-retest and intersubject variability in measurements of vestibular function. Recently, improved methods have been developed for more consistent testing of vestibular function in animals treated with aminoglycosides. Makoto Igarashi and David Jensen point out the value of behavioral ataxiametric tests in the early detection of vestibular dysfunction.

The central nervous system influences the function of the vestibular end organ. In an effort to explore this relationship, Bernard Cohen has examined the central and peripheral components of nystagmus in response to rotation. The methods that he describes could ultimately lead to information on the site or sites of the ototoxic action of aminoglycosides. Cohen emphasizes, however, that it is essential to understand the normal physiology of the vestibular system before we can examine the ototoxic pathophysiology. Vicente Honrubia and his group, in their analysis of the slow and fast components of nystagmus, have contributed further to elucidation of the physiologic mechanisms involved. The studies by David Anderson, which show changes in the output of the first-order neurons after streptomycin administration, provide a direct demonstration of the toxic potential of aminoglycosides for the vestibular sense organs.

8. Vestibulotoxicity Experiments in Animals

Makoto Igarashi and David W. Jensen

Numerous studies have described the ototoxic effects on vestibular and cochlear end organs in a variety of experimental animals after the administration of various kinds of antibiotics, especially aminoglycosides. These previous works are well summarized in chapters by Hawkins and Preston [3] and Hawkins [2]. In our laboratory, we have developed behavioral ataxiametric procedures for squirrel monkeys and cats, and we have applied such methods to assess the vestibulotoxicity of aminoglycosides. In this chapter, we describe three studies in this category: streptomycin toxicity in the squirrel monkey, and comparative toxicity of netilmicin and gentamicin in the squirrel monkey and the cat.

Streptomycin Toxicity in the Squirrel Monkey

In an early study on squirrel monkeys [7], we produced temporary vestibular suppression by streptomycin administered systemically. In eight monkeys, the drug was injected intramuscularly, 70 mg/kg per day, in a cycle with 3 weeks of single daily injections and about 4 weeks without drug; the cycle was then repeated until the vestibular function was suppressed. The vestibular function was evaluated by a caloric threshold test (detection of nystagmus onset by stepwise reduction of water temperature), a motion sickness test (the occurrence of emesis as an indicator) in a Slow Rotation Room, and a body balance maintenance test on a narrow rail. These three vestibular tests show similar temporal manifestations of functional suppression. The three tests were not necessarily performed on the same day, however. Also, as is seen in the decline in caloric threshold of one representative animal (Fig. 8-1), dysfunc-

The second and third parts of this report were supported by a Schering Corporation research grant, and by NINCDS grants NS-07237 and NS-10940. The original work in the first part of this chapter was supported by NASA Order No. R-93.

The authors express their sincere gratitude to Mark Simon, Lars Walberg, Jeff Walne, Joel Levy, Indira Lanig, and June Brown for their technical assistance in the work described in the third part of this report.

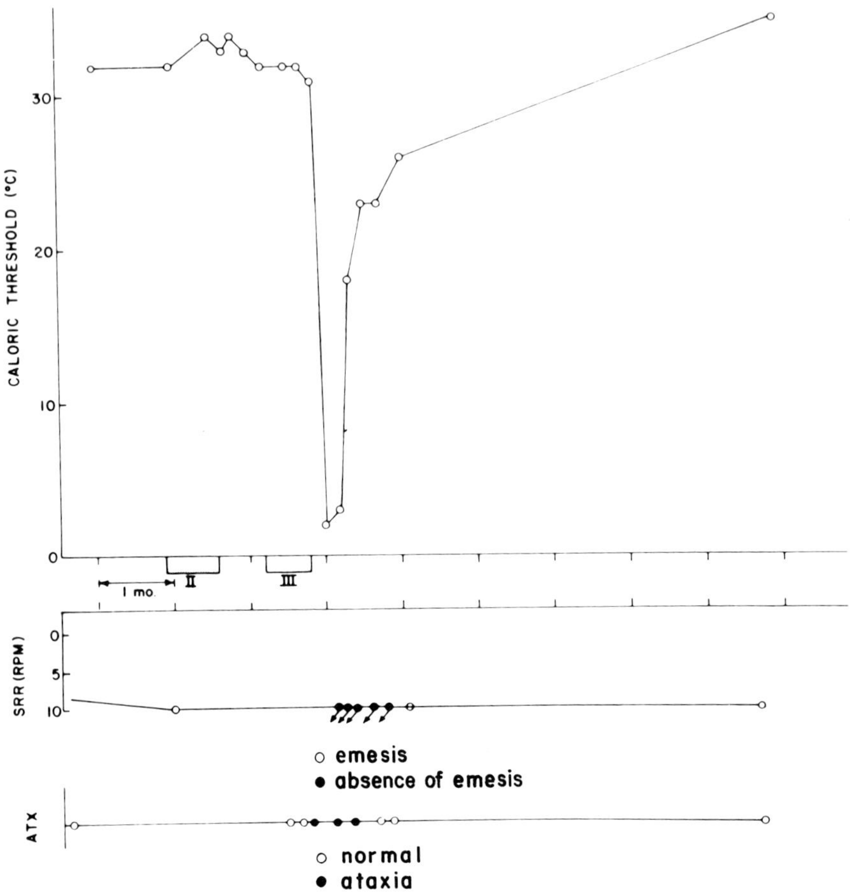

Figure 8-1. Course of caloric threshold (top), susceptibility to emesis in Slow Rotation Room (middle), and ataxia on a rail (bottom) after injection of a total of 3,350 mg streptomycin. The Slow Rotation Room turned at 10 rpm. Roman numerals II and III below the horizontal line indicate the course of streptomycin treatment. (Reproduced from M. Igarashi, M. E. McLeod, and A. Graybiel, Clinical pathological correlations in squirrel monkeys after suppression of semicircular canal function by streptomycin sulfate. *Acta Otolaryngol.* [Suppl. 214]1, 1966.)

tion of the semicircular canal developed so rapidly that it was not possible to evaluate which of the three tests was the most sensitive in detecting the initial manifestation of vestibular dysfunction. Such evaluation may be possible if the drug is administered in doses causing much slower development of vestibular dysfunction.

Streptomycin injections were discontinued at the time of vestibular suppression, but all tests were continued. Six months after suppression, the results of all three tests were back within the normal range in all eight animals. Monkeys were killed upon functional recovery, and the inner ear end organs were examined by light microscopy. In the case shown in Fig. 8-1, the pathologic hair cell changes were moderate in the cristae ampullares, minimal in the maculae, and moderately severe in the cochlea, with no damage to spiral ganglion cells. Four of the eight animals showed clear loss of hair cells and various degrees of pathologic change in the sensory epithelia of all three cristae ampullares. No animal had clear hair cell loss in the maculae, however, showing that streptomycin destroyed the cristae ampullares prior to involving the maculae. In all of the four animals with damage to the cristae ampullares, the caloric threshold 6 months after the suppression was within the normal range. This result indicates that the remaining sensory hair cells (type II hair cells, as there was a propensity for type I hair cell damage) were able to regain the normal level of crista ampullaris function required to provoke caloric nystagmus. If other nystagmus parameters were to be examined in detail, however, some abnormality might be detected.

Comparative Toxicity of Gentamicin and Netilmicin in the Squirrel Monkey

In another study [5], we compared the toxicity of netilmicin and gentamicin in squirrel monkeys. In this series, we gave 30 or 60 mg/kg per day of gentamicin or netilmicin to a total of 16 animals (8 each) until the animals showed severe ataxia or became moribund. Except for one, all gentamicin-treated monkeys developed severe ataxia. Since we have observed that some monkeys treated chronically with gentamicin at high doses exhibit malaise, weakness, and behavioral changes, possibly caused by renal failure or other systemic effects, we could not determine whether gentamicin-induced locomotor ataxia was solely of vestibular origin. At the time ataxia developed, neither the frequency nor the duration of post-rotatory nystagmus (0–200 degrees/sec stimulus, with 1 degree/sec^2 acceleration) was altered significantly. But two of the eight gentamicin-injected monkeys did show a slight prolongation of post-rotatory nystagmus duration, indicating a possible reduction of central inhibition. If we had analyzed other parameters of vestibular nystagmus, we might have seen other alterations as well.

Netilmicin was found to be less toxic than gentamicin, and the netilmicin-treated monkeys could tolerate daily injections over a longer period. Of the four monkeys receiving netilmicin, 60 mg/kg per day, two developed severe ataxia and one developed slight ataxia. Reduction in frequency and duration of post-rotatory nystagmus tended to parallel the severity of gait ataxia. Both of these changes appear to reflect vestibular suppression. These results led us to the general conclusion that, if the drug is not very toxic, vestibular dysfunction can be detected by both the ataxia and post-rotatory nystagmus tests; however, when the drug is more toxic, systemic effects can occur concomitantly with, or even before, vestibular toxicity, and may preclude vestibular testing. The difference in ototoxicity may partly reflect the difference in nephrotoxicity and the resulting differences in drug accumulation.

After this experiment, we developed a method of measuring overground locomotor deviation in squirrel monkeys. We trained squirrel monkeys to shuttle between two end-boxes connected by an enclosed runway. The platform was equipped with a longitudinal array of pressure sensors beneath the floor for measurement of gait deviations [4].

In order to use this method to evaluate aminoglycoside toxicity, in the next study [6] we administered gentamicin (25, 50, and 75 mg/kg) and netilmicin (50, 75, and 100 mg/kg) to squirrel monkeys in single daily doses (four monkeys for each dose level and four receiving saline injections as controls) over a 3-week period or until the animals became moribund. Gentamicin-treated animals developed ataxia, even at the lowest dose. Again, ataxia may have been due in part to systemic toxicity. The majority survived for 6 to 14 days. In contrast, nine of twelve monkeys in the netilmicin-injected group tolerated the full 21-day course of injections. When the locomotor deviation ratios (the total number of deviations before the last injection, divided by the average number of deviations during 5 days of trials before injection) were compared, the group receiving 100 mg/kg per day showed a higher ratio than the groups receiving 75 and 50 mg/kg per day. The deviation ratio was still within the normal limit (less than 1) in the group treated with 75 mg/kg per day. This result indicates that vestibular ataxia was developing gradually in the high-dose group. The finding that netilmicin is less ototoxic than gentamicin in squirrel monkeys is in accord with the result in guinea pigs [1]. Saline-injected animals showed no change.

Comparative Toxicity of Netilmicin and Gentamicin in Cats

Using another experimental approach, we compared the righting reflex of cats after administration of netilmicin or gentamicin. We constructed a device to hold a cat in a supine position with a bomb-bay-door type of support. The cats were dropped from a level 1 meter above the floor. A high-speed camera installed 2.4 meters away took cinematographic records at a speed of 200 frames per second. Two to three drop tests were performed daily before injections.

Both drugs were given in single daily doses of 60 mg/kg. There were four cats in each group, and one control cat was given saline injections. Doses were administered daily until, in the examiner's judgment, signs of ataxia could be detected either in the righting reflex or in overground locomotion. After that time, the cats were continuously tested without further drug injection, in our

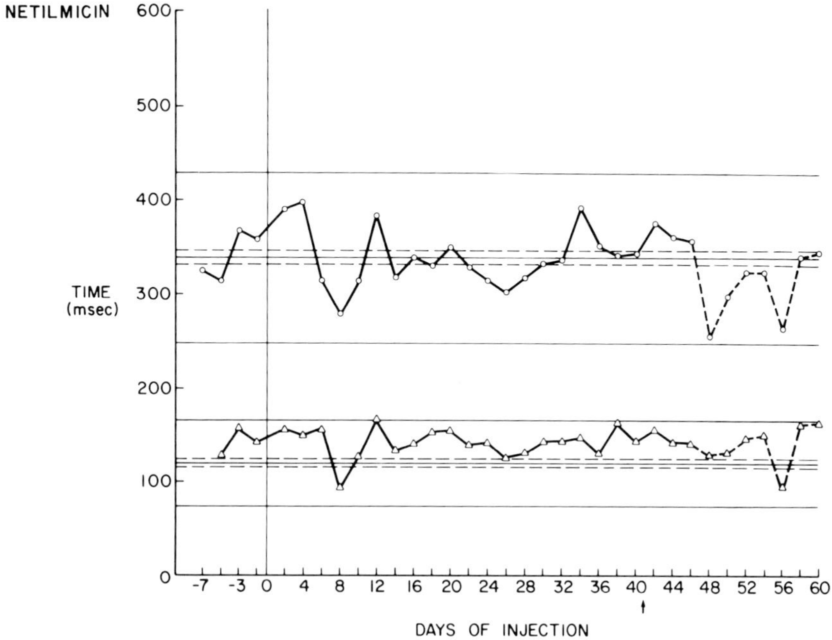

Figure 8-2. Effect of daily netilmicin injections on time course for 90-degree head rotation (open triangles) and 180-degree body rotation (open circles) after the initiation of drop. Injections of netilmicin were continued until day 41 (arrow). Interrupted lines connecting circles and triangles indicate reduced number of samples. Solid and dashed horizontal lines represent ±1 standard deviation (——) and ±1 standard error of mean (-------), based on preinjection data for animals in all three treatment groups.

effort to investigate whether functional compensation would occur. Times (in msec) for 90-degree head rotation, 90-degree body rotation, and 180-degree body rotation and the time for complete limb stretch were studied in frame-by-frame analysis of the film records. Figures 8-2 through 8-4 show the times (ordinate) required for cats to achieve 90-degree head and 180-degree body rotations after netilmicin, gentamicin, and control saline injections. In these figures, complete failures of 90-degree head rotation or 180-degree body rotation were counted as 600 msec. All preinjection cats righted themselves without difficulty. Development of righting impairment in the gentamicin group was rapid. The averaged results for four animals each in the gentamicin and netilmicin groups indicated that gentamicin was more toxic than netilmicin.

After an average of 41 days of injections, the netilmicin-treated cats failed to develop a righting reflex disturbance or overground locomotor ataxia, and the injections were discontinued. The saline-injected cat did not show any change, and after 42 days, the injections were also stopped. On the other hand, gentamicin-treated cats developed functional abnormalities at an average of 14.8 days, and at that time the injections were stopped. The number of injec-

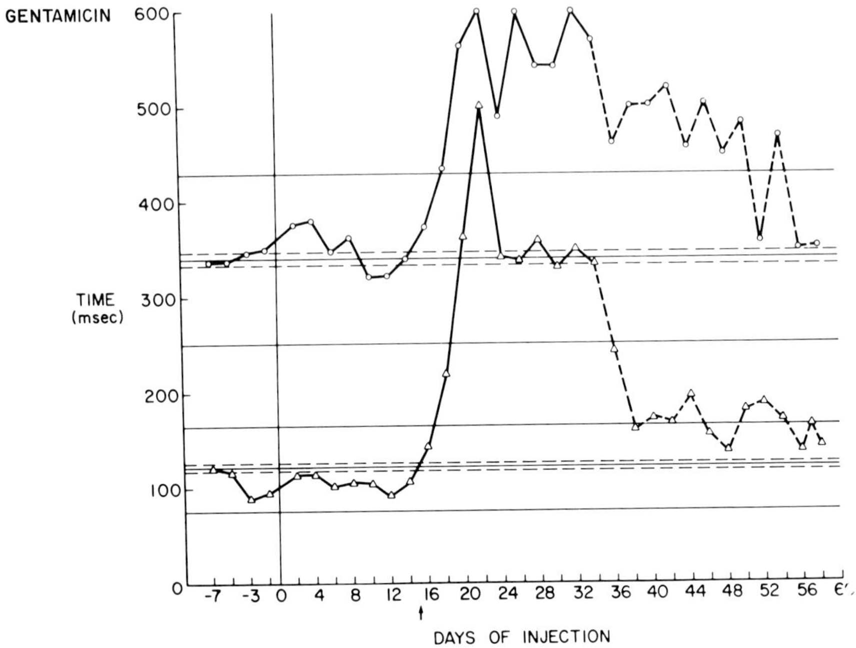

Figure 8-3. Effect of daily gentamicin injections on head rotation and body rotation (see Fig. 8-2). The injections were stopped on the 15th day (arrow), as abnormalities in righting and ataxia were detected. Further development of righting disturbance and subsequent recovery of function can be seen.

tion days before manifestation of symptoms generally agreed with the results of Waitz et al. [11], which showed that ataxia appeared after an average of 12.2 days of treatment in five cats receiving gentamicin, 60 mg/kg per day.

Head and body rotations became slower at almost the same time during the course of gentamicin administration. The slopes of the curves for slowing along days were nearly parallel, indicating that, at least in the initial decrement of performance, slowing of the righting reflex basically involved slowing of the head rotation, without any additional slowing of the body rotation. Righting impairment continued to develop until about 1 week after the cessation of injections, and then a gradual recovery was observed. Head-turning returned to a faster speed slightly earlier than body-turning; however, the reduced number of testable animals might have obscured the significance of this difference. The netilmicin-treated cats did not show slowed head- and body-turning, but instead made some sloppy landings. Netilmicin could have a strong neuromuscular blocking action, which would account for this, but this possibility has not been examined. Similar to overground gait deviation in squirrel monkeys, righting disturbance in cats results from both vestibular dysfunction (for spatial orientation) and systemic effects (for rotation and

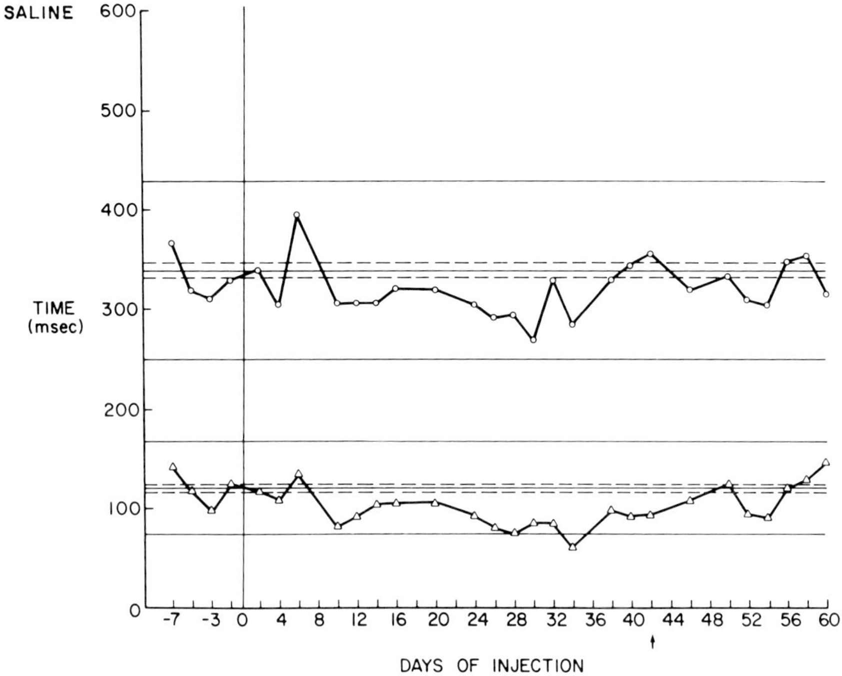

Figure 8-4. Effect of daily saline injections on head rotation and body rotation (see Fig. 8-2). The injections were discontinued after the 42nd day (arrow).

landing). The parameter affected earliest, i.e., slowing of 90-degree head rotation, is perhaps most representative of the macular function [9, 12].

We also analyzed the head position, the head-body angle, and the upper torso–lower torso open angle [8, 10] of the cats treated with gentamicin or netilmicin. All of these parameters clearly indicated that gentamicin-treated cats were more disoriented than those receiving netilmicin. For example, normally righting cats maintained a very consistent head position along the direction of fall. Disorientation was quite obvious in gentamicin-injected cats, as shown by their inability to maintain a steady head position. Netilmicin-treated cats maintained a relatively steady, but not always normal, head position. Just prior to landing after righting, the upper torso and lower torso formed a 100- to 200-degree angle in normal cats, whereas the angle was very obtuse in disoriented cats: the trunk was not properly ventroflexed at the time of landing.

The initial motor actions associated with righting reflexes are generally considered to reflect macular dysfunction; therefore, if these drugs are initially toxic to the crista ampullaris, a disturbance in the righting reflex could be a slightly delayed sign of developing ototoxicity.

Comments

As we have discussed, behavioral ataxiametric tests were found to be a useful tool for evaluation of the development of vestibular toxicity in squirrel monkeys and cats treated with aminoglycoside antibiotics in doses that were not highly toxic. Through our past animal experiments, we have learned that, if vestibular dysfunction is detected at an early stage, if renal function is not impaired, and if drug administration is discontinued at that time, vestibular function can recover, even though some morphologically detectable end organ damage may have developed. Because the ototoxic effect of some antibiotics, e.g., streptomycin, gentamicin, tobramycin, and viomycin, develops earlier in the vestibule than in the cochlea [2, 13], vestibular function tests may play an important role in preventing the subsequent development of irreversible cochlear damage.

References

1. Brummett, R. E., Fox, K. E., Brown, R. T., and Himes, D. L. Comparative ototoxic liability of netilmicin and gentamicin. *Arch. Otolaryngol.* 104:579, 1973.
2. Hawkins, J. E., Jr. Drug Ototoxicity. In W. D. Keidel and W. D. Neff (Eds.), *Auditory System—Clinical and Special Topics. Handbook of Sensory Physiology*, Vol. V/3. Berlin: Springer, 1976. P. 707.
3. Hawkins, J. E., Jr., and Preston, R. E. Vestibular Ototoxicity. In R. F. Naunton (Ed.), *The Vestibular System.* New York: Academic, 1975. P. 321.
4. Igarashi, M. Squirrel monkey platform runway test. *Acta Otolaryngol.* 77:284, 1974.
5. Igarashi, M. Vestibular ototoxicity in primates. *Audiology* 12:337, 1973.
6. Igarashi, M., Levy, J. K., and Jerger, J. Comparative toxicity of netilmicin and gentamicin in squirrel monkeys (*Saimiri sciureus*). *J. Infect. Dis.* 137:476, 1978.
7. Igarashi, M., McLeod, M. E., and Graybiel, A. Clinical pathological correlations in squirrel monkeys after suppression of semicircular canal function by streptomycin sulfate. *Acta Otolaryngol. Suppl.* 214:1, 1966.
8. Kane, T. R., and Scher, M. P. A dynamical explanation of the falling cat phenomenon. *Int. J. Solids Struct.* 5:663, 1969.
9. Melvill Jones, G., and Watt, D. G. D. Macular control of landing from unexpected falls in man. *J. Physiol.* 219:729, 1971.
10. Rademaker, G. G. J., and Ter Braak, J. W. G. Das Umdrehen der fallenden Katze in der Luft. *Acta Otolaryngol.* 23:313, 1935.
11. Waitz, J. A., Moss, E. L., Jr., and Weinstein, M. J. Aspects of the chronic toxicity of gentamicin sulfate in cats. *J. Infect. Dis.* 124:S125, 1971.
12. Watt, D. G. D. An otolith-originating vestibulospinal reflex response to sudden falls in the cat. *DRB Aviation Medical Research Unit Reports.* Vol. IV: 140, 1975.
13. Wersäll, J., Lundquist, P-G., and Björkroth, B. Ototoxicity of gentamicin. *J. Infect. Dis.* 119:410, 1969.

Discussion of Chapter 8

Dr. Federspil: Do you have an explanation for the discrepancy between the morphologic changes and the functional changes in the vestibular disturbances?

Dr. Igarashi: In my first squirrel monkey experiment, we saw clear evidence of damage in the hair cells of the crista ampullaris. However, when we measured caloric thresholds, we did not see any change 6 months after the treatment with streptomycin. Therefore, even if moderate hair cell damage was present, the remaining hair cell population was sufficient to regain the level of normal function of the crista ampullaris, at least as indicated by the caloric threshold. Systemic compensation plays an important role too.

9. Stored Neural Activity in the Vestibulo-Ocular Reflex and the Response to Vestibular Testing

Bernard Cohen and Theodore Raphan

The integrity of the vestibular apparatus has traditionally been tested by measurement of eye movements made in response to rotation about a vertical axis in darkness or during caloric stimulation. A step in angular velocity causes a quick deflection of the cupula, which slowly returns to its resting position, whereas caloric stimulation causes a prolonged deflection that persists for a minute or more.

Usually, it is assumed that these tests mainly evaluate the function of the peripheral sensory end organ, and that there is little transformation of the signal before it impinges on the oculomotor system. There is substantial evidence, however, that an important part of the nystagmus response to steps in angular velocity is caused by the operation of a central mechanism that holds or stores activity related to slow-phase eye velocity. This storage mechanism is activated by cupula deflection, whether induced by angular acceleration or caloric stimulation, and it continues to drive the eyes after the cupula has returned to its resting position. It is activated not only by the vestibular system, but also by the visual system. For an understanding of the normal as well as the pathologic reaction of the vestibular system, it is important to account for both the central and peripheral components of the response.

This research was done primarily on monkeys, but we have also found evidence for central storage of activity in man. We will first consider the question of which part of the response to a step in velocity is caused by the contribution of the sensory end organ and which part is caused by the addition of central neural circuitry. Goldberg and Fernández [3, 4] recorded unit activity in the vestibular nerve of the monkey in response to steps of acceleration. They showed that the neural activity from the cupula of the semicircular canals rises to its steady-state level with a dominant time constant of about 5 seconds.

This work was supported by USPHS Research Grant NS-00294, by an Academic Investigator Award to Theodore Raphan from the National Eye Institute, EY 00157, and by Cane Center Grant EY 01867.

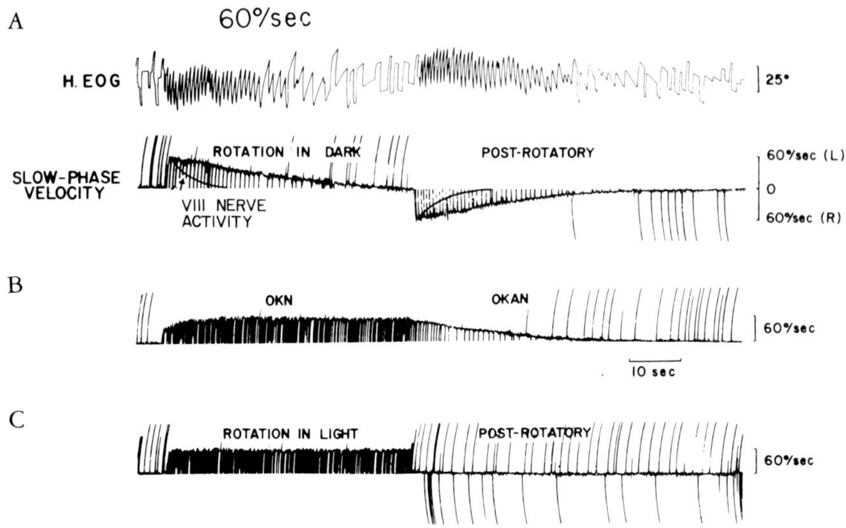

Figure 9-1. Vestibular nystagmus, optokinetic nystagmus (OKN), and optokinetic after-nystagmus (OKAN) in a monkey. In A, the nystagmus was induced by a step of angular velocity of 60°/second in darkness. In B, the OKN drum rotated at 60°/second. In C, the monkey was rotated in light, causing both vestibular and optokinetic stimulation. The top trace in A is the horizontal electro-oculogram (H.EOG). The remaining traces show slow-phase eye velocity. The poststimulus responses in A through C were recorded in darkness. The solid curves in the slow-phase velocity trace of A show the approximate time course of the decline in activity in the eighth nerve in response to a step in velocity. In A, per-rotatory nystagmus in darkness dies away and is followed by post-rotatory nystagmus when the step in velocity is terminated. In B, surround rotation induces OKN with a rapid and then a slow rise to a steady-state level. At the end of stimulation, there is a slight fall in slow-phase velocity, followed by a steady decline during OKAN. In C, rotation in light is associated with a sudden rise of slow-phase velocity to a maximum value. This value is maintained for the duration of the stimulus. Since the activity from the labyrinth dies away quickly during constant-velocity rotation (A), the persistence of the response is caused by optokinetic activation. At the end of the period of stimulation in C, the animal was suddenly stopped and put into darkness; little or no post-rotatory nystagmus was produced by stored central activity. (Modified from T. Raphan et al., Velocity storage in the vestibulo-ocular reflex arc [VOR]. *Exp. Brain Res.* 35:229, 1979.)

When the acceleration is terminated and the animal's head velocity is maintained at a constant value, the neural activity returns to its resting level with a time constant of 5 seconds. This means that, during continuous rotation, vestibular nerve activity will have declined to within 15 percent of its resting level in 10 seconds. Consequently, any significant nystagmus that continues for 10 or 15 seconds after the onset of rotation in darkness must be the result of prolongation by central neural mechanisms.

The contrast between the peripheral and central time course of activation in response to rotation in the dark is shown in Fig. 9-1A. The solid curves labeled "VIII Nerve Activity" under the slow-phase velocity envelope show the approximate time course that the eye velocity would follow if the oculomotor system were being driven only by activity caused by cupula deflection during a step in velocity. It is apparent that the nystagmus lasts considerably longer than this activity.

The central storage mechanism is also activated by the visual system during optokinetic nystagmus (OKN) [1]. The stored activity is manifested as optokinetic after-nystagmus (OKAN) that persists after optokinetic stimulation has ended (Fig. 9-1B). The decline in slow-phase velocity is similar during per- and post-rotatory nystagmus and during OKAN (Figs. 9-1A and B). This is one indication that the stored activity elicited by vestibular and optokinetic stimulation arises in a common storage element [11].

When rotation takes place in light (Fig. 9-1C), initially the nystagmus is caused by activity that arises as a result of cupula deflection. Maintenance of the response is dependent, however, on OKN that is elicited by the relative motion between the subject and the surround. After rotation in light, there is no post-rotatory nystagmus, even if the animal is now in darkness (Fig. 9-1C). This indicates that the stored activity, accumulated during the per-rotatory period, has summated with activity caused by cupula deflection to cancel the post-rotatory response [6, 11, 15]. We recently analyzed and modeled OKN, OKAN, and vestibular nystagmus by using an integrator located in the vestibulo-ocular reflex (VOR) to represent the central storage mechanism [1, 11]. If the integrator is common to both OKN and vestibular nystagmus, the model can predict all of these responses.

Just as the stored activity elicited by rotation in light has the capability to cancel post-rotatory nystagmus, the presence of a stationary surround can cause discharge of the stored central activity and reduce eye velocity [11]. The suppression mechanism is a visual-oculomotor response to inappropriate movement of the eyes. If the eyes are moving in darkness in response to vestibular stimulation and the stationary surround is exposed, eye movements are inappropriate in that they obscure clear vision and are therefore suppressed.

An experiment that illustrates this suppression mechanism is shown in Fig. 9-2. In darkness, slow-phase eye velocity during vestibular nystagmus induced by a step in velocity decays with a time constant of 15 to 20 seconds (Fig. 9-2A). In light (Fig. 9-2A, downward arrows), the time constant of the decay is only about 5 seconds. The difference in gain and time course can be ascribed to discharge of stored central activity by fixation suppression and to

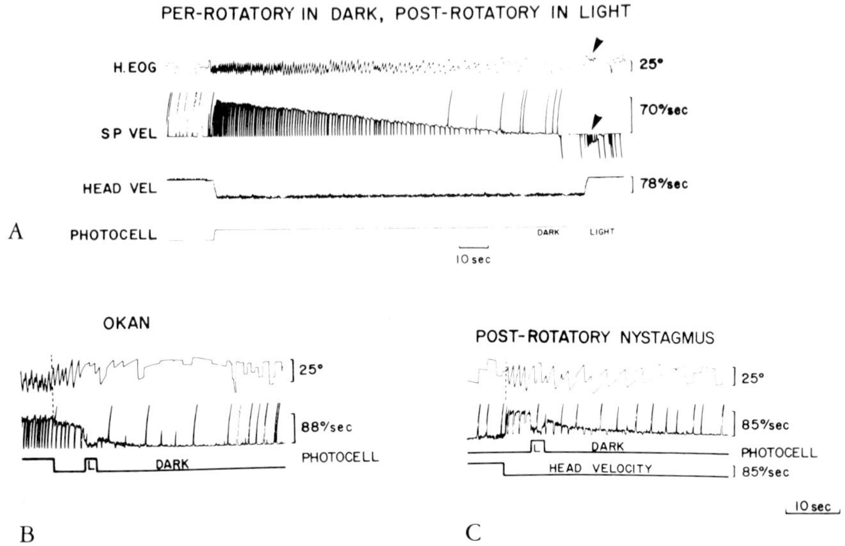

Figure 9-2. A. Eye movements induced by a step of angular velocity in the dark and in light. The per-rotatory step was given in darkness, whereas the post-rotatory step was given in light. The duration of the response in light was shorter, and the peak velocity reached during the post-rotatory response was smaller. The latter is marked by arrows. B and C. A short period of visual fixation was given during OKAN (B) and post-rotatory nystagmus (C); this is marked by the L in the photocell trace. The slow-phase velocity declined when the stationary visual field was exposed. The recovery velocity attained after the animal was again placed in darkness after the short period in light was less than if there had been no period of fixation. This demonstrates that stored activity had been lost during the period of fixation. (From B. Cohen et al., Quantitative analysis of the velocity characteristics of optokinetic nystagmus and optokinetic after-nystagmus. *J. Physiol. (Lond.)* 270:321, 1977; and T. Raphan et al., Velocity storage in the vestibulo-ocular reflex arc [VOR]. *Exp. Brain Res.* 35:229, 1979.)

activation of direct visual pathways; these counteract vestibular activity projecting to the oculomotor system [5, 11].

Figure 9-2A shows the effect of total discharge of the central storage mechanism by a long period of fixation. If a shorter period of exposure to a stationary visual surround is used, the post-rotatory response is partially suppressed (Fig. 9-2C). Since all available evidence indicates that the peripheral labyrinth is not affected by the presence of light or by eye movements [5], the partial discharge of the activity responsible for the nystagmus shown in Fig. 9-2C must have been brought on by a loss of activity in central structures. A considerable body of evidence suggests that the mechanism for suppression is mediated through the flocculus [2, 5, 7, 14]. Consistent with the idea that the same storage mechanism is activated by optokinetic as by vestibular stimulation, the loss of stored activity during OKAN induced by short periods of visual fixation (Fig. 9-2B) is similar to that during post-rotatory nystagmus (Fig. 9-2C).

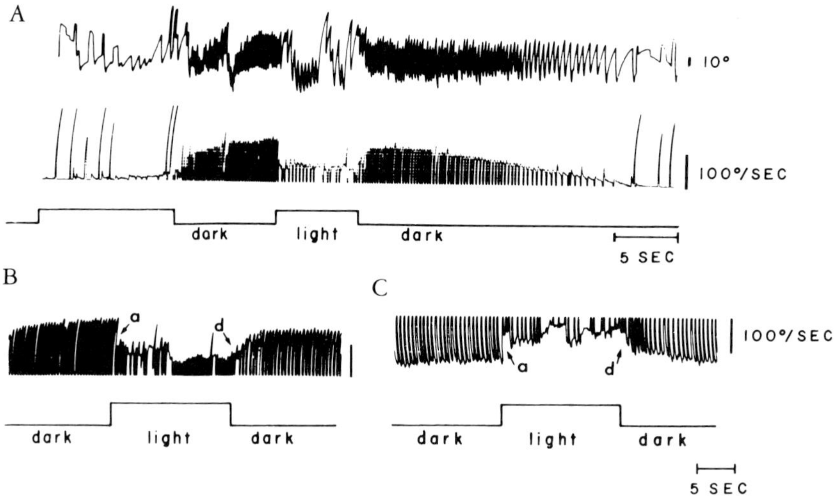

Figure 9-3. A, B, C. Effects of visual fixation on caloric nystagmus in three monkeys. When the animals were exposed to a stationary visual environment during the culmination of caloric nystagmus, there was a sudden drop in slow-phase velocity (B,a; C,a). At the end of the period of light, there was a slow rise back toward the steady-state level (B,d; C,d). The maximum velocity of the nystagmus was lower after the period of light. The top trace in A is the horizontal EOG. The second trace in A and the traces in B and C are rectified slow-phase velocity. (Modified from S. Takemori and B. Cohen, Visual suppression of vestibular nystagmus in rhesus monkeys. *Brain Res.* 72:203, 1974.)

Additional evidence that activity is stored in the VOR comes from studies on visual-vestibular interaction during caloric nystagmus [13]. With the introduction of a caloric stimulus, the cupula is deflected, and there is a buildup of nystagmus (Fig. 9-3A). If the lights are turned on while the nystagmus is in progress, the nystagmus is rapidly suppressed (Fig. 9-3B,a and C,a). When the lights are turned off again, slow-phase velocity rises more slowly than it fell (Fig. 9-3B,d and C,d). This shows that, in addition to rapid suppression of eye velocity by the visual system during caloric nystagmus, there is suppression of a more slowly activated mechanism that also participates in the response. Presumably, the rapid drop in eye velocity when the lights are turned on is due to activation of direct pathways from the visual system that immediately counteract the ongoing nystagmus.* There is also a slower loss of stored activity. When the animal is put into darkness after a period of fixation, the direct visual pathways are inactivated, and the storage mechanism is then

*These direct pathways are also probably responsible for the rapid rise in eye velocity at the beginning of OKN (Fig. 9-1B) and for the slight rapid drop at the beginning of OKAN (Fig. 9-1B and ref. 1).

slowly charged to the level of the eighth nerve activity induced by the caloric stimulus.

A mechanism for storage of activity related to slow-phase eye velocity similar to that associated with horizontal nystagmus is present in vertical nystagmus, with one striking exception. Nystagmus in the horizontal plane is usually symmetric to the right and to the left, but there is marked asymmetry in vertical nystagmus for movements in the upward and downward directions [8, 9, 12]. During vestibular nystagmus induced by steps in angular velocity, the time constant of decay for the slow-phase velocity of upward nystagmus is much shorter than that for downward nystagmus (Fig. 9-4C). The decay time constant of upward nystagmus is close to that of activity in the vestibular nerve [3, 4], suggesting that little or no storage is associated with upward nystagmus. Consistent with this, there is little or no upward OKAN in most monkeys (Fig. 9-4B). Downward OKN, OKAN, and downward vestibular nystagmus are similar to those found for movements in the horizontal plane, however (Figs. 9-4A and C).

Visual-vestibular interaction reflects this asymmetry in stored activity for movements in the upward and downward directions. After rotation in light that elicits downward nystagmus, there is little or no post-rotatory upward nystagmus (Fig. 9-4D). Presumably, the stored activity for nystagmus in the downward direction had summed with the post-rotatory upward response to cancel it. In the reverse situation, however, in which upward nystagmus is elicited in light, the downward poststimulus nystagmus, recorded in darkness (Fig. 9-4E), is as vigorous as if the preceding nystagmus has been induced in darkness (compare Fig. 9-4C and E).

One of the major functions of the VOR is to compensate for head movement; it acts to hold the angle of gaze stable in space. The stored activity that has been demonstrated in the VOR aids ocular compensation in several ways. First, it lengthens the time constant of the vestibular response as compared to that of the eighth nerve activity. This allows the VOR to have a better low-frequency response in the absence of vision than if there had been no storage. That is, the gain of the VOR is closer to one, and the phase of the response is closer to 180 degrees for low-frequency head movements. Second, the stored activity smooths and maximizes the velocity of the eyes during movements made in response to optokinetic stimulation. Third, the stored activity provides a mechanism whereby after-responses to prolonged rotation are abolished or markedly attenuated. Finally, the storage mechanism serves as a focus for establishing visual-vestibular interactions, and it plays an important role in helping the vestibular system generate a signal in the vestibular nuclei that closely represents movement of the organism in space.

This last point is shown in the studies of Waespe and Henn [16 through 18], who recorded the activity of single cells in the vestibular nuclei of alert monkeys. In response to steps of velocity, all neurons in the vestibular nuclei had time constants of decline in their firing rates that approximated the slow-phase envelopes shown in Fig. 9-1A. In none of the neurons did the firing rates decay at the time constant of the cupula. The sample studied included neurons that

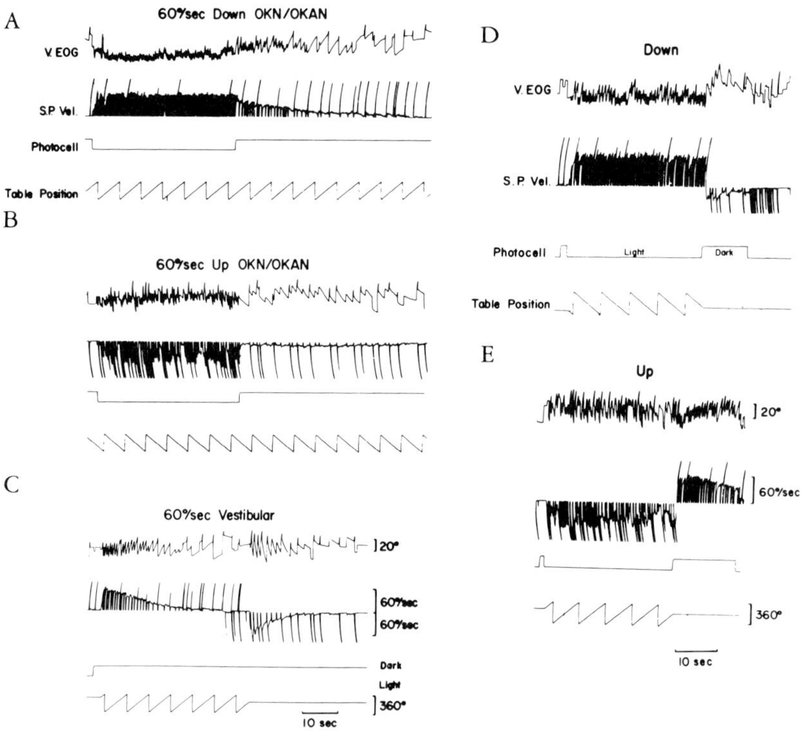

Figure 9-4. Downward and upward optokinetic and vestibular nystagmus in a monkey. A. Downward OKN was regular and was followed by strong OKAN. B. In contrast, upward OKN was irregular and was followed by weak OKAN. C. Vestibular stimulation with the animal lying on its side and rotating about a vertical axis in darkness. Note the shorter upward than downward nystagmus. D and E. Steps of velocity with the animal in light. The post-rotatory response was recorded in darkness. The presence of light caused the nystagmus to be maintained at the velocity of rotation. At the end of rotation in light (D), the upward post-rotatory nystagmus was significantly weaker than after rotation in darkness (compare C and D). In E, the per-rotatory nystagmus in light was in the upward direction. The nystagmus velocity was irregular and poorly maintained, as during OKN in light (B). Following rotation in E, the post-rotatory nystagmus in the downward direction was as vigorous as it had been when the animal was rotated in darkness (C). This demonstrates that there was little or no effect of stored activity during upward nystagmus in light to counteract the downward post-rotatory nystagmus. (From V. Matsuo et al., Asymmetric velocity storage for upward and downward nystagmus. *Brain Res.* 176:159, 1979.)

received direct activation from neurons in the vestibular nerve, indicating that the stored activity is manifested at the first level of information processing in the vestibular nuclei. Virtually all of the neurons in the vestibular nuclei that they encountered responded to rotation of the visual surround by increasing or decreasing their firing rates when the direction of motion of the visual surround was appropriate to that experienced during head movement. Moreover, the neurons continued to fire during OKAN, indicating that stored activity was driving the neurons in the vestibular nuclei after the end of stimulation.

In regard to the ototoxicity of aminoglycosides, the effects of end-organ damage are likely to be shown most sensitively in the response to head rotation at high frequencies. Stored activity makes relatively minor contributions to the total response under this condition. On the other hand, the storage mechanism contributes significantly to both the phase and gain of compensatory eye movements at lower frequencies of rotation [10]. It also makes a significant contribution to both the gain and the duration of the caloric response. Little information is available about vertical caloric nystagmus in man, but if there is a similar lack of stored activity for nystagmus in the upward direction, then upward and downward caloric nystagmus in human subjects should reflect differences in the dynamic response properties. Overall, it seems certain that a better understanding of the various components that form the oculomotor response to vestibular testing is essential for the design of tests that can most quickly and efficiently demonstrate the destructive effects of ototoxic medication.

References

1. Cohen, B., Matsuo, V., and Raphan, T. Quantitative analysis of the velocity characteristics of optokinetic nystagmus and optokinetic after-nystagmus. *J. Physiol. (Lond.)* 270:321, 1977.
2. Dichgans, J., von Reutern, G. M., and Römmelt, U. Impaired suppression of vestibular nystagmus by fixation in cerebellar and noncerebellar patients. *Arch. Psychiatr. Nervenkr.* 226:183, 1978.
3. Fernández, C., and Goldberg, J. M. Physiology of peripheral neurons innervating semicircular canals of the squirrel monkey. II. Response to sinusoidal stimulation and dynamics of peripheral vestibular system. *J. Neurophysiol.* 34:661, 1971.
4. Goldberg, J. M., and Fernández, C. Physiology of peripheral neurons innervating semicircular canals of the squirrel monkey. I. Resting discharge and response to constant angular accelerations. *J. Neurophysiol.* 34:635, 1971.
5. Henn, V., Cohen, B., and Young, L. R. Visual-Vestibular Interaction in Motion Perception and the Generation of Nystagmus. Neurosciences Research Program Bulletin. 18:4, 1980. Pp 457–651. Cambridge, Mass.: MIT Press.
6. Jung, R. Die Registrierung des postrotatorischen und optokinetischen Nystagmus und die optisch-vestibuläre Integration beim Menschen. *Acta Otolaryngol. (Stockh.)* 36:199, 1948.
7. Lisberger, S. G., and Fuchs, A. F. Response of flocculus Purkinje cells to adequate vestibular stimulation in the alert monkey: Fixation versus compensatory eye movements. *Brain Res.* 69:347, 1974.
8. Matsuo, V., Cohen, B., Raphan, T., de Jong, V., and Henn, V. Asymmetric velocity storage for upward and downward nystagmus. *Brain Res.* 176:159, 1979.

9. Money, K. E., and Scott, J. W. Functions of separate sensory receptors of nonauditory labyrinth of the cat. *Am. J. Physiol.* 202:1211, 1962.
10. Raphan, T., and Cohen, B. The Role of Integration in Oculomotor Control. In B. Zuber (Ed.), *Models of Oculomotor Behavior and Control.* West Palm Beach, Fla.: CRC Press, 1981 (in press).
11. Raphan, T., Matsuo, V., and Cohen, B. Velocity storage in the vestibulo-ocular reflex arc (VOR). *Exp. Brain Res.* 35:229, 1979.
12. Takahashi, M., and Igarashi, M. Comparison of vertical and horizontal optokinetic nystagmus in the squirrel monkey. *Otorhinolaryngol.* 39:321, 1977.
13. Takemori, S., and Cohen, B. Visual suppression of vestibular nystagmus in rhesus monkeys. *Brain Res.* 72:203, 1974.
14. Takemori, S., and Cohen, B. Loss of visual suppression of vestibular nystagmus after flocculus lesions. *Brain Res.* 72:213, 1974.
15. Ter Braak, J. W. G. Untersuchungen über optokinetischen Nystagmus. *Arch. Neerl. Physiol.* 21:309, 1936.
16. Waespe, W., and Henn, V. Neuronal activity in the vestibular nuclei of the alert monkey during vestibular and optokinetic stimulation. *Exp. Brain Res.* 27:523, 1977.
17. Waespe, W., and Henn, V. Vestibular nuclei activity during optokinetic after-nystagmus (OKAN) in the alert monkey. *Exp. Brain Res.* 30:323, 1977.
18. Waespe, W., and Henn, V. The velocity response of vestibular nucleus neurons during vestibular, visual, and combined angular acceleration. *Exp. Brain Res.* 37:337, 1979.

Discussion of Chapter 9

Dr. R. A. Butler (The University of Chicago, Chicago, Illinois): Do you conceive of storage as having a neurologic center?

Dr. Cohen: Yes. We are now doing microelectrode studies to try to find evidence for storage on a cellular level. One can see the effects of storage in the neurons of the vestibular nuclei just one synapse away from the peripheral end organ. During rotation in light, the unit activity jumps to some level, presumably due mainly to the direct input from the vestibular system, and then is maintained despite the fact that the cupula is no longer deflected.

We know that a number of lesions will cause a loss of optokinetic after-nystagmus—for example, bilateral labyrinthectomy, section of the vestibular commissural fibers, and lesions of the prepositus. On the other hand, one is relatively certain that the storage is due to neural circuitry involving the vestibular nuclei. It does not depend on the vestibular cerebellum. We know that because storage persists if the vestibular cerebellum is removed. We don't have any more information about this problem at present.

10. Slow and Fast Components of Nystagmus: Two Systems with Different Characteristics

Vicente Honrubia, Jeffrey W. Birns, and Clifford G. Y. Lau

The vestibulo-ocular reflex has been assessed experimentally and clinically by evaluation of the characteristics of the slow component of nystagmus, but only by measurements of eye velocity. Other aspects of the nystagmus reaction, such as the fast component (amplitude, velocity, or position), that could be affected in certain abnormal conditions are not evaluated routinely. Fast components, in particular, because of their brevity and high speed, could be sensitive indicators of central nervous system malfunction. Unfortunately, our knowledge about the properties and mechanism of production of fast components is limited at present.

In this chapter, we summarize the results of several investigations into the properties of the slow and fast components of vestibular nystagmus, done with the hope of contributing to their understanding and to their use for the evaluation of vestibulo-ocular reflex function.

Lorente de Nó [9] made a fundamental contribution in his pioneering work on the vestibular system when he identified a circuit of interneurons, located in the reticular formation, which is responsible for producing fast components. Most of the anatomic information was obtained from Golgi-stained material. Drawings made from such material are reproduced in Fig. 10-1. Lorente de Nó was able to identify two types of input to the oculomotor neurons. The first consists of fibers in the middle longitudinal fasciculus (m.f.l.), whose cells of origin are located in the vestibular nuclei. This input corresponds to the elementary ocular reflex arc [4, 9]. The second input consists of fibers running parallel to the m.f.l., but with their neurons of origin in the parapontine reticular formation. This organization of the vestibulo-ocular reflex (Fig. 10-1) has been widely accepted, although the precise location and connections of the neurons responsible for the fast component still remain to be elucidated.

Numerous experimental and clinical observations support the notion that an independent group of neurons controls the production of fast components of nystagmus [6, 9]. Under a variety of circumstances, for example, under the

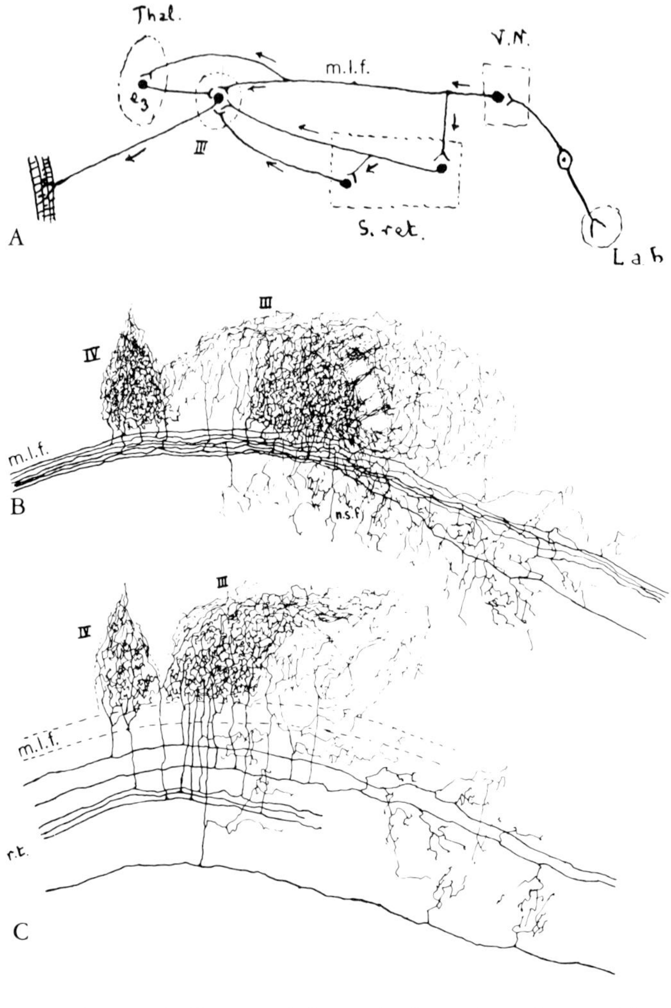

Figure 10-1. A. Schematic diagram of the vestibulo-ocular reflex arc. The existence of interneurons in the reticular formation (S. ret.) has been postulated to be responsible for the production of fast components. (Lab = labyrinth; V.N. = vestibular nuclei; Thal. = thalamus; III = third nucleus.) B. Drawing of Golgi-stained neural plexus showing the input of axons in the middle longitudinal fasciculus (m.l.f.) to the third and fourth nuclear complexes. C. Illustration to demonstrate the existence of a second bundle of fibers (r.t.) parallel to the m.l.f. The cell bodies of origin for the r.t. fibers were located in the adjacent reticular formation. (Modified from R. Lorente de Nó [personal courtesy], vestibulo-ocular reflex arc. *Arch. Neurol. Psychiatry* (*Chicago*) 30:245, 1933.)

influence of depressant drugs (anesthetics, barbiturates) or as a result of certain pathologic conditions, nystagmus changes to a compensatory movement. This is the pure vestibular response, whose presence, while the other response disappears, suggests that there are indeed two groups of neurons, each group being responsible for the production of one component of nystagmus. Accurate measurements designed to ascertain in detail the relationship between the fast- and slow-component systems and to demonstrate that changes in one aspect of the nystagmus (i.e., the slow component) occur independently of changes in the other (i.e., the fast component) are not available, however.

Recently, the development of techniques for automatic and accurate recording of eye movement has made it possible to investigate some of the characteristics of the fast component, including the dependence of the initiation of this component on the position and velocity of the eye during nystagmus induced by stimulation of the horizontal semicircular canals [5, 7, 8]. These techniques were used in the present experiments, which we conducted on rabbits. In investigations on the relationship between the initiation of the fast component and eye position, the capability of neck reflexes to modify the eye position in the orbit in these animals was particularly useful [2]. We administered halothane, a quick-acting and reversible anesthetic gas, to modify both slow and fast components pharmacologically and to elucidate the interdependence of the two systems.

Methods

Horizontal eye movement responses were measured in adult Dutch rabbits with a "search coil" technique similar to that developed by Robinson [10]. This method allows for very stable and accurate recording of eye movements. Several weeks prior to the tests, a magnetic coil consisting of four turns of fine wire was implanted under the eye muscles and the globe of the left eyeball. An acrylic crown with a metal bolt for restraining the animal was implanted at the same time. We calibrated the eye movement by first positioning the body of the rabbit, and thus the plane of the search coil, parallel to the direction of the magnetic field created by the field coil. In this position, no voltage is induced in the search coil. From a computer program we obtained a calibration factor which we used to calibrate the nystagmus record after it was digitized, to determine the change in eye displacement in degrees. The accuracy of calibration was evaluated from measurements of the voltage induced by rotation of a search coil mounted on a plastic holder which simulated an eyeball. The platform was mounted on a rate table (Inland 800), thus allowing accurate rotations at various frequencies and peak velocities.

The signal representing the angular displacement of the eye was simultaneously displayed on a polygraph, stored on magnetic tape, and digitized on-line with a PDP-11/15 minicomputer system. Techniques used for the collection, display, and analysis of data have been described previously [7, 11].

For experiments in which halothane was administered, an airtight, lightweight, clear Plexiglas chamber was placed around the animal. Plastic tubing conducted the anesthetic gas mixture from the anesthesia machine outside the chamber to a gas input port positioned in the midline directly above the animal's head. The chamber was closed posteriorly with a large plastic bag, which was taped into position. An outlet for the gas was fashioned near the animal's feet, and gas leaving the chamber was removed by an electric fan. The volume within the chamber was 7.7 liters. Halothane (Fluothane) was vaporized in a copper kettle vaporizer mounted on a standard anesthesia machine. All mixtures of vaporized halothane were administered with an oxygen flow of 2 liters per minute.

Results

Dependence of Fast Components on Eye Position and Velocity During Slow Component

During sinusoidal rotation of the head in the dark with low stimulus velocity, the eye response has a sinusoidal trajectory. At higher velocities, nystagmus sets in. The eye trajectory is interrupted at irregular intervals by corrective saccades (fast components) that restrict the range of eye movement within the orbit (Fig. 10-2).

In six animals exposed to the same frequency and to the range of stimuli shown in Fig. 10-2, the position of the eye was recorded at the times of the

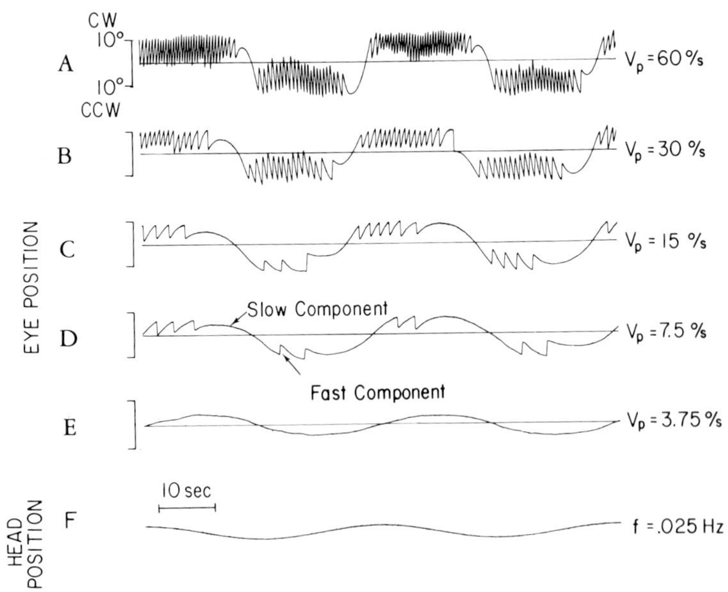

Figure 10-2. Examples of rabbit eye movement response to sinusoidal head rotation in the dark at various peak velocities, indicated to the right of the tracings. Eye calibrations (±10 degrees) are shown at the left of each tracing. The 0.025-Hz stimulus frequency is indicated at the bottom.

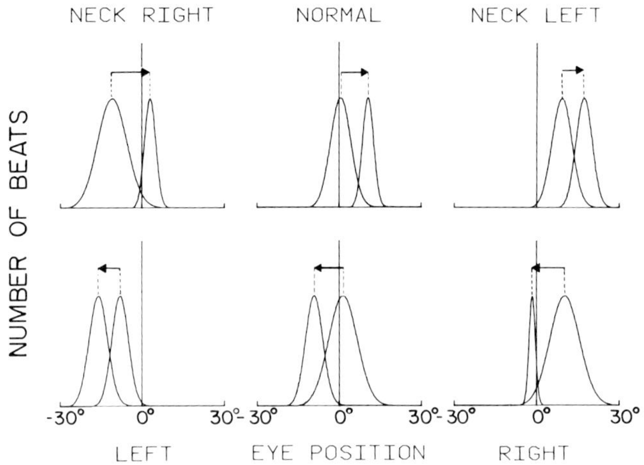

Figure 10-3. Normalized eye histograms, showing the distribution of points of initiation and termination of the slow component of nystagmus beating from left to right (top) and from right to left (bottom). The direction of each arrow indicates the direction of the slow-component motion. The plots in the center were obtained during stimulation with the body and head aligned normally. The plots on the left were obtained with the body deviated 30 degrees in the counterclockwise direction, and those on the right, with the body deviated 30 degrees in the clockwise direction. The first maneuver closes the angle of the head and neck toward the left side, the second maneuver toward the right side.

start and end of the slow components. Graphs showing the distribution of these points in the orbit under three different experimental conditions are given in Fig. 10-3. Leftward slow components start at 1.36 ± 5.19 degrees from the center and end at −9.18 ± 3.16 degrees. Rightward slow components start at 0.61 ± 3.69 degrees and end at 10.64 ± 2.01 degrees. (The range of normal eye movement is approximately 20 degrees.)

To investigate the dependence of the distribution of these starting and end points on both eye position and velocity, we prepared graphs like those in Fig. 10-4. The ordinate indicates eye velocity at the beginning and end of the slow component, and the abscissa, the position of the eye at the same instant. In Fig. 10-4, data points obtained from the six rabbits used in the study are combined. The upper scatter plots correspond to data for the rightward slow component, and those at the bottom, to the leftward slow component. Lines describing the relationship of each of the two nystagmus reactions within a cycle were obtained by least-square regression analysis. The lines describing the behavior of the points for the end of the slow component (ESC) are almost vertical; the slopes are 0.04 ± 0.04 and 0.06 ± 0.04 degree per degree/second during leftward and rightward slow components, respectively. The slopes of the points for the start of the slow component (SSC) are −0.19 ± 0.08 and −0.16 ± 0.10 degree per degree/second for the leftward and rightward slow components, respectively. Since the lines describing the behavior of the ESC points

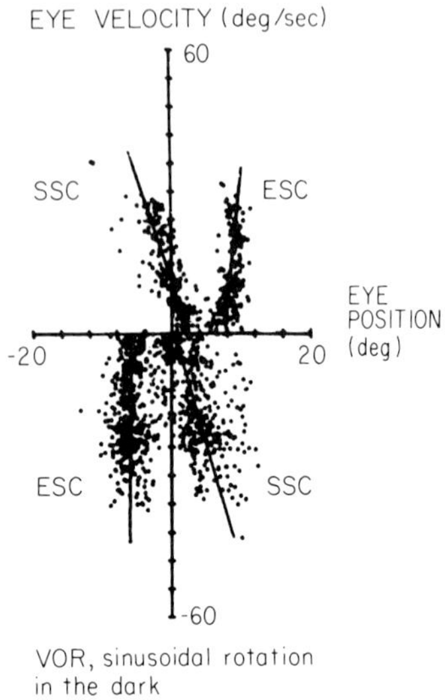

Figure 10-4. Example of VOR data points in the phase plane for one rabbit. (SSC = start of slow component; ESC = end of slow component.) The abscissa indicates eye position and the ordinate, eye velocity. The linear regression lines are drawn through the corresponding data points. (Slopes in text are given in deg per deg/sec.)

represent the point of initiation of fast components, the data show that the initiation of the fast components is dependent chiefly on eye position, rather than on eye velocity. It appears that there is a positional "threshold" for the initiation of fast components.

Influence of Neck Reflex on the Threshold of the Fast Component

If the so-called threshold of the fast component corresponds to an absolute orbital position, and if vestibular nystagmus is induced after a change in the eye position at rest as a result of neck postural reflexes [2], one would expect the pattern of eye movement during physiologically induced vestibular nystagmus (i.e., the location of the fast-component threshold) to remain the same. To evaluate this hypothesis, we induced nystagmus at three different angular positions of the body and neck relative to the head.

An example of the resulting nystagmus reactions is shown in Fig. 10-5. The tracings in row B were obtained with the head and torso aligned; in A, the torso was rotated 30 degrees toward the animal's left side, and in C, 30 degrees toward the right. This rotation, as expected, caused a compensatory change in the resting position of the eyes. During vestibular stimulation, the mean eye position of the nystagmus can be seen in Fig. 10-5 to take place on the side opposite the torso location (to the right in A and to the left in C). The symmetric nystagmus in curve B became asymmetric when the neck was flexed. When the slow component has the direction of the tonic eye deviation, its amplitude is smaller. Measurements of the eye velocity during the slow

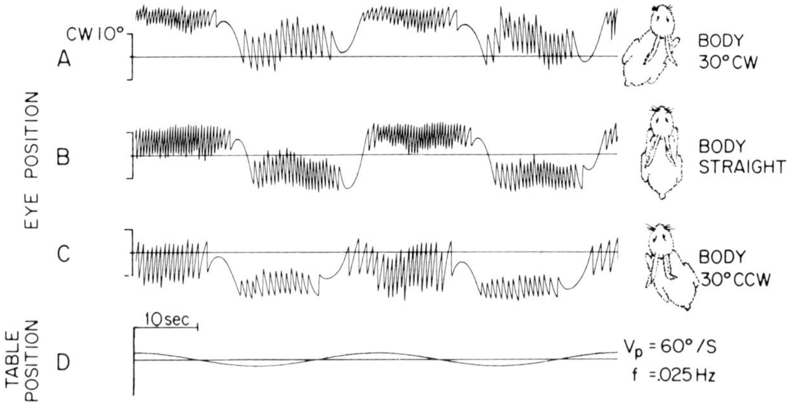

Figure 10-5. Examples of rabbit eye movements in response to sinusoidal head rotation in the dark during static neck bending. The two most significant effects of stimulating the neck receptors are (1) to produce a positional shift of the eye as well as nystagmus motion toward the side opposite the direction of neck bending, and (2) to produce an increase in the amplitude of the nystagmus, whose slow component moves in the direction opposite to that of the tonic deviation. The slow components to the right are greater when the neck is turned to the right; the slow components to the left are greater when the neck is turned to the left.

component, however, showed that the gain of the reflex remains unchanged. The only change was in the overall position of the nystagmus reaction, which was shifted in the direction of the tonic deviation.

The graphs on the left and right sides of Fig. 10-3 summarize the results of measurements of the eye position at the beginning and end of the slow component when the neck and body deviate to the right and left, respectively. (Data for the rightward slow component are at the top and for the leftward component, at the bottom.) The locations of the end points of the slow component remain within a restricted region in the orbit, but their mean position depends on the experimental conditions. Therefore, the so-called threshold of the fast component does not depend on an absolute orbital position.

Effect of Halothane on the Threshold of Fast Components

The vestibulo-ocular reflex was found to be highly sensitive to the effect of halothane. Visually detectable changes in nystagmus occurred within 2 minutes after 9% halothane in oxygen began to be introduced into the chamber enclosing the rabbit (Fig. 10-6). After 9 minutes of halothane administration, the range of eye movements was approximately double that before the anesthetic was given.

Figure 10-7 shows the results of measurements of four parameters of nystagmus in three animals. The effect of the drug was minimal on the slow-component velocity and amplitude, but it was significant on the fast components. The distance between the points of initiation of the fast components

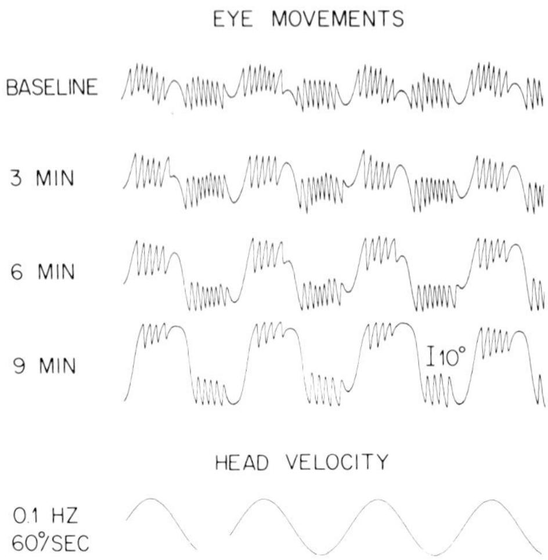

Figure 10-6. Eye movement recordings obtained at 3, 6, and 9 minutes after the administration of halothane into the chamber enclosing the animal. During activation of the vestibulo-ocular reflex, the range of eye movements widens as the period of halothane respiration is increased.

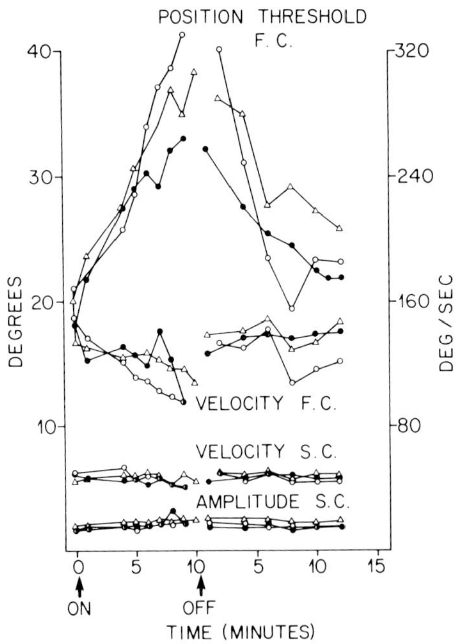

Figure 10-7. Graph indicating the effect of halothane on four parameters of nystagmic movements: the amplitude and velocity of the slow component (S.C.), the velocity of the fast component (F.C.), and the range of eye movement. The symbols △, ●, and ○ each correspond to one animal. The times of beginning and termination of halothane administration are indicated by arrows. The ordinate on the left shows degrees of eye deviation and that on the right, velocity of eye movement.

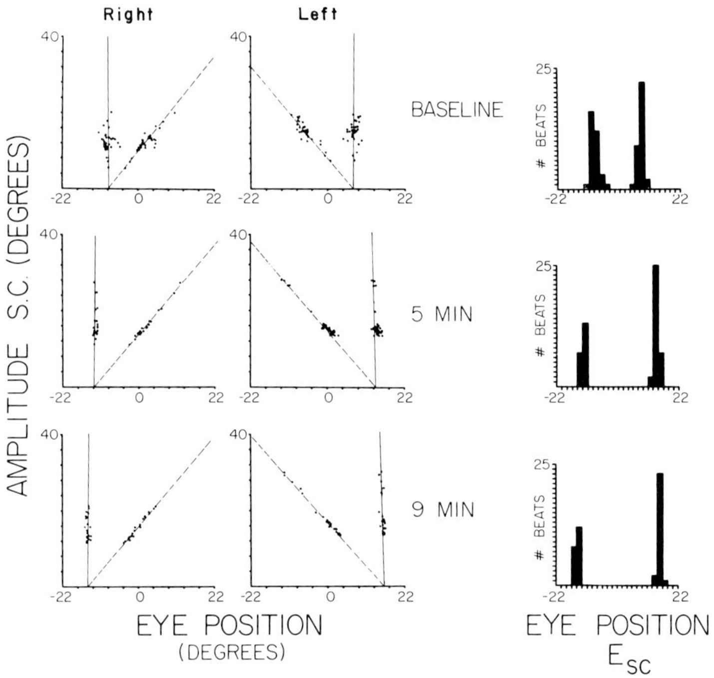

Figure 10-8. Composite plot illustrating the changes in the eye position during nystagmus following halothane administration. The plots on the left indicate the relationship between the amplitude of the slow component (ordinate) and the eye position at the start and at the end of the slow component (abscissa). The dashed lines are the least-square regression curves fitted to the data points. The lines indicating the relationship between the position of the eye at the start of the slow component and the amplitude of the slow component are approximately at a 45-degree angle with the vertical lines. The lines indicating the relationship between the eye position at the end of the slow component (E_{SC}) and the amplitude of the nystagmus are practically vertical. These lines move toward the periphery of the orbit after halothane administration. (Times after halothane administration are shown between graphs.) Histograms indicating the distribution of the E_{SC} points in the orbit are shown on the right side.

increased to approximately 40 degrees. There was a decrease in the average velocity of the fast component from approximately 150 degrees per second to 100 degrees per second. The effect of the anesthetic on the so-called threshold of the fast component is further illustrated in Fig. 10-8. The graphs on the left indicate the dependence of the ESC and SSC points of the slow component (abscissa) on the amplitude of the slow component (ordinate). Data for rightward nystagmus are shown on the left, and for leftward nystagmus, on the right. The data were collected before (top) and at 5 and 9 minutes after the administration of the gas, as indicated. Least-square regression lines are shown for each set of points. In the three plots, the ESC lines are almost vertical, since the location of the fast-component threshold continues to depend mostly on orbital position (abscissa). The location of these points changes, however, as shown in the histograms on the right side. As expected, the lines describing the dependence of the SSC on the amplitude of the slow component are at about a 45-degree angle with the lines of the ESC points. Since all of the slow components finish at the same place in the orbit, it follows that, the greater the slow-component amplitude, the greater the distance of the point of initiation of the slow component (SSC) from the vertical ESC line. Apparently, regardless of the shift in the position of the threshold of the fast component, the mechanisms that produce fast components operate with the same controls that regulate their behavior before the anesthesia.

The differential effect of the drug on each of the parameters strongly suggests that the neurons responsible for the production of fast components are different from those controlling the production of slow components.

Comments

The differential effect of the anesthetic on the fast-component neurons supports the notion that these neurons are independent of those producing slow components, and that they are among the long chains of interneurons in the reticular formation; hence their greater sensitivity to anesthesia. Certain drugs, anesthetics in particular, have been shown first to impair the transmission of impulses through the interneuronal chains [1]. Perhaps the effect is the same in all neurons; but because the number of synapses in the fast-component is greater than that in the slow-component circuits, the effects appear to be more obvious in the former.

The fast-component threshold restricts the range of eye movement to a small angular deviation around the center of the orbit. It is reasonable to assume that, under these conditions, all muscles of the eye participate optimally in the production of nystagmus.

As was shown in man [8], the initiation of fast components in the rabbit is quite insensitive to the velocity of the head or that of the eye during the preceding slow component. Hence the threshold of the fast component is not directly dependent on vestibular nerve impulses, which reflect mostly the velocity of the head [3, 12]. Furthermore, under the influence of neck reflexes or under the initial effect of halothane, the eye velocity during the slow component does not change, whereas the position of the threshold of the fast component changes significantly. It is therefore quite plausible that the neurons controlling the production of fast components do not receive direct vestibular input. From where does the fast-component neuron receive commands to inhibit the motor neurons at the end of the slow components? It is reasonable to assume that these fast-component neurons react to the same signal that activates the motor neurons, whose firing reflects mostly the eye position. The membrane of these fast-component neurons presumably has a long time constant and hence a high threshold. These neurons may require large numbers of action potentials, arriving synchronously at the synapses, for activation. Once the threshold is reached, they fire briefly to inhibit the motor neurons.

The motor neurons, however, could simultaneously be under the influence of other reflexes, such as tonic reflexes, which can bias the eye position, causing the nystagmus to take place in a different range of orbital positions. The result is that the pattern of nystagmus production remains the same except for the influence of the bias on the overall eye position; hence the observed changes in the location of fast-component thresholds. These assumptions remain to be elucidated, however. An increased understanding of the properties and mechanism of fast-component production may eventually enable us to understand how fast components are generated.

References

1. Brazier, M. H. B. The Action of Anesthetics on the Nervous System with Special Reference to the Brain Stem Reticular System. In J. F. Delafresnaye (Ed.), *Brain Mechanisms and Consciousness.* Oxford, Eng.: Blackwell, 1954. Pp. 163–199.
2. deKlein, A. Recherches quantitatives sur les positions compensatoires de l'oeil chez le lapin. *Arch. Neerl. Physiol.* 7:138, 1922.
3. Fernández, C., and Goldberg, J. M. Physiology of peripheral neurons innervating semicircular canals of the squirrel monkey. II. Response to sinusoidal stimulation and dynamics of peripheral vestibular system. *J. Neurophysiol.* 34:661, 1971.
4. Graybiel, A. M. Some Patterns of Connectivity in the Central Nervous System. In H. Asanuma and V. J. Wilson (Eds.), *Integration in the Nervous System, A Symposium in Honor of David P. C. Lloyd and Rafael Lorente de Nó.* Tokyo: Igaku-Shoin, 1979. Pp. 69–96.
5. Honrubia, V., Baloh, R. W., Lau, C. G. Y., and Sills, A. W. The pattern of eye movements during physiologic vestibular nystagmus in man. *Trans. Am. Acad. Ophthalmol. Otolaryngol.* 84:ORL339, 1977.
6. Janeke, J. B., Jongkees, L. B. W., and Oosterveld, W. J. Selective suppression of the fast phase of labyrinthine nystagmus by phentanyl (fentanyl). *Acta Otolaryngol.* 68:468, 1969.
7. Lau, C. G. Y. Modeling of visual-vestibular interaction and the fast components of nystagmus. University of California, Santa Barbara, Ph.D. Thesis, 1978.
8. Lau, C. G. Y., Honrubia, V., and Baloh, R. W. The pattern of eye movement trajectories during physiological nystagmus in humans. In *Proceedings of the 6th Extraordinary Meeting of the Bárány Society,* London, September 11–15, 1977.
9. Lorente de Nó, R. Vestibulo-ocular reflex arc. *Arch. Neurol. Psychiatry* (*Chicago*) 30:245, 1933.
10. Robinson, D. A. A method of measuring eye movement using a scleral search coil in a magnetic field. *I.E.E.E. Trans. Biomed. Eng.* 10:137, 1963.
11. Sills, A. W., Honrubia, V., and Kumley, W. E. Algorithm for the multi-parameter analysis of nystagmus using a digital computer. *Aviat. Space Environ. Med.* 46:934, 1975.
12. Skavenski, A. A., and Robinson, D. A. Role of abducens neurons in vestibulo-ocular reflex. *J. Neurophysiol.* 36:724, 1973.

Discussion of Chapter 10

Dr. Cohen: It seems to me that you have shown two independent thresholds for the fast component of nystagmus; one threshold can be changed by various manipulations, and the second is fixed and related to eye velocity. In other words, no matter what the eye position was, it appeared that the amplitude of the beat was strictly dependent on the velocity of the eyes, whereas the "trigger" position shifted back and forth across the beating field depending on whether you had the neck turned or whether other manipulations were done.

Dr. Honrubia: I must not have explained our findings properly. In our experience, the threshold is independent of the eye velocity. The fact that all the slow components terminate in the same location in the orbit can be interpreted as indicating that there must be some neurons in the central nervous system that know that the eye got to that particular position. However, the point where all the slow components always end, which is about 10 degrees from the center of the orbit, is not the absolute orbital position. We like to think about the threshold as an operational threshold that can be manipulated.

Dr. Cohen: Does the slow-component velocity vary with eye position? You gave various frequencies of stimulation. Did the slow-component velocity depend at all on where in the orbit you triggered the beat?

Dr. Honrubia: No. We have been able to investigate the VOR system mainly in terms of the velocity of the slow components within certain ranges of orbital positions. The slow component is independent of the position of the eye in the orbit. This has also been verified in human subjects.

Dr. L. Eviatar: Did you infer that the reticular activating system controls mainly the fast component? If so, why would a person who is drowsy have both components of the nystagmus depressed? Someone who is about to fall asleep will have a gradual decrease of both components of nystagmus until they disappear, no matter what stimulus is used.

Dr. Honrubia: I hope you didn't misunderstand me. The two components of nystagmus are not completely independent of each other, nor can one system proceed without the other. What I said was that one system has a greater sensitivity, and that, if you give a drug such as halothane, you will eventually affect the two systems. Halothane acts earlier on the fast component, and its later and greater effect is on the slow component. The fast-component system receives input from the slow-component system. They are dependent and interrelated, but the neurons involved in producing each component show a difference in sensitivity to different experimental manipulations.

Dr. C. W. Hart (Northwestern University, Chicago, Illinois): I have been studying spontaneous nystagmus in patients with their eyes closed. They are requested to deviate their eyes to either side by looking in the direction of their thumb. The nystagmus usually follows Alexander's law; when they look to the right, the slow-phase velocity and amplitude are larger, and when they look to the left, the slow-phase velocity and amplitude become less. How do you explain that in the light of your observations?

Dr. Honrubia: Let's suppose there is a point of termination of the slow component somewhere toward the center of the orbit. What you do by changing the gaze of the subject is actually shifting, or introducing a position bias on, the internal mechanism that is generating the spontaneous vestibular nystagmus. I postulate that this bias shifts the range of the eye movements, but that the threshold remains in the same place, and every time the eye reaches that position it will produce a fast component.

11. The Early Effects of Streptomycin on First-Order Vestibular Neurons in the Gerbil

David J. Anderson

Behavioral, anatomic, electrophysiologic, and biochemical data in the literature attest to the effects of streptomycin on the vestibular system in a number of animal species. The precision with which the sequence of observable events leading to aminoglycoside ototoxicity can be determined depends on the technique used. Investigators have generally concerned themselves with events occurring during the course of systemic drug therapy. With most quantitative techniques, one can sample these events with a temporal resolution of the order of hours or days.

Our own work follows the lead of those investigators who are interested chiefly in the detail of events taking place in the first few minutes of exposure of sensory cells to a drug. We intend to show that, under certain conditions, profound neurophysiologic changes can occur in the output of the vestibular first-order neurons in the critical few minutes after the direct administration of streptomycin to the middle ear.

Our experiments confirm that there is an early component to the ototoxic effect of streptomycin on the vestibular system, and that the changes that result can be analyzed with the statistical parameters commonly used in electrophysiologic studies of single vestibular neurons.

Background

Reports on the effects of streptomycin and other drugs on the vestibular sensory epithelia are numerous, but a line of progress can be traced by means of a few selected studies. A recent review by Hawkins [5] cites the major contributions in this area. Physiologic and anatomic experiments on the effects of streptomycin were reported by Wersäll and Hawkins [17] in a study that combined measures of ataxia and per-rotatory nystagmus with histologic findings. Differential effects on type I and type II hair cells were observed, and the authors suggested that studies of hair cell populations should be carried out.

Possible physiologic differences between the two types of cells were taken into consideration only in later experiments, but anatomic investigations became increasingly detailed. Duvall and Wersäll [2] provided evidence that the sites of streptomycin action were the plasma membrane of the sensory cell and the membrane component of the mitochondria. In subsequent studies, animals were given long-term exposure to streptomycin, and their inner ears were examined histologically several days after the final dose [7, 15]. These studies confirmed earlier conclusions as to the differential sensitivity of the two types of hair cells.

Wersäll and Flock [16] studied the early effects of streptomycin on the lateral line organ of the teleost fish *Lota vulgaris.* They found that the microphonic potential could be abolished by the local application of streptomycin and restored after washout of the antibiotic. The effect of the application occurred at 3 to 10 minutes, whereas 80 to 90 percent restoration could be achieved 2 minutes after washout. The rate at which changes occurred suggested to the investigators that locally applied streptomycin affected primarily the surface membrane of the hair cell. These same rapid rates of disruption and restoration of activity in response to application and removal of streptomycin were observed by Harada et al. [4], who used an isolated frog ampullar receptor. In this study, they recorded neural activity rather than the microphonic potential, but included no quantitative measurements of the discharge patterns. Valli et al. [13], who used a similar frog preparation, reported very rapid onset and washout of d-tubocurarine effects. Recently, Gallais has quantified the effects on the rate of discharge of frog primary vestibular fibers as a function of time after administering a number of aminoglycosides [3].

Studies on the concentration of ototoxic drugs in the inner ear fluids have also been carried out. Voldrich [14] used a guinea pig preparation to establish the rates of accumulation of streptomycin, kanamycin, and neomycin in the inner ear after intramuscular injections. Four hours were required for the concentration to reach a maximum, whereas more than 24 hours were required for removal of the drug. Stupp et al. [12] reported similar time constants after subcutaneous injection of these drugs. Balogh et al. [1], von Ilberg et al. [6], and Portmann et al. [9] used autoradiographic techniques to determine the sites in the inner ear where radioactive streptomycin appears within minutes after administration.

A new technique for perfusion of the inner ear of mammals with ototoxic drugs was introduced by Schnieder [10]. Two glass capillaries are inserted in the basal coil of the cochlea, one in the scala vestibuli and the other in the scala tympani. In this way, the perilymph can be exchanged completely in less than 10 minutes. Nuttall et al. [8] (see Chap. 3) used this technique to study the action of ototoxic drugs on the cochlear potentials and obtained excellent quantitative results.

Methods

We have had consistent success for some time in using the gerbil as an experimental animal for investigations on the first- and second-order vestibular neurons [11]. The animal is anesthetized with 15 mg of Vetalar administered intramuscularly, followed by 25 mg of urethane injected intraperitoneally. Additional 4-mg doses of Vetalar are given as required. The trachea is cannulated, and the pinnae are removed with the skin overlying the posterior region of the skull. In addition, the bulla is exposed and opened for later introduction of the drug solution. We use external ear canal and tooth fixation points to secure the animal on a gimbaled animal holder mounted above the center of rotation of our stimulation table. A cranial opening is made above the cerebellum, which is removed by gentle suction under direct visual control until the vestibular nerve with Scarpa's ganglion is exposed. Throughout the experiment, the temperature of the animal is maintained between 35° and 39°C.

The electrode we use for recording from cell bodies is a 10- to 15-megohm sodium-chloride-filled micropipette. The amplifier is a Grass P-16, operated with the driven shield and with capacity compensation, and set to have a gain of 100 and a frequency pass band between 0.3 and 3.0 kHz. Stimulation is applied to the semicircular canals by rotation of the stimulation table, which is driven by a torque motor-linear DC amplifier combination.

When the preparation is complete, a micropipette is introduced by micromanipulation into a portion of the nerve where horizontal vestibular neurons are likely to be found. Discharge patterns of a small number of neurons are recorded and analyzed before the drug is introduced, to assure that the vestibular system is healthy. When a neuron is located that appears to be typical of Scarpa's ganglion cells and yields stable data on spontaneous and driven response over several minutes of recording, the drug is introduced directly through the opening in the bulla, in such a way as to place it in the region of the round window. When the initial thermal transients caused by introduction of fluid into the middle ear have faded, a systematic series of recordings is made for as long as single-neuron recordings of high quality persist. Sequences of tests consisting of a measurement of spontaneous activity and a sensitivity test are administered at a rate of one sequence every 5 minutes. Since we have no method of reversing the effects of the drug once it has been administered, we can obtain data from only one neuron per animal. Therefore, we are very careful to select high-quality recordings.

Stimulus Delivery and Data Collection

For all the experiments, the stimulus delivery system shown in Fig. 11-1 was used. For the driven-activity trials, a preset counter determines the number of cycles of the table. The frequency and amplitude of the cycles are determined by function generator and attenuator settings. The usual stimulation consists of 5 cycles of a 0.5-Hz sine wave at an amplitude determined by the sensitivity of the neuron to horizontal angular acceleration. Spontaneous activity data are recorded under the same conditions, except with the table control signal turned off.

After amplification and frequency band selection, the vertical deflection circuits of a Tektronix 565 oscilloscope normalize the neural spike signal before it is recorded on analog tape. If on-line computer analysis is being used,

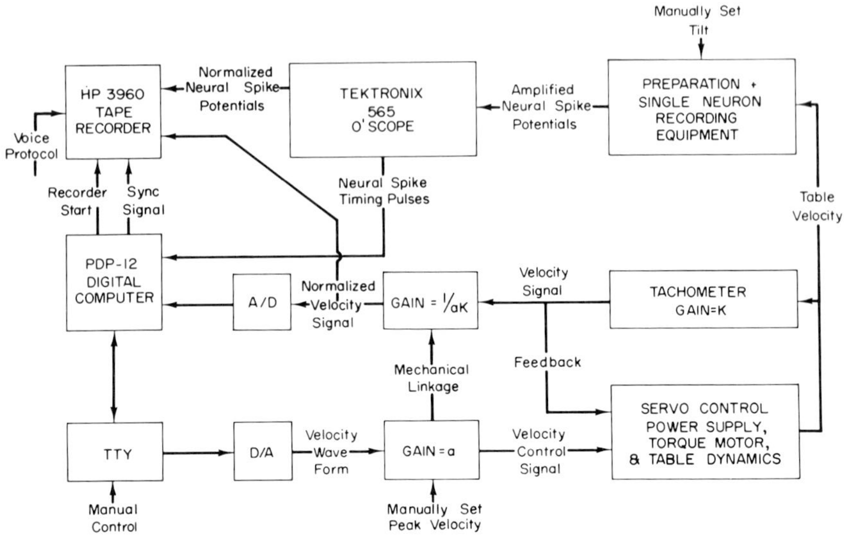

Figure 11-1. Stimulus delivery and data analysis are provided by an integrated data system with a computerized velocity-controlled rate table. Recorder data are observed on-line as well as preserved for off-line analysis.

the trigger circuits of the oscilloscope discriminate single neural discharges from the background noise. Synchronization signals, the rate table tachometer output, and a voice protocol are recorded with the spike train on an HP-3960 tape recorder for later analysis.

The recorded neural discharges were processed by digital computer analysis. The data are summarized in histograms of three types.

Poststimulus histograms are used on-line to show the general responsiveness of a cell to the stimuli applied. In the case of spontaneous activity, the poststimulus histogram is used to assure that the data being recorded are stable. The "bursting" type of Scarpa's ganglion neuron, which has been recorded under conditions of streptomycin intoxication, is most easily illustrated by such a histogram.

The interval histogram is used for analysis of spontaneous activity. From the general appearance of this histogram, we evaluate some types of abnormality that may be present in the neural firing pattern. If the histogram is monomodal, various quantities can be computed that summarize the discharge statistics across the entire population of recorded neurons. The statistics we used to quantify the discharge patterns are the mean intervals of discharge and coefficient of variation.

When periodic stimuli are delivered to the preparation, we use a version of the poststimulus histogram called the "period histogram" to illustrate the results. A feature of the stimulus waveform serves to reset the time to the origin of the poststimulus histogram. The period histogram is thus an average over all of the stimulus periods of the sampled output waveform. The primary information extracted from the period histogram is the sensitivity and phase with respect to the stimulation waveform. When the neuron discharges continuously over the whole period of the stimulus wave, the amplitude ratio and phase are most easily obtained by computation of the discrete Fourier series of the histogram sequence, followed by use of the magnitude of the first component for the computation of sensitivity. If the neuron has a near-zero resting discharge rate, or if it is sufficiently sensitive to reduce its discharge rate to zero during a portion of the cycle, a nonlinear fitting process must be employed by which the sensitivity and phase are determined. These techniques have been perfected, and the calculations can be performed with little more effort than is required for the linear case. Since the stimulation frequency is in the flat band of the gain versus velocity curve for semicircular canal neurons, we find it convenient to express gain in terms of action potentials per second per degree per second.

Results

The vestibular neurons studied in this series are of both the regular and irregular types, in both of which systematic changes occur, reducing the gain and spontaneous activity of the system. The first effects are usually seen at about 20 minutes after the introduction of the drug into the bulla. For regular neurons, there is an increase in the coefficient of variation with a simultaneous reduction in the spontaneous rate, followed by a reduction in the gain or sensitivity. In the case of irregular neurons, the spontaneous discharge rates and the sensitivity can be found as for regular neurons, but the changes in the coefficient of variation are less noticeable. Figure 11-2 illustrates the usual course of events for a regular neuron. Beyond the trends mentioned above, the sensitivity increases slightly before it begins to decrease; this is a typical finding for both regular and irregular neurons.

Comments

We have studied the early toxic effects of streptomycin on vestibular neurons, as recorded from Scarpa's ganglion of the gerbil. The drug was introduced directly into the tympanic cavity. The presumed path of drug transport is diffusion through the round window membrane. In early experiments, when the drug had been introduced several days before the electrical recordings were made, either the neurons were found to be normal, indicating failure of drug transport to the site of action, or the recordings failed to yield the normal dense population of operating neurons, indicating that the time of interaction had passed and that few active neurons remained. Introduction of a drug solution while recordings from a single neuron are in progress may be followed by modifications in the discharge patterns for that neuron. Typical changes are a reduction of spontaneous activity, an increase in the coefficient of

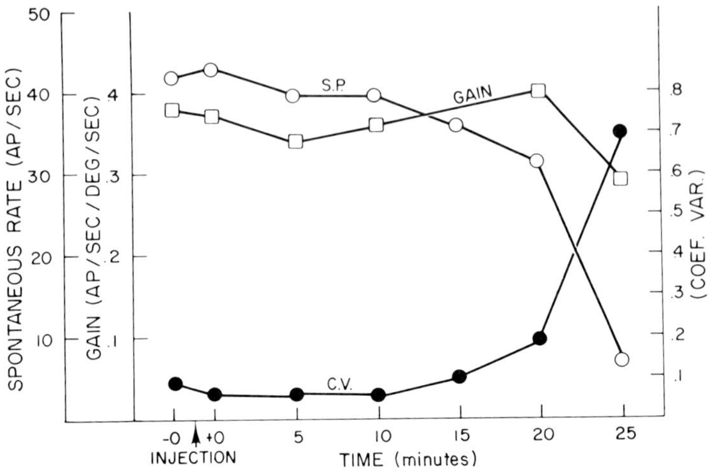

Figure 11-2. Three parameters are plotted as a function of time in minutes, showing the postinjection effects of streptomycin. (AP = action potential; S.P. = spontaneous rate; C.V. = coefficient of variation.)

variation in interspike intervals, and a decrease in sensitivity to angular acceleration.

References

1. Balogh, K., Hiraide, F., and Ishii, D. Distribution of radioactive dihydrostreptomycin in the cochlea—an autoradiographic study. *Ann. Otol. Rhinol. Laryngol.* 79:641, 1970.
2. Duvall, A. J., and Wersäll, J. Site of action of streptomycin upon inner ear sensory cells. *Acta Otolaryngol.* 57:581, 1964.
3. Gallais, A. Comparative study of the influence of aminoglycoside antibiotics on the activity of the horizontal semicircular canal in the frog. *Acta Otolaryngol.* 88:88, 1979.
4. Harada, Y., Musso, E., and Mira, E. Action of streptomycin, dihydrostreptomycin, neomycin, and kanamycin on the ampullar receptors of the frog. *Acta Otolaryngol.* 64:327, 1967.
5. Hawkins, J. E., Jr., and Preston, R. E. Vestibular Ototoxicity. In R. F. Naunton (Ed.), *The Vestibular System.* New York: Academic, 1975. Pp. 321–349.
6. von Ilberg, C., Spoendlin, H., and Arnold, W. Autoradiographical distribution of locally applied dihydrostreptomycin in the inner ear. *Acta Otolaryngol.* 71:159, 1971.
7. Lindeman, H. H. Regional differences in sensitivity of the vestibular sensory epithelia to ototoxic antibiotics. *Acta Otolaryngol.* 67:177, 1969.
8. Nuttall, A. L., Marques, D. M., Stockhorst, E., and Schacht, J. Neomycin effects on cochlear microphonics and phospholipid metabolism. *J. Acous. Soc. Am.* 57[Suppl. 1]:S60, 1975.
9. Portmann, M., Darrouzet, J., and Coste, C. Distribution within the cochlea of dihydrostreptomycin injected into the circulation. An autoradiographic and electron microscopic study. *Arch. Otolaryngol.* 100:473, 1974.

10. Schnieder, E. A contribution to the physiology of the perilymph. Part I: The origins of perilymph. *Ann. Otol. Rhinol. Laryngol.* 83:76, 1974.
11. Schneider, L. W., Anderson, D. J. Transfer characteristics of first and second order lateral canal vestibular neurons in gerbil. *Brain Res.* 112:61, 1976.
12. Stupp, H., Rauch, S., Sous, H., Brun, J. P., and Lagler, F. Kanamycin dosage and levels in ear and other organs. *Arch. Otolaryngol.* 86:515, 1967.
13. Valli, P., Taglietti, V., and Rossi, M. L. Effects of d-tubocurarine on the ampullar receptors of the frog. *Acta Otolaryngol.* 78:51, 1974.
14. Voldrich, L. The kinetics of streptomycin, kanamycin, and neomycin in the inner ear. *Acta Otolaryngol.* 60:234, 1964.
15. Watanuki, K., and Meyer zum Gottesberge, A. Toxic effects of streptomycin and kanamycin upon the sensory epithelium of crista ampullaris. *Acta Otolaryngol.* 72:59, 1971.
16. Wersäll, J., and Flock, A. Suppression and restoration of the microphonic output from the lateral line organ after local application of streptomycin. *Life Sci.* 3:1151, 1964.
17. Wersäll, J., and Hawkins, J. E., Jr. The vestibular sensory epithelia in the cat labyrinth and their reactions to chronic streptomycin intoxication. *Acta Otolaryngol.* 54:1, 1962.

Discussion of Chapter 11

Dr. Wersäll: Dr. Flock and I have put gentamicin on the lateral line organ in order to study the effect of this drug on the activity of single fibers. Gentamicin reduced the activity of these single fibers to a zero level, but the activity recovered after rinsing of the lateral line organ with a potassium-enriched medium. The decrease occurred both during stimulated activity and while the lateral line organ was at rest.

Dr. C. Fernández (The University of Chicago, Chicago, Illinois): Do you have any hypothesis as to the nature of the process underlying the regularity of units and the relationship between this physiologic property and the type of sensory cells?

Dr. Wersäll: I would suggest that the regular fibers innervate a large number of cells in such a way that the randomized transmitter release from the separate cells will coincide into a system that will give a regular discharge rate. One would expect that, with the slope of the curve in the figure, the release of transmitter substance will decrease to the point where the action potential will stop and you will get a randomized system, and then you will get an irregular system. If this hypothesis is correct, every regular fiber should, after some exposure to the drug, become irregular.

Dr. Brummett: What drug concentrations are you using?

Dr. Anderson: In some cases we didn't know how much drug we were putting into the bulla. This was a pilot study, and we were merely trying to get an idea of the effects of the drug.

Histopathology

Soon after ototoxicity had first been observed in patients treated with streptomycin, experimentalists confirmed the ototoxic effects of this drug on animals. Later, similar effects were observed with neomycin and kanamycin. Comparable expectations of ototoxicity with gentamicin, and with aminoglycosides introduced subsequently, were realized in histopathologic studies on animals even before the start of clinical trials. Current histopathologic techniques of cochlear surface preparation with light microscopy and both transmission and scanning electron microscopy, as described by Joseph Hawkins and Lars-Göran Johnsson and by Jan Wersäll, not only permit screening of new aminoglycosides for their ototoxic potential, but also aid in the determination of the mechanism of their toxicity. The technique devised by Matti Anniko permits the development of isolated mouse otocysts in culture. His system enables him to observe ototoxic effects of aminoglycosides on organogenesis, which may have important implications for intrauterine toxicity. It may also facilitate efficient screening of new aminoglycosides.

12. Histopathology of Cochlear and Vestibular Ototoxicity in Laboratory Animals

Joseph E. Hawkins, Jr., and Lars-Göran Johnsson

The most impressive changes that occur in the tissues of the inner ear in response to the ototoxic action of the aminoglycoside antibiotics are found in Corti's organ, in the ampullar cristae, and in the maculae of the utricle and saccule. The destruction and disappearance of sensory cells and other elements of these neuroepithelia can readily be seen by light microscopy, as first demonstrated in conventional serial sections of celloidin-embedded temporal bones from experimental animals treated with streptomycin [2, 3, 15, 21].

The method of cochlear reconstruction from serial sections [8, 22] can be used for evaluation of ototoxic injuries in laboratory animals such as the guinea pig [4], but the method of microdissection and surface preparations (whole mounts) of inner ear tissues stained with osmium tetroxide [5, 6, 7, 9] avoids the delays that are inherent in the processes of decalcification and celloidin embedding. This method has other advantages as well, since it permits a quick survey, with the dissecting microscope, of Corti's organ and its innervation. Furthermore, it makes possible a detailed, quantitative assessment of the extent and severity of hair cell loss in the form of a cytocochleogram, which is based on a count of hair cells over the whole length of the basilar membrane. Reports based on its use in the study of aminoglycoside ototoxicity in guinea pigs include publications by Hawkins and Engström [11], Kohonen [19], and Ylikoski et al. [26]; in cats, by Hawkins, Johnsson, and Aran [13]; and in monkeys, by Stebbins et al. [24] and Hawkins et al. [17].

This chapter is concerned mainly with the changes that can be seen by light microscopy in the cochlear and vestibular tissues of commonly used laboratory animals, i.e., guinea pigs, cats, and monkeys, as a result of daily parenteral

This work was supported by Research Grants NS 05065, NS 05077, and NS 12706, and by Program Project Grant NS 05785 from the National Institute of Neurological and Communicative Disorders and Stroke.

Technical assistance by Bonnie Bower, Julie Davis, and Pamela Henry is gratefully acknowledged.

administration of one or another of the aminoglycoside antibiotics. Changes seen at the electron-microscope level are considered in the chapter by Wersäll. Inner ear pathology in patients who had received antimicrobial therapy with aminoglycosides is described in Chapter 27.

Materials and Methods

The animals used included guinea pigs, both albino and pigmented, cats, macaque monkeys of various species, and patas monkeys (*Erythrocebus patas*). Many of the monkeys had been trained for behavioral audiometry (see Chap. 1).

The aminoglycosides were amikacin, gentamicin, kanamycin, neomycin, netilmicin, sisomicin, streptomycin, and dihydrostreptomycin. They were administered in aqueous solutions, subcutaneously in the guinea pigs and cats, and intramuscularly in the monkeys. In the case of streptomycin and dihydrostreptomycin, the daily doses, on a body weight basis, were similar to those that had previously been used in the treatment of human tuberculosis. For the other aminoglycosides, the doses were several times greater than those recommended for clinical use.

Guinea pigs were killed by decapitation, the temporal bones were removed, and the inner ear tissues were fixed by perilymphatic perfusion with 1 percent OsO_4 solution. The monkeys were anesthetized with ketamine, and the inner ear was fixed in situ after the middle ear had been opened through the mastoid antrum. Microdissection of the temporal bones was carried out in 70 percent alcohol, as described by Hawkins and Johnsson [12]. The entire length of the basilar membrane and the organ of Corti was removed in segments and mounted in glycerol for light microscopy, as were the spiral ligament and stria vascularis. In all cases, complete hair cell counts were made and cytocochleograms were plotted.

Examination and photomicrography were carried out with the Wild-Heerbrugg M-5 Stereomicroscope and the Wild-Heerbrugg M-20 Research Microscope. The vestibular organs were either embedded in araldite and examined as "thick" sections (approximately 1 μm) by light microscopy, or prepared for scanning electron microscopy and photographed with a JEOL JSM-U3 scanning electron microscope.

Results

The appearance of the basal turn of the left cochlea of a behaviorally trained monkey treated with neomycin, 50 mg/kg per day IM for 8 days, is seen in Fig. 12-1A. For this ear, the audiogram showed a partial loss of hearing above 2 kHz and a complete loss above 15 kHz. Throughout the first quadrant of the basal turn, as seen in Fig. 12-1A, the organ of Corti had disappeared except for a few small islands of supporting cells that had survived. In the second quadrant, the typical pattern of light and dark longitudinal bands, representing the organ of Corti, is still present. Above this point, except for a very small area of

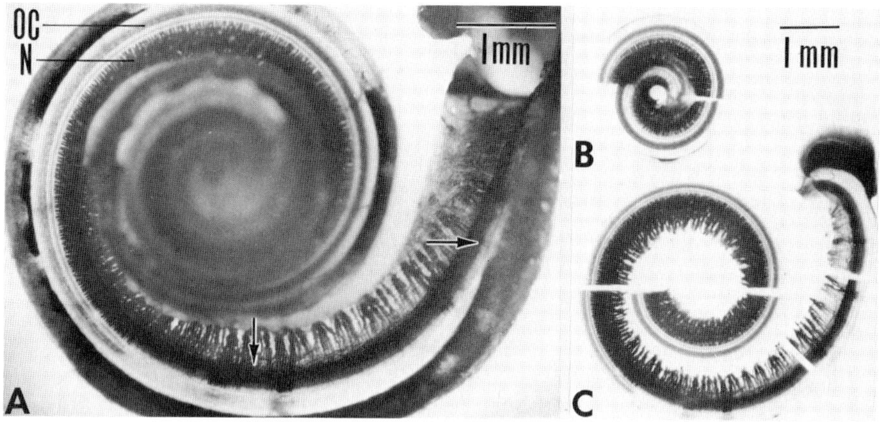

Figure 12-1. Left cochlea of monkey M-18, treated with neomycin, 50 mg/kg per day IM for 8 days. A. Basal turn exposed. Organ of Corti is absent in first quadrant, except for small islands of supporting cells (vertical arrow). (OC = organ of Corti, with pattern of light and dark longitudinal bands; N = myelinated cochlear nerve fibers in osseous spiral lamina.) Note degeneration of nerve fibers (horizontal arrow) wherever OC is missing. At right, entire length of osseous spiral lamina and basilar membrane has been dissected from the cochlea. B. Apical turn and upper portion of middle turn. C. Basal turn and lower portion of middle turn. Nerve degeneration of apex in B. OsO_4.

degeneration less than 1 mm, the pattern of nerve fibers in the osseous spiral lamina is complete, extending peripherally to the habenula perforata, where it appears to have a serrated border. Wherever the organ of Corti is absent, the nerve fibers have begun to degenerate, and the serrated border is no longer seen. Only where the small islands of supporting cells are still present do the fibers reach the habenula. Figure 12-1B shows that the innervation at the apex has also become sparse because of degeneration secondary to hair cell loss in this region.

For reasons still not adequately understood, the hair cells at the extreme basal end of Corti's organ are most often affected by the ototoxic action of the aminoglycosides, and the initial injury is usually concentrated there. Scattered loss of individual hair cells, however, may be found elsewhere. The specimen illustrated in Fig. 12-2 was taken from the lower basal turn of another monkey (M-16), which was described by Stebbins et al. [24]. The animal had been treated with neomycin, 100 mg/kg per day IM for 5 days, and had a hearing loss at frequencies above 15 kHz. Complete loss of outer (OHC) and inner (IHC) hair cells was seen in the first 2 to 3 mm of Corti's organ, but the great majority of the hair cells were present above 5 mm. In this photomicrograph from the 15- to 16-mm region, one OHC is missing from the first row and two are missing from the third row. Such scattered losses are not uncommon in untreated control animals, at least among guinea pigs and cats. In this case, the phalangeal "scars" do not look new; they may, in fact, antedate the aminoglycoside treatment. The row of IHC is intact.

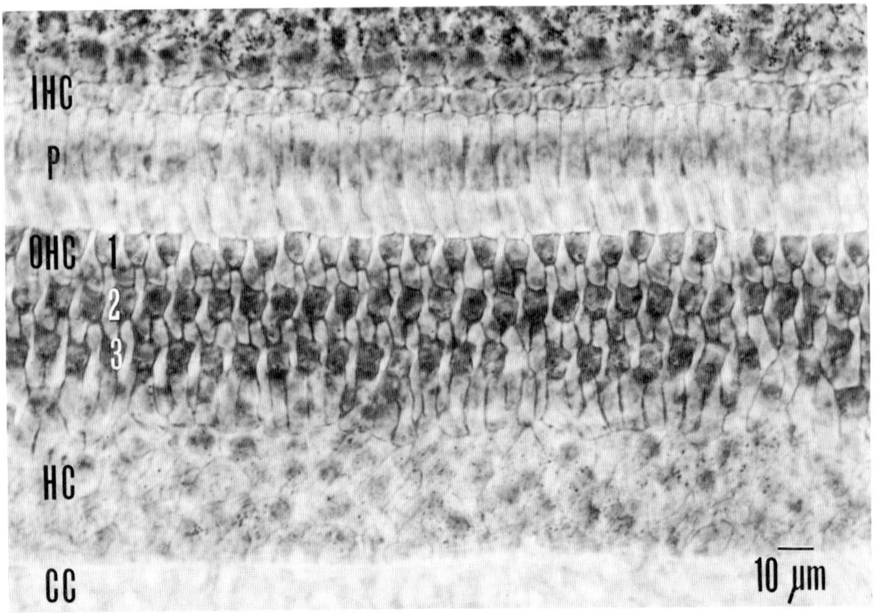

Figure 12-2. Loss of three outer hair cells in lower basal turn of monkey M-16, treated with neomycin, 100 mg/kg per day IM for 5 days. (IHC = inner hair cells; P = pillar cells; OHC = outer hair cells; HC = Hensen cells; CC = Claudius cells.) OsO_4, phase contrast.

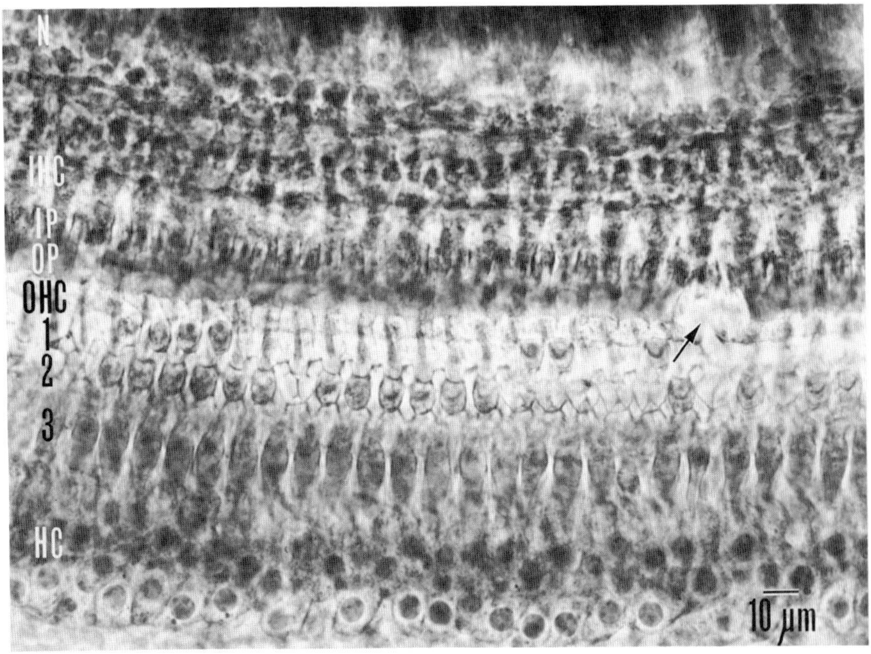

Figure 12-3. Loss of outer hair cells from second turn in guinea pig treated with kanamycin, 200 mg/kg per day SC for 14 days, and killed 1 week later. Phalangeal "scars" in OHC rows 1 and 2. Two outer pillar cells are missing (arrow). (N = nerve fibers near habenula perforata; IHC = inner hair cells; IP = inner pillars; OP = outer pillars; OHC = outer hair cells; HC = Hensen cells.)

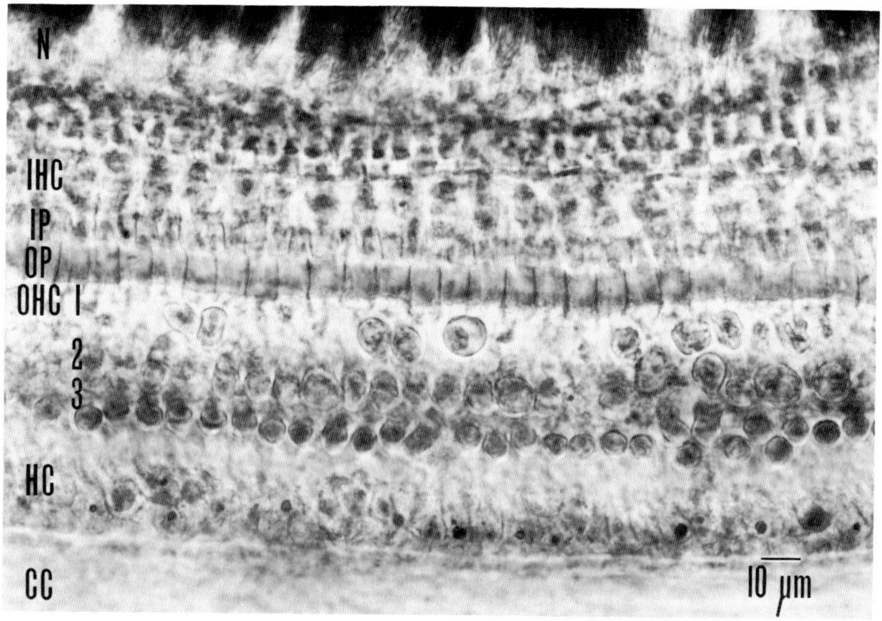

Figure 12-4. Loss of outer hair cells from second turn in guinea pig treated with gentamicin, 135 mg/kg per day SC for 10 days, killed 1 day later. Remaining OHC bodies are swollen and distorted. Focus below reticular lamina. (N = nerve fibers near habenula perforata; IHC = inner hair cells; IP = inner pillars; OP = outer pillars; OHC = outer hair cells; HC = Hensen cells; CC = Claudius cells.)

The type of hair cell loss often regarded as characteristic of the guinea pig cochlea after kanamycin treatment is illustrated in Fig. 12-3, which shows a portion of the second turn. The animal had received 200 mg/kg per day for 14 days and had been kept for 1 week after the period of treatment. Loss of OHC from the first row is greater than that from the second. Typical phalangeal scars of recent origin are seen in both rows. Those of the first row are formed by expansion of the phalangeal processes of the head plates of the outer pillars, those of the other rows by the phalangeal plates of the Deiters cells. The inverted Y (row 2) clearly marking the junctions of these elements indicates that they have been formed recently. Two outer pillar cells have also disappeared. The third-row OHC and the IHC are all present.

A similar distribution of hair cell loss is seen in Fig. 12-4, taken from the second turn of a guinea pig cochlea that had received gentamicin, 135 mg/kg per day for 10 days, and had been kept for 24 hours after treatment. In this case, the plane of focus is below the reticular lamina. Cell bodies of the remaining OHC of rows 1 and 2 are swollen and distorted, but those of row 3 and of the IHC are little affected.

Complete loss of OHC from the second turn of a sisomicin-treated guinea pig is shown in Fig. 12-5. The animal had received sisomicin, 135 mg/kg per

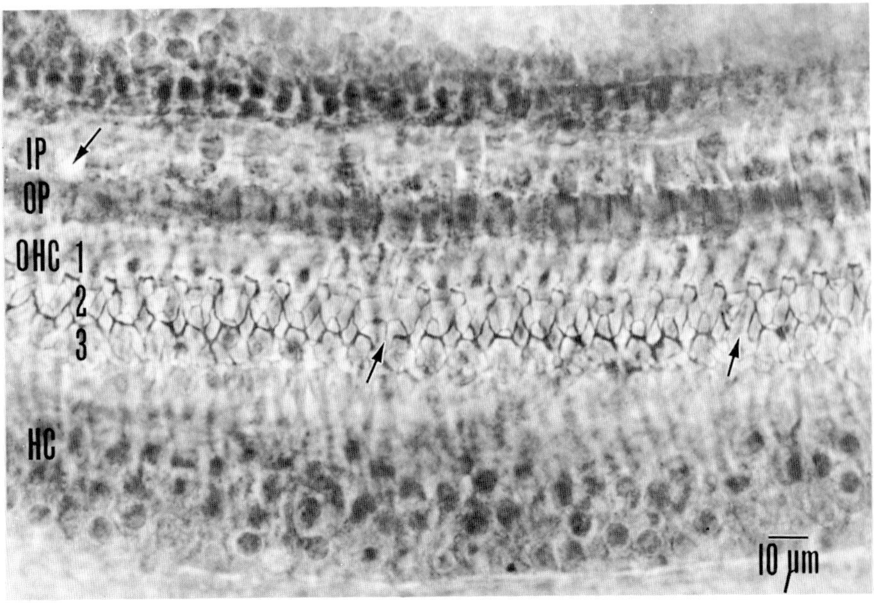

Figure 12-5. Loss of outer and inner hair cells from second turn in guinea pig treated with sisomicin, 135 mg/kg per day SC for 14 days, killed 1 day later. Irregular scarring is indicated by lower arrows. One inner pillar is missing (upper arrow). (IP = inner pillars; OP = outer pillars; OHC = outer hair cells; HC = Hensen cells.)

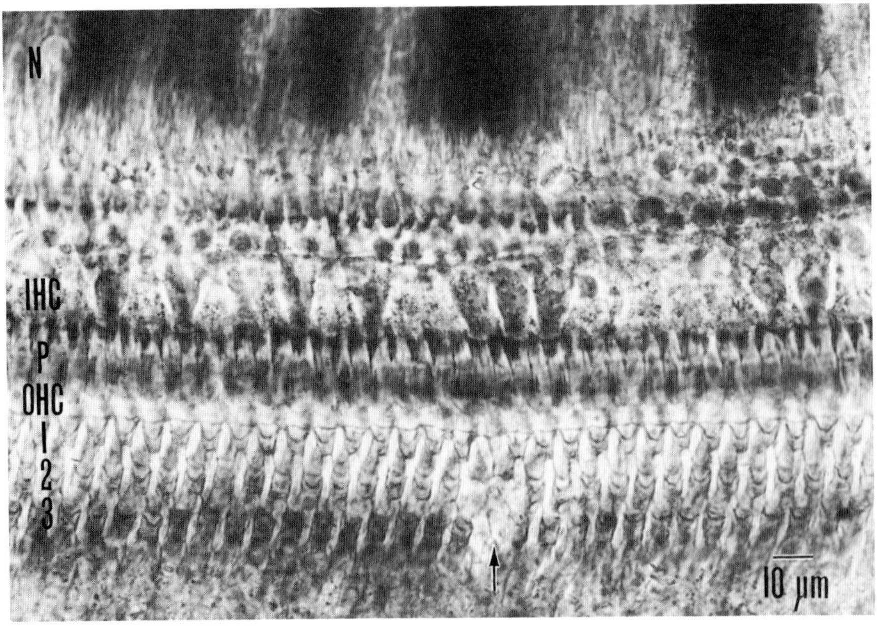

Figure 12-6. Loss of inner hair cells from second turn in cat treated with gentamicin, 80 mg/kg per day SC for 20 days. A few outer hair cells are missing (arrow). Note correspondence between loss of IHC and degeneration of nerve fibers. (N = nerve fibers near habenula perforata; IHC = inner hair cells; P = pillar cells; OHC = outer hair cells.)

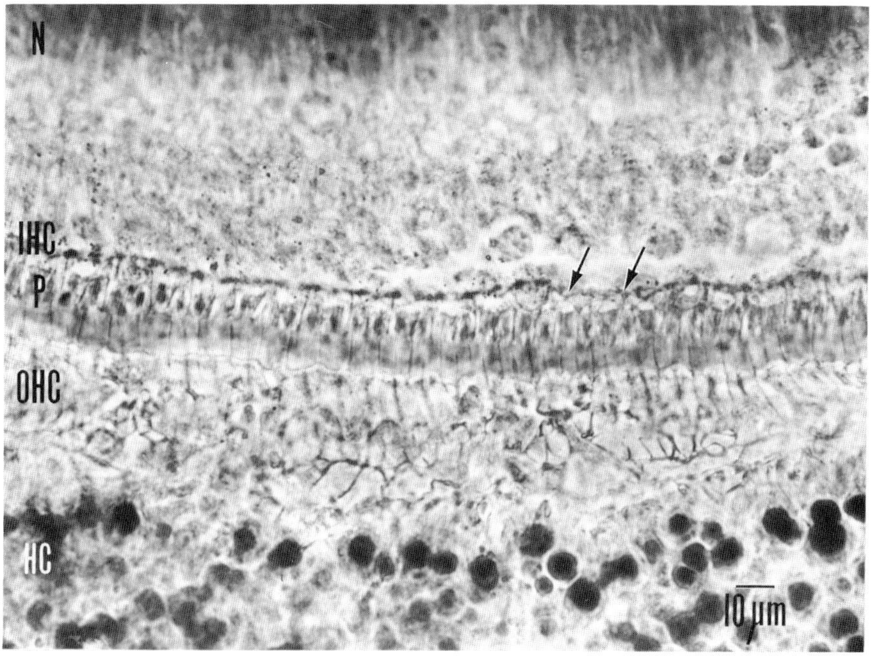

Figure 12-7. Loss of most inner as well as outer hair cells from third turn in guinea pig treated with kanamycin, 400 mg/kg per day SC for 14 days, and killed 1 week later. Note the scars of IHC (arrows) and irregular scarring of OHC. (N = nerve fibers near habenula perforata; IHC = inner hair cells; P = pillar cells; OHC = outer hair cells; HC = Hensen cells.)

day for 14 days, and was killed 24 hours after the last dose. Below the middle of the second turn, both OHC and IHC were completely absent. The phalangeal scars seen in the photomicrograph in row 2 are of recent origin, and not all are completely formed or as clearly defined as they would have been a few days later. The rest of the IHC bodies and nuclei are seen above the rows of head plates of pillar cells, from which one inner pillar is missing.

Selective loss of IHC from the second cochlear turn of a gentamicin-treated cat is shown in Fig. 12-6. The antibiotic had been given in a dose of 80 mg/kg per day for 20 days. Except in a single area of scarring involving no more than six cells, the OHC are all present in the region shown. Loss of OHC was seen in the basal turn, and there was complete loss of Corti's organ from the extreme basal end of the basilar membrane, the so-called hook. This specimen shows another feature not usually seen in the guinea pig, monkey, or man. The myelinated nerve fibers of the osseous spiral lamina have degenerated wherever the IHC have disappeared, but they are clearly still present where the IHC remain.

Extensive loss of IHC from the third turn in a kanamycin-treated guinea pig, together with the irregular healing of the reticular lamina after destruction of

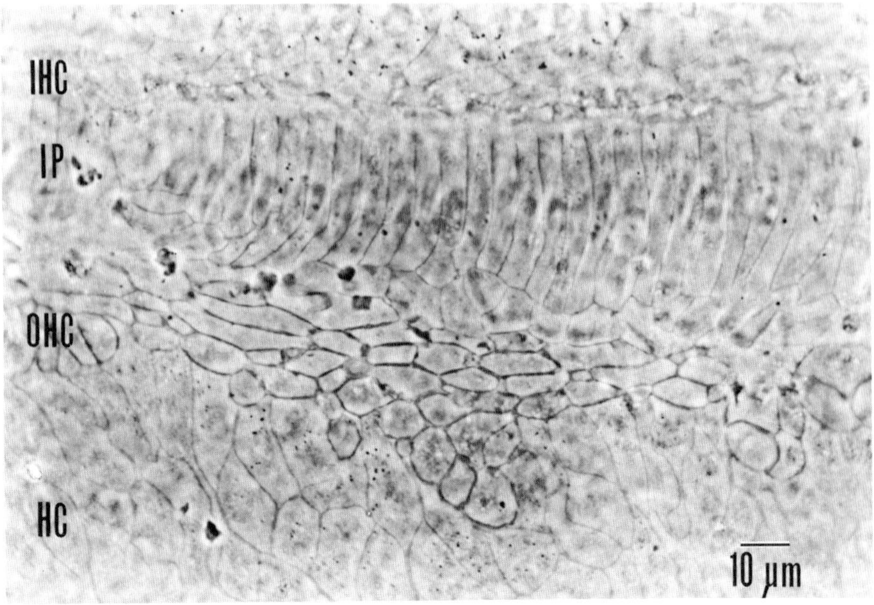

Figure 12-8. Irregular healing of reticular lamina in monkey M-21 treated with neomycin, 50 mg/kg per day IM for 15 days, and killed 4 months later. (IHC = inner hair cells; IP = inner pillars; OHC = outer hair cells; HC = Hensen cells.)

OHC, is shown in Fig. 12-7. This animal had received kanamycin, 400 mg/kg per day SC for 14 days, and was kept for 1 week after treatment. Typical IHC scars are seen, but two or three of the cuticular plates have not been replaced by scars. The disordered state of the reticular lamina over the OHC is evidence of the severity of the ototoxic process. Even though the majority of the IHC were still present elsewhere in this cochlea, except at the apex and the extreme base, the presence of IHC could hardly have been expected to give a valid or reliable picture of IHC potentials in the absence of the OHC.

Disordered scarring of the reticular lamina, including the head plates of the pillar cells, is typical of neomycin ototoxicity. Figure 12-8 shows a portion of the upper middle turn from a monkey (M-21) that had received neomycin, 50 mg/kg per day IM for 15 days. The audiogram at 15 weeks showed hearing only at 0.5 to 2.0 kHz, with threshold shifts of 80 to 90 dB. In the photomicrograph, neither OHC nor IHC is present, and the regular mosaic pattern of the reticular lamina is completely lost.

In severe ototoxicity, localized "lesions" of the organ of Corti may occur in which all of the sensory and supporting elements have disappeared. This condition is illustrated in Fig. 12-9, taken from the lower middle cochlear turn of a patas monkey that had received dihydrostreptomycin, 100 mg/kg per day IM for 75 days, and was killed 3 months later. The patas is the only animal species we have found thus far that exhibits the well-known human cochlear ototoxic-

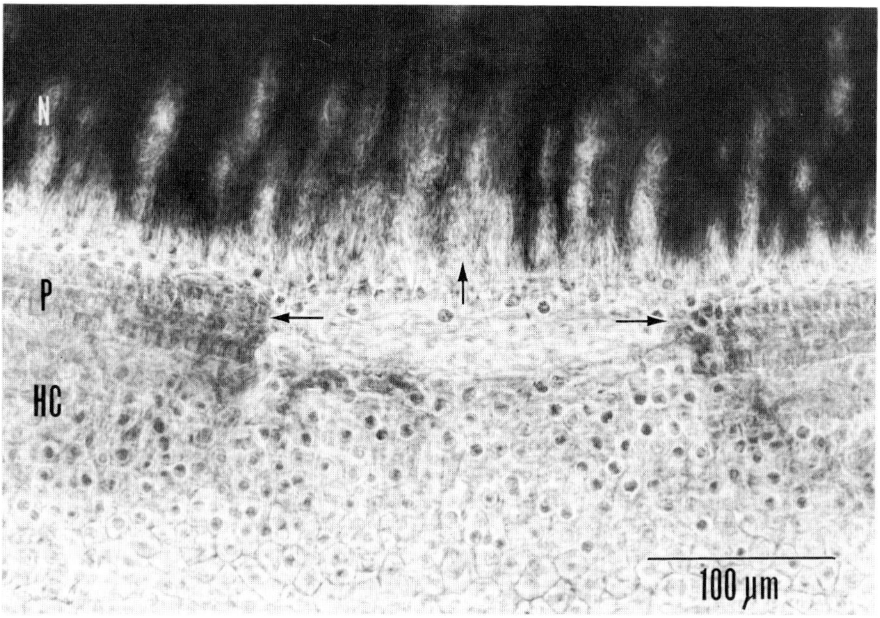

Figure 12-9. Organ of Corti "lesion" in the lower middle turn, left ear, of patas monkey M-62 treated with dihydrostreptomycin, 100 mg/kg per day IM for 75 days, and killed 3 months later. Note interruption of pillar cell rows and complete absence of organ of Corti between horizontal arrows. Incipient nerve fiber degeneration (vertical arrow). (N = nerve fibers near habenula perforata; P = pillar cells; HC = Hensen cells.)

ity of this aminoglycoside. Hearing had been lost at all frequencies except those below 0.5 kHz, and only a few OHC remained in the apical turn. In the region of the lesion, where all supporting cells have disappeared, an incipient degeneration of the myelinated nerve fibers can be discerned.

After treatment with dihydrostreptomycin, the lower basal turn of the cochlea often shows long portions with complete absence of Corti's organ. Figure 12-10 illustrates this condition in a specimen taken from the cochlear "hook" of another patas monkey treated with dihydrostreptomycin. The drug had been given in a dose of 20 mg/kg per day for 90 days, and the monkey was killed 4 months after the last dose. The basilar membrane is covered by a layer of large, flat, polygonal epithelial cells replacing the organ of Corti, with only occasional rests of supporting cells remaining. The peripheral ends of the cochlear neurons in the osseous spiral lamina have begun to degenerate, so that they are no longer visible at the habenula perforata near the inner margin of the basilar membrane.

Cytocochleograms

The extent and severity of ototoxic injury to the cochlea can best be expressed in the form of a cytocochleogram, based on a complete count of the hair cells

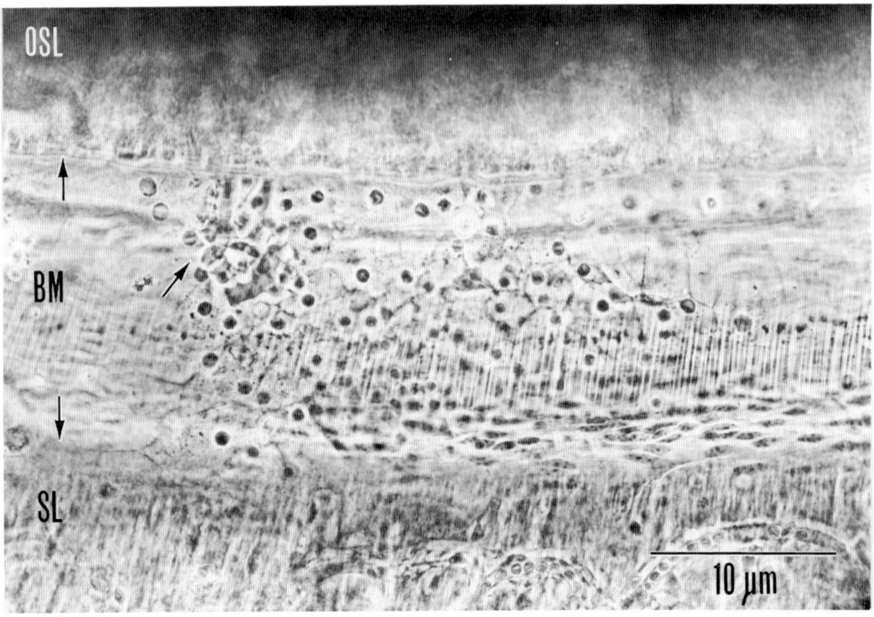

Figure 12-10. Destruction and disappearance of organ of Corti in lower basal turn ("hook") of patas monkey M-92 treated with dihydrostreptomycin, 20 mg/kg per day IM for 90 days. An "island" of degenerated supporting cells is still present (oblique arrow). (OSL = osseous spiral lamina, with nerve fibers degenerated; BM = basilar membrane [between vertical arrows]; SL = spiral ligament.)

present and missing in each row of IHC and OHC, over the whole length of Corti's organ. The percentage of hair cells remaining in each row is plotted millimeter by millimeter. Examples illustrating the effects of large subcutaneous doses of amikacin, netilmicin, and sisomicin in guinea pigs are shown in Figs. 12-11 through 12-14.

The typical early effect of an aminoglycoside on the outer hair cells of the lower basal end of the organ of Corti is demonstrated in the cochlea of an amikacin-treated guinea pig in Fig. 12-11. Only slight losses of inner hair cells were observed in that region and near the apex. That this restricted loss, seen only 24 hours after 2 weeks of treatment, would probably have proved to be progressive is seen in Fig. 12-12, representing the cochlea of another animal that received almost the same treatment, but was kept for 2 weeks before being killed. Here there is extensive loss of OHC, greatest in row 1 and least in row 3, but only a slightly increased loss of IHC near the apex.

Figure 12-13 shows an essentially normal population of IHC and OHC in a guinea pig that had received netilmicin, 150 mg/kg per day for 15 days, and had been kept for 4.5 months after receiving medication. Small numbers of sensory cells missing from the upper turns can often be recorded in normal control animals and may not represent the result of ototoxic injury.

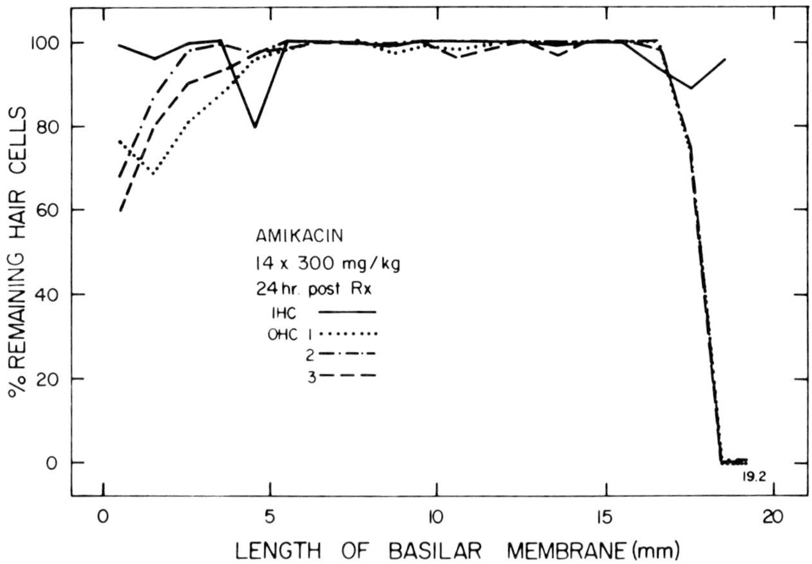

12-11

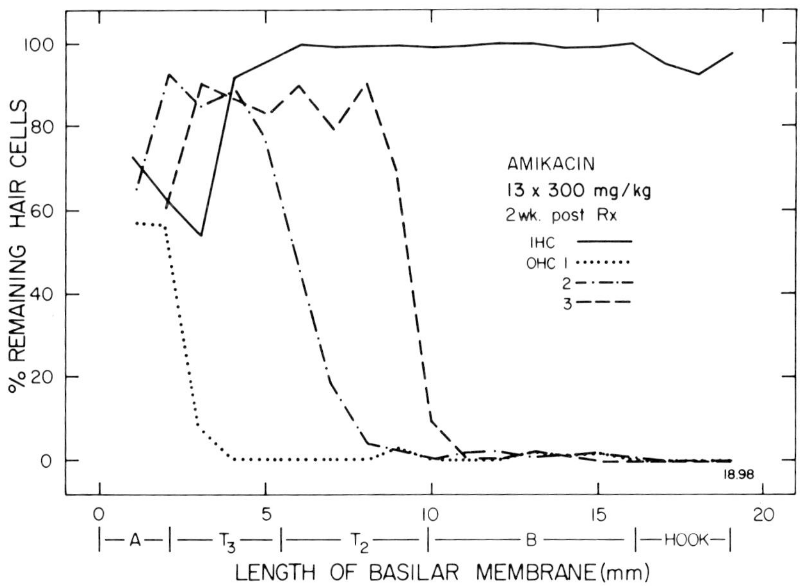

12-12

Figures 12-11 through 12-14. Cytocochleograms, showing various degrees of hair cell loss after treatment with different aminoglycosides.

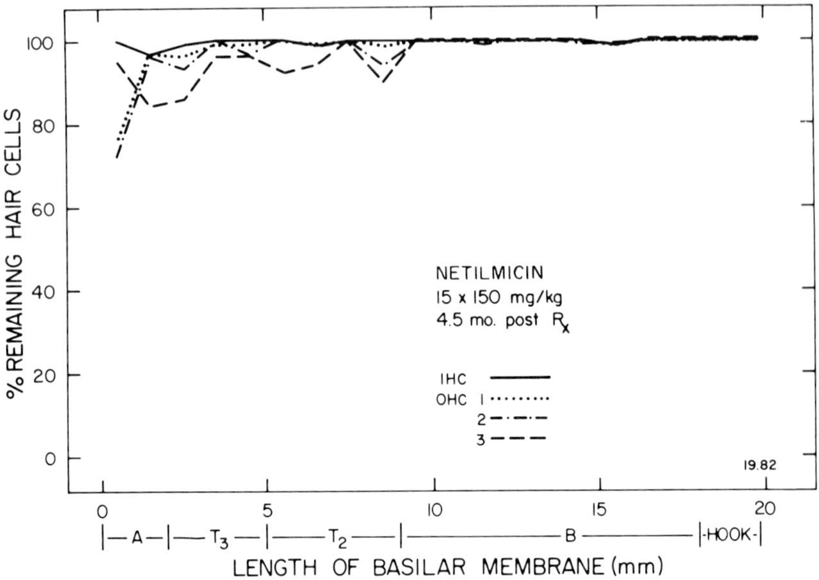
100
80
60
40
20
0
% REMAINING HAIR CELLS
NETILMICIN
15 x 150 mg/kg
4.5 mo. post Rx
IHC
OHC 1
2
3
19.82
0
5
10
15
20
|—A—|—T3—|——T2——|————B————|-HOOK-|
LENGTH OF BASILAR MEMBRANE (mm)

12-13

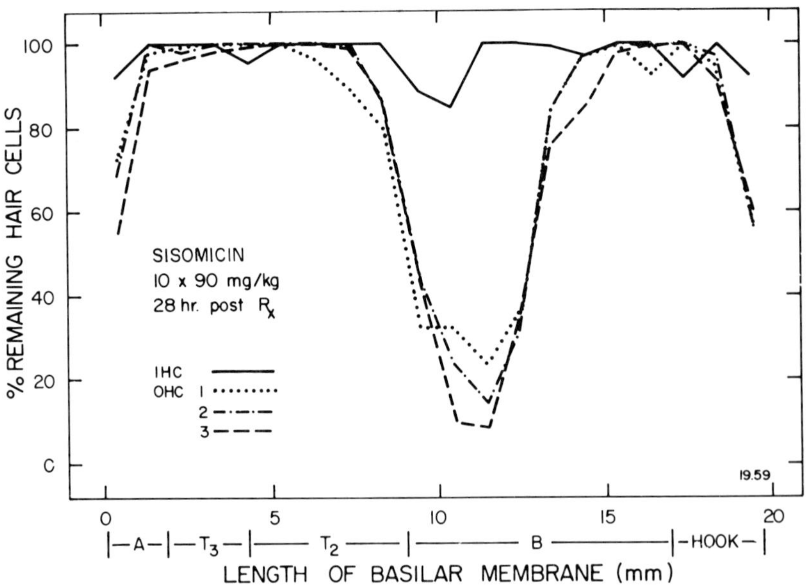
100
80
60
40
20
0
% REMAINING HAIR CELLS
SISOMICIN
10 x 90 mg/kg
28 hr. post Rx
IHC
OHC 1
2
3
19.59
0
5
10
15
20
|—A—|—T3—|—— T2 ——|———— B ————|—HOOK—|
LENGTH OF BASILAR MEMBRANE (mm)

12-14

Although it is usually stated that the hair cells at the extreme basal end of the organ of Corti are the first to be affected by an aminoglycoside, the ototoxic process gradually advancing from the base toward the apex, a selective loss, especially of outer hair cells in the upper basal and lower second turns, is sometimes found in guinea pigs. Injury of this type is seen in animals killed shortly after treatment with appropriately large doses of sisomicin, as illustrated in Fig. 12-14. Variants of this pattern have been found also after gentamicin treatment. This is a sufficiently frequent occurrence to indicate that an orderly progression of ototoxic damage from base to apex is not invariably the rule.

Effects on Other Cochlear Tissues

SPIRAL LIGAMENT

In the guinea pig, the changes observed in the spiral ligament after aminoglycoside treatment are generally limited to the suprastrial region, i.e., the thin portion of the ligament above the stria vascularis and the insertion of Reissner's membrane. These changes affect the superficial cells of the ligament and its suprastrial capillaries. The superficial cells often appear shrunken and sometimes disappear, leaving openings that seem to communicate with the perivascular spaces of the underlying capillaries.

The fact that some of these suprastrial capillaries are themselves injured suggests that there is an angiotoxic component in aminoglycoside ototoxicity. An affected capillary may collapse upon itself and appear as an intravascular strand linking two normal-appearing vessels, or it may disappear entirely, leaving an avascular channel (AVC). The latter is formed simply by the remaining perivascular space (PVS), which presumably continues to be filled with plasma. It forms a communication between the perivascular spaces of two or more other capillaries (Fig. 12-15). The AVCs, which have been described elsewhere [14], are also found in the spiral ligament and in certain other inner ear tissues of normal guinea pigs, presumably as a result of the same process of gradual devascularization that occurs in the human labyrinth with maturity and aging [18]. They appear to be more numerous after injury by ototoxic drugs or by noise, and they are associated with presbycusis in the human ear. Since the walls of these channels are the same as those of perivascular spaces, and since all endothelial elements have disappeared from them, the term *vessels lacking blood corpuscles* [1] is incorrect and misleading.

STRIA VASCULARIS

In the stria vascularis, both the marginal cells and the strial capillaries may be affected. Small vacuoles may appear in limited areas, or there may be patches of strial atrophy. The strial capillaries, normally larger in diameter than those of the spiral ligament, may be constricted, and the marginal cells become pale, having lost their osmiophilic character. These changes are illustrated in Fig. 12-16, which shows the stria from the basal turn of a guinea pig treated with

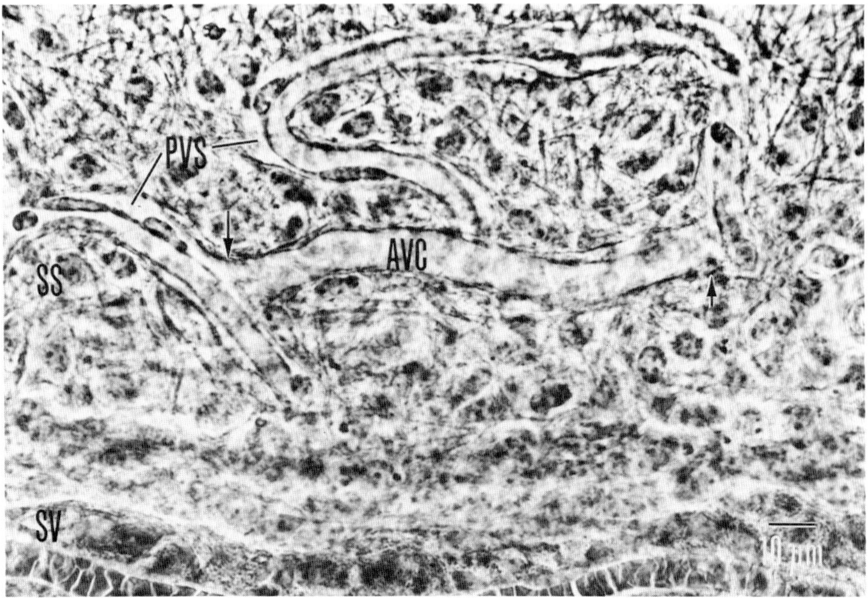

Figure 12-15. An avascular channel (AVC) in the suprastrial (SS) portion of the spiral ligament, third turn, from a guinea pig treated with sisomicin, 135 mg/kg per day SC for 10 days. The ends of the AVC (arrows) communicate with the perivascular spaces (PVS) of capillaries. (SV = upper margin of stria vascularis.)

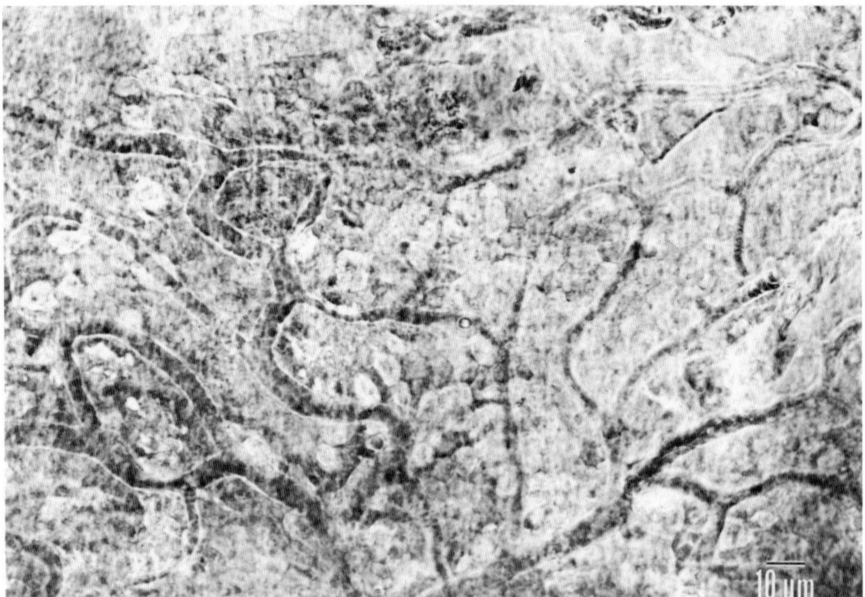

Figure 12-16. Stria vascularis from basal cochlear turn of a guinea pig treated with gentamicin, 100 mg/kg per day SC. Strial capillaries are irregularly constricted. Note vacuole formation and loss of osmiophilia in marginal cells.

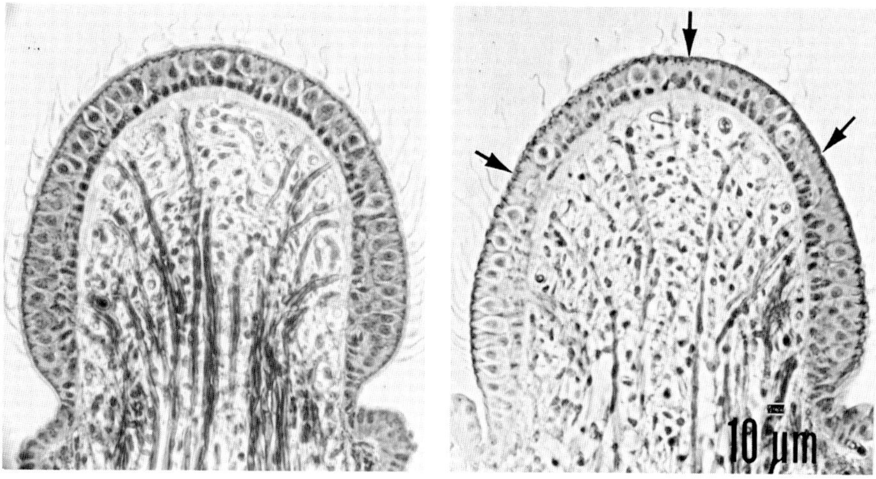

A B

Figure 12-17. Cross sections of ampullar cristae from two squirrel monkeys treated with gentamicin, 40 mg/kg per day IM. A. Four days: neuroepithelium is essentially normal. B. Four weeks: loss of hair cells from top and upper slopes of crista (arrows).

gentamicin, 100 mg/kg per day SC for 3 weeks. In monkeys kept for 1 to 2 years after treatment with neomycin, the stria may become completely atrophic, its capillaries reduced to a few degenerated strands.

Vestibulotoxic Effects

Although the vestibular end organs can be dissected out and mounted as surface preparations [12, 20], they are not particularly well suited to this form of analysis because of their thickness and the opacity of the underlying layer of nerve fibers when these are stained with OsO_4. The ampullar cristae can best be embedded in epon or another suitable medium and examined by light microscopy as "thick" sections. Figure 12-17 shows cross sections of the horizontal ampullae from two squirrel monkeys treated with gentamicin, 40 mg/kg per day, one for only 4 days and the other for 4 weeks. In the 4-day specimen, a full complement of hair cells can be seen with their ciliary bundles, but the 4-week specimen shows a loss of 50 percent of the sensory cells and cilia, mainly from the top of the crista and the upper slopes. On the lower slopes, the hair cells are still present on both sides.

The most instructive surface views of the effects of aminoglycosides on the cristae and the otolith organs can be obtained by scanning electron microscopy. Figure 12-18 shows the horizontal crista from a patas monkey treated with dihydrostreptomycin. Extensive loss of ciliary bundles has occurred, so that much of the surface of the crista appears bare. The surface of the superior crista (Fig. 12-19) shows many scars where hair cells have disappeared, but other cells are still present, with bundles of cilia, some of which are fused.

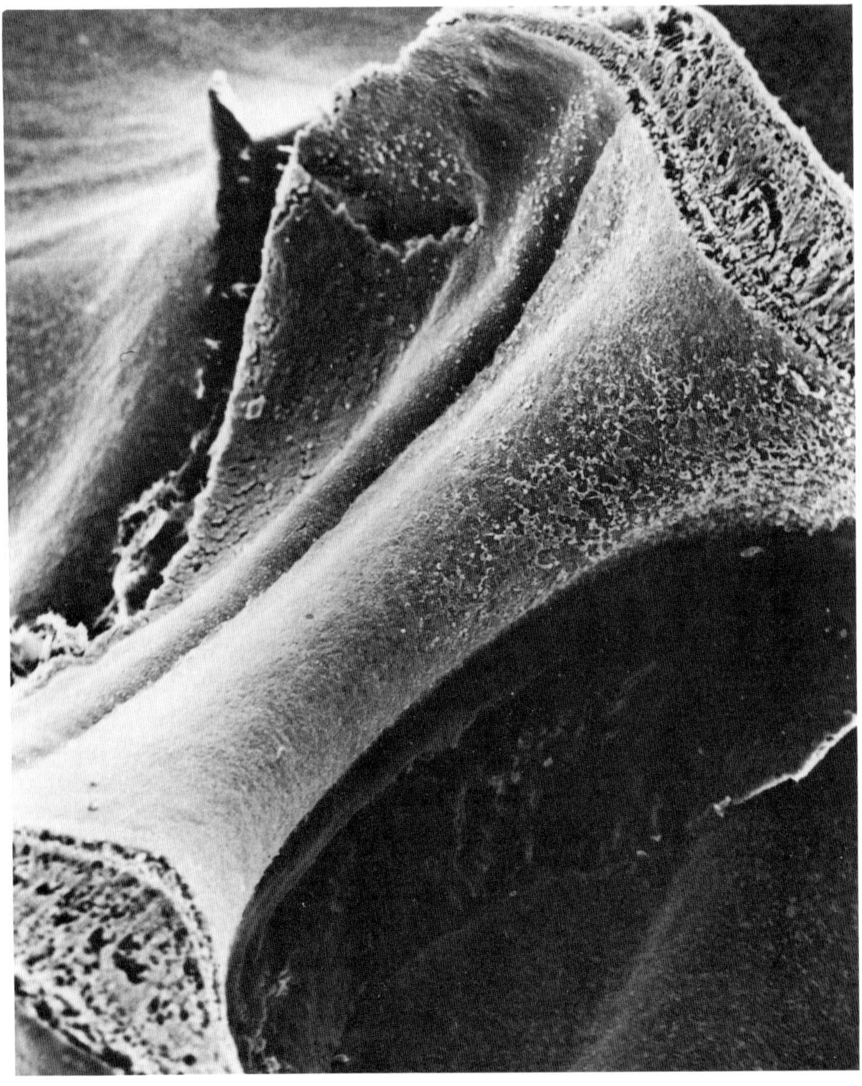

Figure 12-18. Left horizontal crista ampullaris of patas monkey M-44. Dihydrostreptomycin, 100 mg/kg per day IM for 24 days. Few, if any, bundles of cilia remain. Scanning electron microscopy.

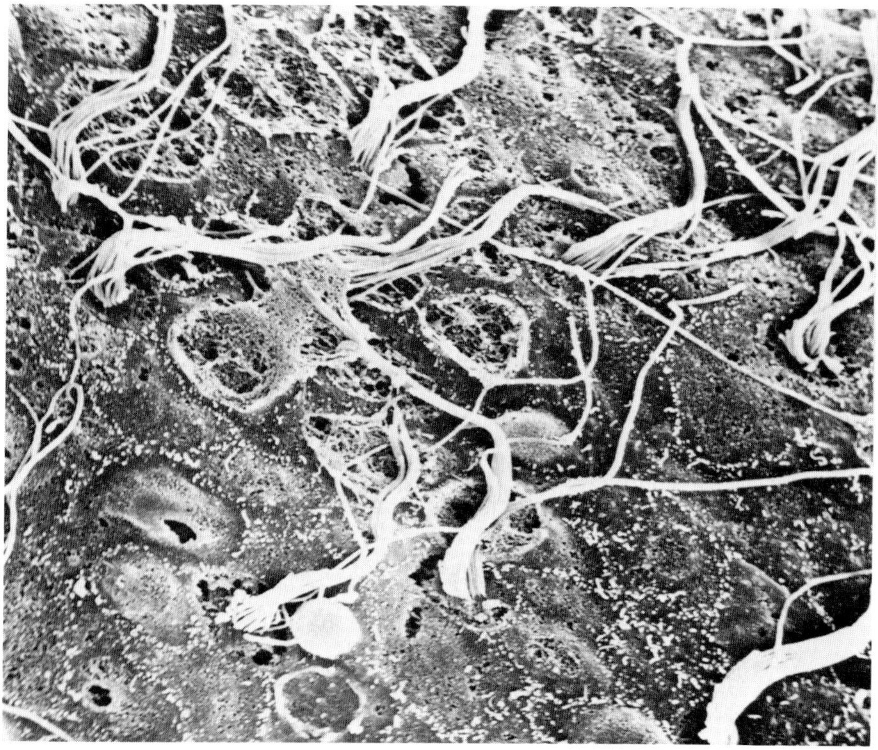

Figure 12-19. Surface of right superior crista of patas monkey M-44, showing scars where hair cells have disappeared, and a few bundles of cilia on the remaining hair cells.

An unusual instance of vestibulotoxic injury by neomycin is illustrated in Fig. 12-20. The monkey (*Macaca nemestrina*) had received 40 doses of neomycin, 25 mg/kg per day IM, a treatment which completely destroyed all hair cells of the organ of Corti and caused widespread degeneration of the cochlear nerve fibers except in the apical turn. The saccule showed loss of cilia, especially along the striola line (S), where the type I sensory cells are normally found [20]. On either side of this crescent-shaped clearing, residual hair bundles indicate that many type II cells had survived.

In addition to the hair cells of the ampullar crista, the dark cells at its base and the cells of the planum semilunatum can be affected by the aminoglycosides. Changes of this kind are not readily seen in surface preparations, but are best demonstrated by transmission electron microscopy [23]. They are particularly striking in the pigeon [16].

Comments

The changes in inner ear tissues illustrated in this chapter occurred in response to aminoglycosides given parenterally in multiple doses, which reached the

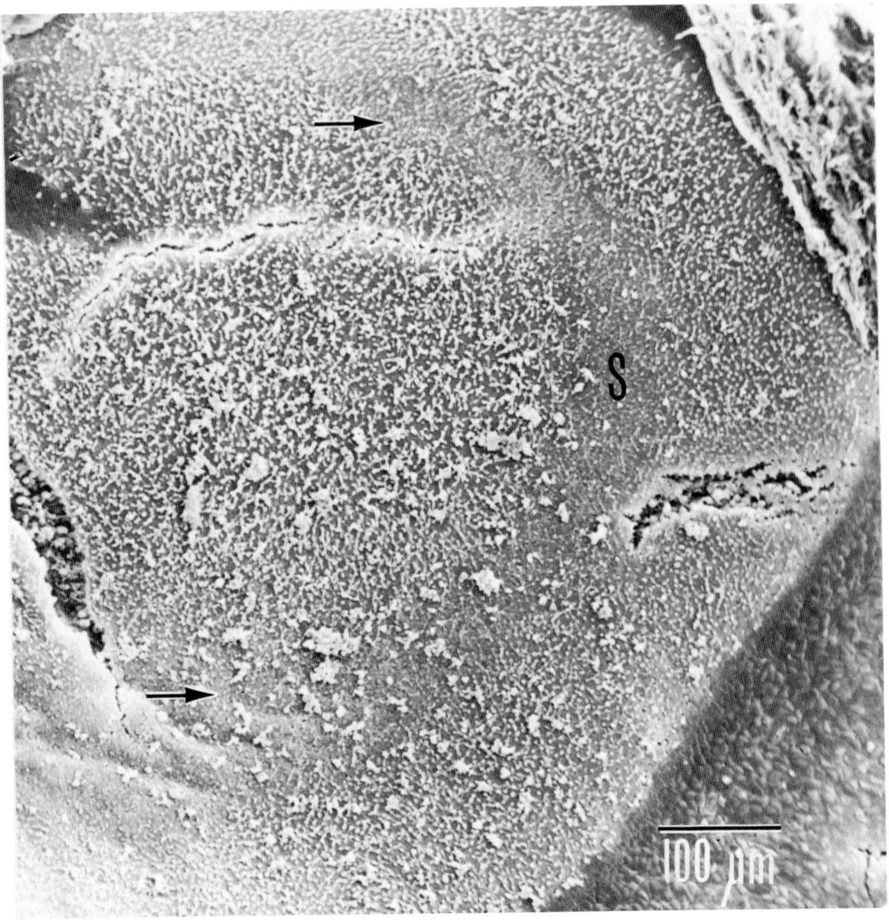

Figure 12-20. Neomycin injury to the saccular macula in a pigtail monkey treated with neomycin, 25 mg/kg per day IM for 40 days. Degeneration of type I cells along the curved striola line S, between the two arrows.

inner ear by way of the bloodstream. When a much smaller single dose is injected into the middle ear cavity, destruction of cochlear and vestibular tissues is more rapid and more nearly complete [25], presumably because of a higher concentration of the drug in the inner ear fluids.

Differences between species in their response to the ototoxic action of the various aminoglycosides are still unexplained, but they may depend more on differences in access to the inner ear fluids, i.e., on the blood-perilymph barrier, than on differences in renal clearance. The peculiar susceptibility of *E. patas* to dihydrostreptomycin [17] extends also to streptomycin, but not to kanamycin. Like dihydrostreptomycin, streptomycin produces hearing loss in patas monkeys when given in doses of 20 mg/kg per day, which had been shown to have little ototoxic effect when used in the treatment of tuberculosis in man for periods of up to 4 months.

Aminoglycosides, and particularly kanamycin, are frequently used to produce experimental cochlear lesions for behavioral and electrophysiological analysis of cochlear function. The tendency of kanamycin to destroy the outer while sparing the inner hair cells makes it particularly appealing for this purpose. It should be clear, however, from examples given above, especially in Figs. 12-3 and 12-7 and in Figs. 12-11 and 12-12, that the dose level and duration of treatment, as well as the length of time the animal is kept alive after treatment, must be chosen with care if the results are to be valid and reliable. For retaining the inner hair cells while destroying the outer, kanamycin, 200 mg/kg per day for 2 weeks, with a recovery or stabilization period of at least 2 weeks after treatment, appears to be optimal. Doses of 300 or 400 mg/kg per day are not recommended because of the greater likelihood of injury to the stereocilia and the intracellular organelles of the inner hair cells [10]. In any event, the extent of hair cell loss cannot be inferred from the dose level and the duration of treatment, but should be determined by complete hair cell counts and cytocochleograms. The inner hair cells should be examined by electron microscopy before they can be regarded as normal.

Although it is easy to generalize about ototoxic phenomena, the temptation should be resisted, since species differences in response to aminoglycosides can set traps for the unwary experimenter and even for the clinician. For example, although kanamycin can differentiate between the inner and outer hair cells in the guinea pig, and dihydrostreptomycin in the patas monkey, in macaques both types of hair cells are affected almost equally by kanamycin [24], whereas neither type of cell responds to a significant extent to dihydrostreptomycin. Dihydrostreptomycin has produced hearing loss in man [22], although it has little or no cochlear toxicity in laboratory animals other than the patas monkey. Streptomycin, which is most often vestibulotoxic in man, shows a strong cochlear toxicity in the patas.

These differences serve to emphasize the importance of choosing more than one type of laboratory animal for evaluating the ototoxicity of new aminoglycosides. Experience suggests that macaque monkeys as well as guinea pigs should be used in such tests. The value of the patas monkey as an experimental model is still not established, but it appears that its special sensitivity may be limited to the streptomycins. For vestibular testing the cat is useful, but the pigeon, which has not been considered here, and the squirrel monkey may offer significant advantages. In both of them, vestibular dysfunction is almost immediately apparent, since it affects the ability of the one to fly and of the other to climb. Histopathologic changes in their vestibular organs are readily visualized by light and electron microscopy. Whatever the experimenter's choice of animal subjects for such tests, the need persists for caution in attempts to predict the ototoxic potential of new aminoglycosides in clinical use.

References

1. Axelsson, A., and Vertes, D. Vascular histology of the guinea pig cochlea. *Acta Otolaryngol.* 85:198, 1978.
2. Berg, K. The toxic effect of streptomycin on the eighth cranial nerve. *Ann. Otol. Rhinol. Laryngol.* 58:448, 1949.
3. Caussé, R. Action toxique vestibulaire et cochléaire de la streptomycine au point de vue expérimental. *Ann. Otolaryngol.* 66:518, 1949.
4. Darrouzet, J., and De Lima Sobrinho, E. Oreille interne, kanamycine et traumatisme acoustique: Etude expérimentale. *Rev. Laryngol. Otol. Rhinol. (Bord.)* 83:781, 1962.
5. Engström, H., Ades, H. W., and Andersson, A. *Structural Pattern of the Organ of Corti.* Stockholm: Almquist and Wiksell, 1966.
6. Engström, H., Ades, H. W., and Hawkins, J. E., Jr. Structure and function of the sensory hairs of the inner ear. *J. Acoust. Soc. Am.* 34:1356, 1962.
7. Engström, H., Ades, H. W., and Hawkins, J. E., Jr. Cytoarchitecture of the organ of Corti. *Acta Otolaryngol. (Stockh.)* [*Suppl.* 188]:92, 1964.
8. Guild, S. R. A graphic reconstruction method for the study of the organ of Corti. *Anat. Rec.* 22:141, 1921.
9. Hawkins, J. E., Jr. Cytoarchitectural basis of the cochlear transducer. *Cold Spring Harbor Symp. Quant. Biol.* 30:147, 1965.
10. Hawkins, J. E., Jr. Condition of the Inner Hair Cells after Aminoglycoside Intoxication. In M. Portmann and J. M. Aran (Eds.), *Inner Ear Biology.* Paris: Colloques INSERM 68, 1977. Pp. 327–334.
11. Hawkins, J. E., Jr., and Engström, H. Effect of kanamycin on cochlear cytoarchitecture. *Acta Otolaryngol. (Stockh.)* [*Suppl.* 188]:100, 1964.
12. Hawkins, J. E., Jr., and Johnsson, L-G. Microdissection and Surface Preparations of the Inner Ear. In C. A. Smith and J. A. Vernon (Eds.), *Handbook of Auditory and Vestibular Research Methods.* Springfield, Ill.: Thomas, 1975. Pp. 5–52.
13. Hawkins, J. E., Jr., Johnsson, L-G., and Aran, J-M. Comparative tests of gentamicin ototoxicity. *J. Infect. Dis.* 119:417, 1969.
14. Hawkins, J. E., Jr., Johnsson, L-G., and Preston, R. E. Cochlear microvasculature in normal and damaged ears. *Laryngoscope* 82:1091, 1972.
15. Hawkins, J. E., Jr., and Lurie, M. H. The ototoxicity of streptomycin. *Ann. Otol. Rhinol. Laryngol.* 61:789, 1952.
16. Hawkins, J. E., Jr., and Preston, R. E. Vestibular Ototoxicity. In R. F. Naunton (Ed.), *The Vestibular System.* New York: Academic, 1975. Pp. 321–349.
17. Hawkins, J. E., Jr., Stebbins, W. C., Johnsson, L-G., Moody, D. B., and Muraski, A. The patas monkey as a model for dihydrostreptomycin ototoxicity. *Acta Otolaryngol.* 83:123, 1977.
18. Johnsson, L-G., and Hawkins, J. E., Jr. Vascular changes in the human inner ear associated with aging. *Ann. Otol. Rhinol. Laryngol.* 81:364, 1972.
19. Kohonen, A. Effect of some ototoxic drugs upon the pattern and innervation of cochlear sensory cells in the guinea pig. *Acta Otolaryngol. (Stockh.)* [*Suppl.* 208], 1965.
20. Lindeman, H. H. Regional differences in sensitivity of the vestibular sensory epithelia to ototoxic antibiotics. *Acta Otolaryngol.* 67:177, 1969.
21. Rüedi, L. Some animal experimental findings on the functions of the inner ear. *Ann. Otol. Rhinol. Laryngol.* 60:993, 1951.
22. Schuknecht, H. F. *Pathology of the Ear.* Cambridge, Mass.: Harvard University Press, 1974.
23. Sparwald, E., Lange, G., and Leupe, M. Veränderungen an den dunklen Zellen der Crista ampullaris nach Streptomycin-Medikation beim Meerschweinchen. *Arch. klin. exp. Ohr.-, Nas.- u. Kehlk.-Heilk.* 199:587, 1971.
24. Stebbins, W. C., Miller, J. M., Johnsson, L-G., and Hawkins, J. E., Jr. Ototoxic hearing loss and cochlear pathology in the monkey. *Ann. Otol. Rhinol. Laryngol.* 78:598, 1969.

25. Wersäll, J., Björkroth, B., Flock,A., and Lundquist, P-G. Experiments on ototoxic effects of antibiotics. *Adv. Oto-Rhino-Laryngol.* 20:14, 1973.
26. Ylikoski, J., Wersäll, J., and Björkroth, B. Hearing loss and cochlear pathology in gentamicin intoxicated guinea pigs. *Acta Pathol. Microbiol. Scand.* [*B*] 241:30, 1973.

13. Structural Damage to the Organ of Corti and the Vestibular Epithelia Caused by Aminoglycoside Antibiotics in the Guinea Pig

Jan Wersäll

Structural damage to inner ear sensory cells, caused by the first aminoglycoside, streptomycin, was demonstrated with light microscopy in cats and guinea pigs [1, 2, 5, 6, 12, 13]. In these early studies, streptomycin was shown to have an unusual selectivity for destruction of cochlear and vestibular hair cells, whereas supporting cells stayed intact for a considerable length of time. With the aid of a combination of electrophysiologic and morphologic methods, it was demonstrated that the primary site of damage is the peripheral sensory organ. Most of the nerve fibers and ganglion cells outside the sensory epithelia remained morphologically and physiologically intact for a period of time, but subsequently many underwent secondary retrograde degeneration [10, 23]. The use of semiquantitative [3, 11] or quantitative techniques [26] for the determination of hair cell degeneration has facilitated studies of localization and progression of cochlear hair cell damage after antibiotic intoxication. In the vestibular system, also, quantitative techniques have facilitated the analysis of the localization and progression of hair cell damage [17]. The introduction of transmission electron microscopy [7, 23] and scanning electron microscopy [21] for analysis of fine structural damage of the inner ear after antibiotic intoxication has provided abundant data on the detailed histopathology of inner ear ototoxicity.

Structural Damage to the Organ of Corti

Pattern of Degeneration

The pattern of degeneration of sensory cells in the organ of Corti (Figs. 13-1 through 13-4) is similar, but not identical, for the various aminoglycoside

This project is supported by Swedish Medical Research Council Project No. 12-720. Much of the background material for the chapter was produced in cooperation with Miss B. Björkroth and Dr. J. Ylikoski. The photographs by B. Hedberg are much appreciated.

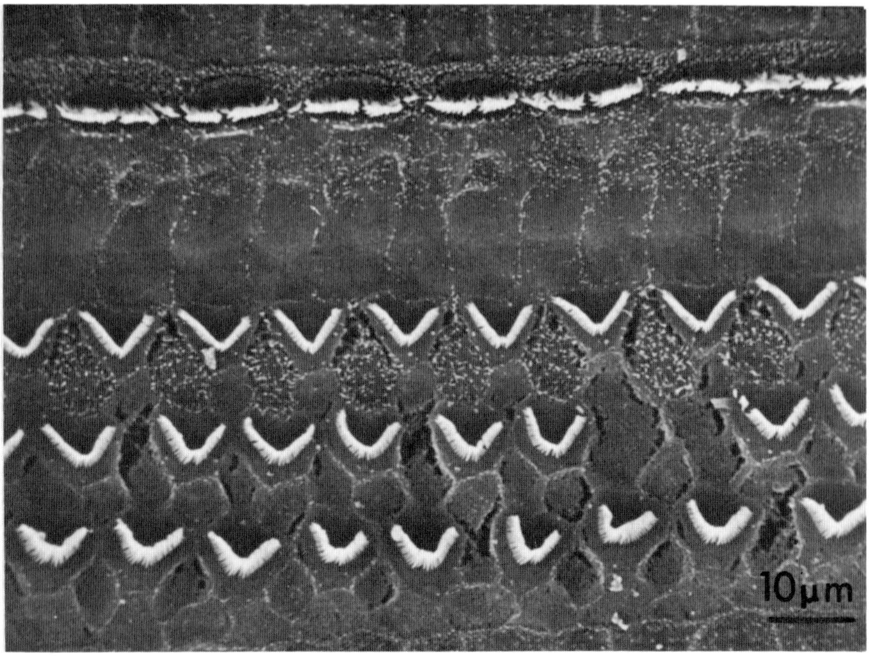

Figure 13-1. Early degeneration of the organ of Corti after amikacin treatment. Degeneration of one cell in the second row of outer hair cells is apparent. Guinea pig cochlea. Amikacin, 100 mg/kg per day (in two divided doses) subcutaneously for 18 days. The animal was killed 30 days after the last dose.

antibiotics. The outer hair cells are generally more sensitive to damage than the inner hair cells, and the first row of outer hair cells closest to the tunnel of Corti is generally more severely damaged than the third row [9, 11, 16, 26]. Most animals show more advanced degeneration in the basal coil of the cochlea, with progressive involvement of hair cells along the basilar membrane toward the apex when the dosage level and duration of treatment are increased [9, 11, 16, 25, 26]. Long-term treatment with low doses leads to scattered degeneration over large areas in the cochlea, whereas short-term treatment with high doses tends to cause damage that is confined to the basal part of the cochlea. An exception to this may be neomycin, which might produce more severe early damage in the apical part of the cochlea. There is, however,

Figure 13-2. Advanced damage to the hair cells of all rows after gentamicin treatment. Guinea pig cochlea, second coil. Gentamicin, 50 mg/kg for 30 days. The animal was killed 30 days after the last dose.

Figure 13-3. Interference contrast survey picture of the organ of Corti, second coil, with moderate hair cell damage. Kanamycin, 400 mg/kg for 6 days. The animal was killed 15 days after the last dose.

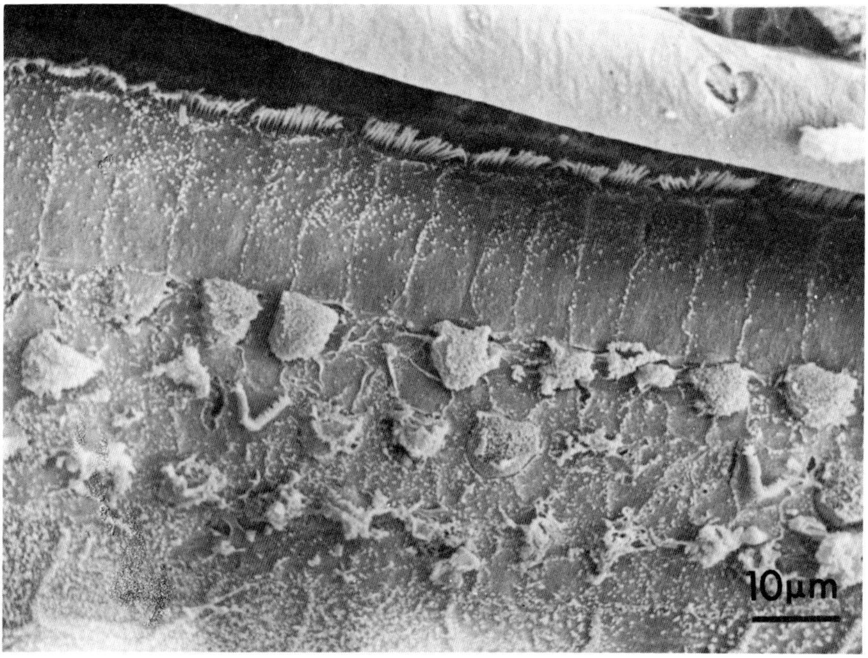

13-2

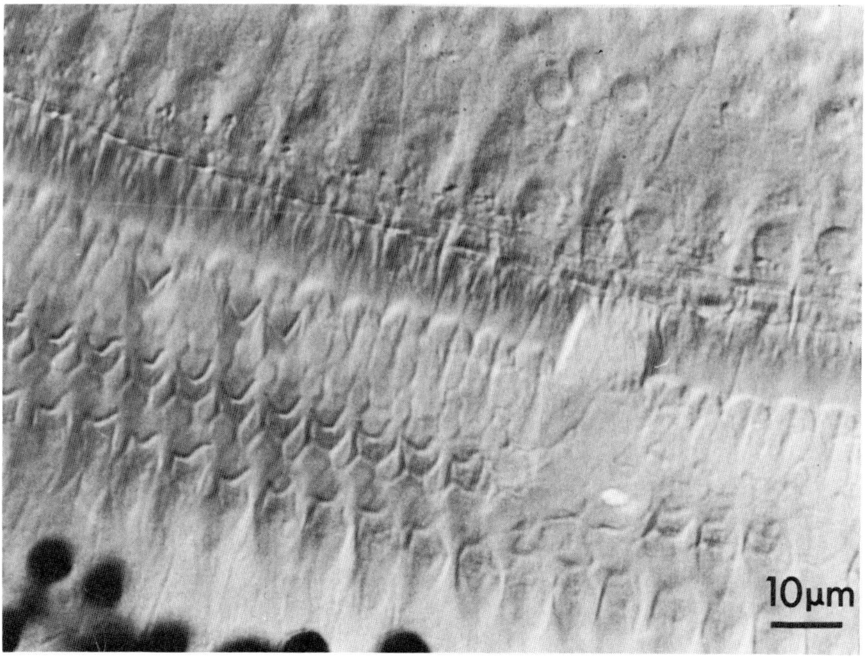

13-3

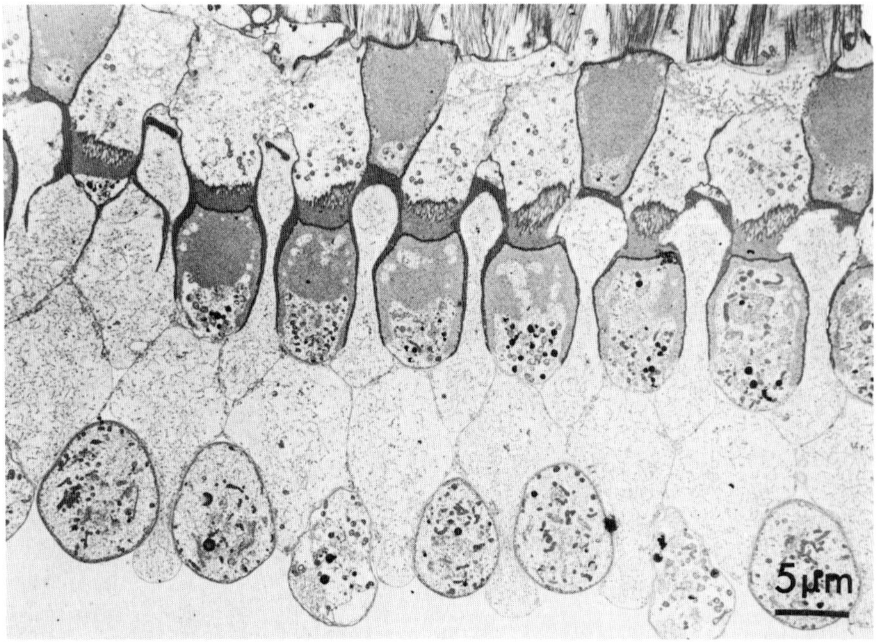

Figure 13-4. Transmission electron micrograph of the same section coil, sectioned parallel to basilar membrane. Deiters cells fill in the spaces between missing hair cells.

considerable variation in the progression of damage and in the percentage of damaged hair cells in the various coils at the same dose schedule [25]. In 5 percent of a series of animals treated with gentamicin, tobramycin, and amikacin, the maximal damage occurred in the upper coil of the cochlea [8].

The sensory cells in the cochlea are generally much more sensitive to damage than are the supporting cells. In general, the cells tend to degenerate in this order: first, second, and third rows of outer hair cells, pillar cells, Deiters cells, and Hensen cells.

Fine Structural Damage of Cochlear Hair Cells

The normal cochlear outer hair cells have a characteristic architecture. The cells are cylindrical, with the nucleus located in the lower third of the cell. The surface facing the endolymph is flat and is supported by a cuticle composed of dense granular substance located immediately below the surface of the plasma membrane. Sensory hairs protruding from the surface are arranged in regular rows forming a V or W. The lateral plasma membranes of the cells are lined down to the nuclear level by concentric layers of fenestrated membranes forming a structure of varying thickness. In osmium-fixed specimens, the plasma membrane itself appears considerably thinner and more irregularly folded than the plasma membrane of the neighboring supporting cells. The mitochondria are found primarily in three regions: immediately below the cuticle, along the fenestrated membranes of the side of the cell, and in the infranuclear region. Fenestrated membranes sometimes form concentrically arranged lamellar structures, the so-called Hensen bodies, between the nucleus and the cuticular region. A number of nerve fibers terminate on the rounded base of the cell. Lysosomes are found below the cuticle among the mitochondria in this region.

The structural changes in the outer sensory cells have a similar appearance, no matter which aminoglycoside is used to produce ototoxicity. The degree of damage depends, however, not only on the dose schedule and total dose, but also on the antibiotic used. The most pronounced changes are found after neomycin treatment, whereas the smallest changes are found after netilmicin treatment.

A typical sign of early damage is an accumulation of dense bodies in the subcuticular region and along the sides of the hair cells. Some of these bodies appear to be lysosomes; the majority of them, however, have a different ultrastructure. They are surrounded by a single membrane and contain a varying number of lamellae. These dense lamellae can be either irregularly (Figs. 13-5 and 13-6) or concentrically arranged in the body. When the lamellae are concentrically arranged, they have the same interspace as densely packed layers of phospholipid. Some of these structures can be identified as phagolysosomes.

As another early sign of cell damage, the interspaces between the pairs of membranes located on the inside of the hair cells become more irregular. Some of the membranes seem to fuse, forming extremely dense single layers. In other areas, the interspace between the membranes increases and the dense substance between the layers disappears. In some cells, large areas may be occupied by accumulations of lamellated bodies, of varying size and structure, surrounded by concentrically arranged lamellar membranes. This indicates degeneration of the membrane substance of the Hensen body, with formation of new phospholipid membranes.

As the degeneration of the cell progresses, the mitochondria begin to disintegrate. Some of the mitochondria accumulate dark substances and form lamellated bodies like those described above. Other mitochondria swell, with degeneration of the inner membranes and dilation of the intermembrane spaces. The ribosomes decrease in number, and the cells become watery in appearance, with large, clear areas lacking any cellular content. Vacuoles of various sizes are formed within the cells, and finally the plasma membrane disintegrates, leaving debris floating freely in the fluid spaces surrounding the sensory cells. An indication of the very slow turnover of the fluid in these spaces is the fact that cell debris with disintegrated mitochondria and remnants of membranes and granules may still be found floating between sensory cells and supporting cells several weeks after the last injection of the antibiotic.

As the number of sensory hairs on the surface of the hair cell decreases, their stability is lost. In some cases, fusion of sensory hairs occurs, forming irregular protrusions from the cell surface. Very often, the cuticle protrudes

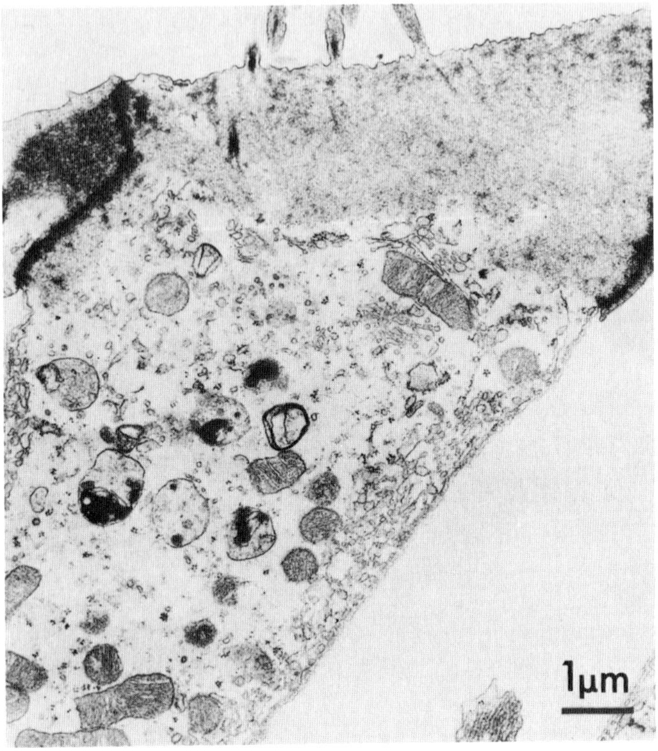

Figure 13-5. Supranuclear part of outer hair cell, demonstrating very slight damage. Netilmicin, 50 mg/kg for 30 days. Irregular bodies with membrane formation can be seen.

over the surface of the supporting cells. As the cuticle disintegrates, the cell debris can move out into the endolymphatic space. Thus, cell debris is often found between remaining sensory hairs in the vicinity of degenerating hair cells.

In sections parallel to the surface of the organ of Corti which are cut at various levels through the hair cells and supporting cells, the progressive changes in the organ of Corti during sensory cell degeneration can be followed. A typical finding is that, during the degenerative phase of one or several outer hair cells, the phalangeal plates of the Deiters cells between them expand. These normally very thin extensions fill in the space formerly occupied by the sensory cells (Fig. 13-4). It is thus unlikely that any defect normally appears in the reticular membrane during the process of sensory cell degeneration. Occasionally, one of the pillar cell heads might degenerate, apparently as a result of the toxic effect of the antibiotic (Fig. 13-3). It has been observed in some specimens that these degenerating pillar cells have left an open space between the membrane of the supporting cells and the remaining pillar cells. Therefore there may be areas where mixing of the endolymph and

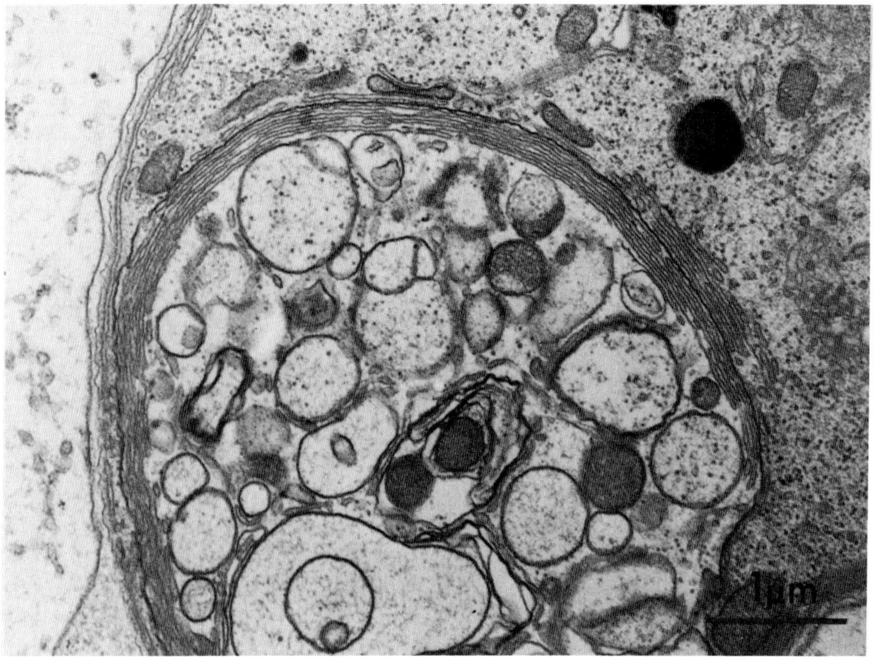

Figure 13-6. Irregular membrane formations in the supranuclear portion of outer hair cell. Third coil of guinea pig cochlea. Gentamicin, 70 mg/kg for 18 days.

fluid of the Nuel space can take place, although it is very difficult to prove that the opening remaining after pillar cell degeneration is not an artifact. In the Hensen cells, Deiters cells, and pillar cell heads, dark bodies and membrane fragments have been found, indicating that these cells have a phagocytic capacity of taking up degenerating fragments of neighboring hair cells. It is very unusual to see any large accumulations of this type of debris in the supporting cells. Therefore, this material is likely to pass rapidly through the supporting cells, into the surrounding endolymphatic space. Such material which has not disintegrated completely in the supporting cells is probably transported by the endolymph to the endolymphatic sac, where it is destroyed by macrophages.

Nuclear swelling can be observed even in the light microscope in otherwise intact sensory cells. This is an indication of nuclear accumulation of fluid and is also apparently an early sign of degeneration of some of the sensory cells. Although this is a common phenomenon in degenerating cells, it does not seem to be a regular occurrence, as the nuclei of some cells with advanced degeneration seem to have a relatively normal appearance.

As the number of degenerating hair cells increases, the major part of the organ of Corti beyond the outer pillar cells is taken up by the Deiters cell bodies (Figs. 13-7 and 13-8). The organ of Corti may remain in this condition for some time, but later on, successive changes in the Deiters cells and a shrinking of the organ of Corti are observed. When the inner hair cells degen-

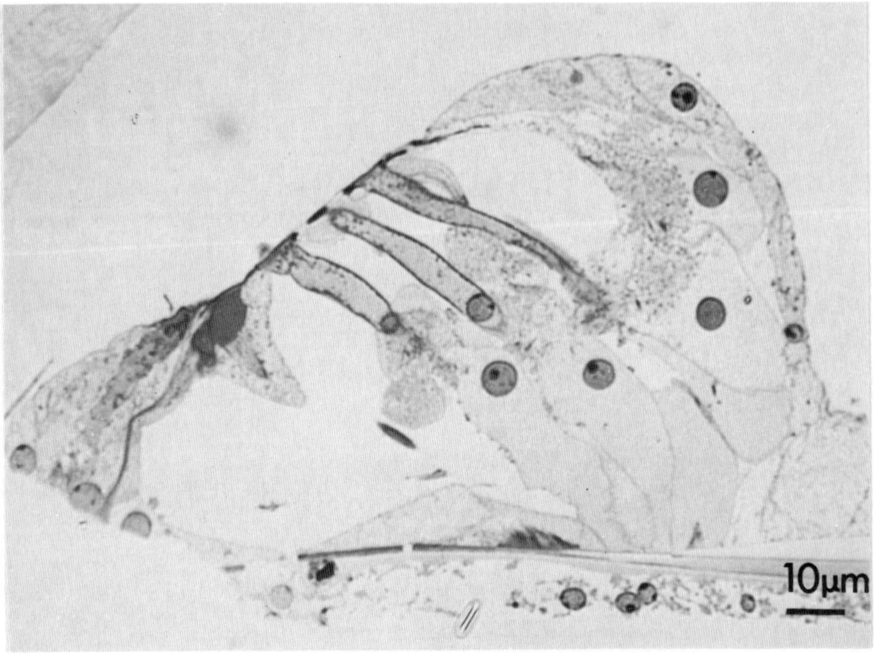

Figure 13-7. Normal sensory cells in upper second coil, guinea pig organ of Corti.

erate, collapse and degeneration of the pillar cells soon follow, and then the Deiters cells and pillar cells degenerate and are absorbed. Finally, the whole organ of Corti disappears, leaving behind a single layer of cells on the basilar membrane.

Degeneration and disintegration of the afferent nerve endings occur very soon after the degeneration of the hair cells. Efferent nerve endings, on the other hand, can be seen between the Deiters cells several weeks after degeneration of the outer hair cells (Figs. 13-9 and 13-10).

The degeneration pattern of the inner hair cells closely resembles that of the outer hair cells, with accumulation of dark membranes, phagolysosomes, vacuolization, nuclear damage, and finally lysis of the plasma membrane and complete cellular disintegration. Sometimes swelling and degeneration of the afferent nerve fibers below the inner hair cells can be seen before the hair cells degenerate. It can be seen in the light microscope that the myelinated nerve

---

Figure 13-8. Severely degenerated organ of Corti from the basal coil of a guinea pig cochlea. All outer hair cells have degenerated. Deiters cells (DC) fill out the area of damaged hair cells. Some inner hair cells (IHC) with nerve endings remain. Kanamycin, 200 mg/kg for 20 days. Survival time, 27 days after end of treatment course.

Figure 13-9. Enlargement of a portion of Fig. 13-8, demonstrating nerve fibers and nerve endings below inner hair cells.

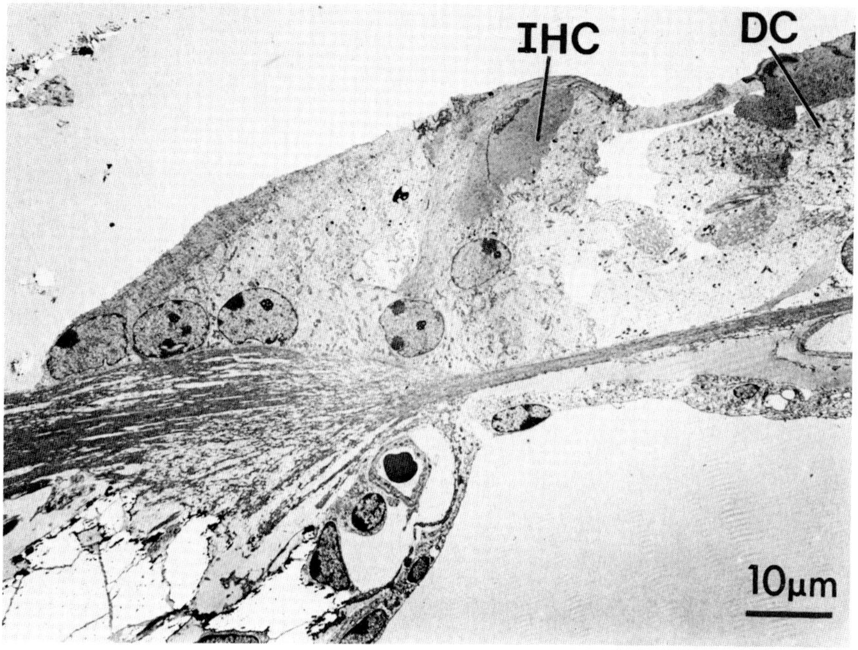

13-8

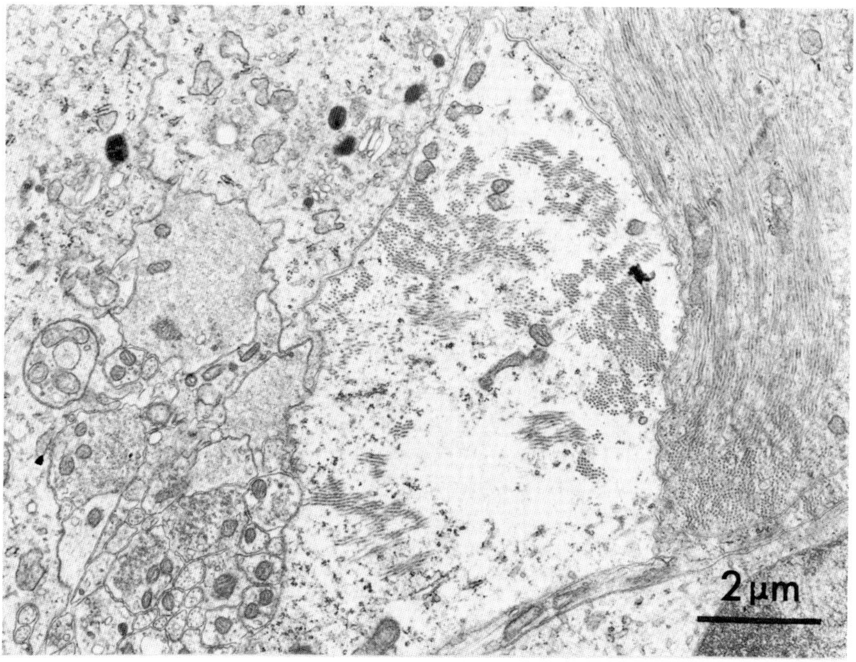

13-9

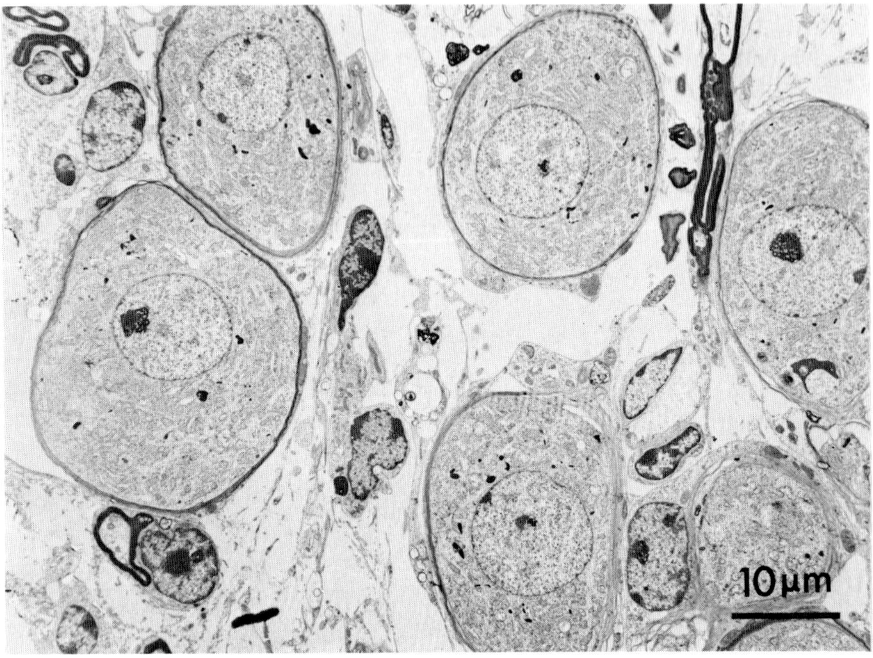

Figure 13-10. More than two-thirds of the ganglion cells remain 2 months after degeneration of most of the outer hair cells and several inner hair cells in the same area (cf. Figs. 13-8, 13-9). Kanamycin, 200 mg/kg for 20 days. Specimen obtained 27 days after last treatment.

fibers to the organ of Corti and their ganglion cells remain intact even several weeks after degeneration of the sensory cells [26], although progressive degeneration eventually occurs. When only the outer hair cells have degenerated, 80 to 90 percent of the nerve fibers and ganglion cells are preserved. In most animals in which all sensory cells were destroyed after antibiotic treatment, the spiral lamina contained less than 20 percent of the normal number of nerve fibers 2 months after the treatment. The number of ganglion cells remaining varied between 10 and 50 percent. Even when the whole organ of Corti was completely destroyed, more than 30 percent of the ganglion cells were still intact in some of the animals. The number of ganglion cells preserved when the whole organ of Corti is destroyed appears to vary widely. The time necessary for degeneration of the majority of nerve fibers and ganglion cells is at least 1 month. In many animals, progressive ganglion cell degeneration apparently takes place for even 2 months or more after damage to the organ of Corti, but none of our animals showed complete loss of all cochlear nerve fibers and ganglion cells.

Structural Damage to Vestibular End Organs

The vestibular sensory epithelia in animals contain two types of sensory cells [20]. A nerve chalice surrounds most of the cell surface of the type I sensory

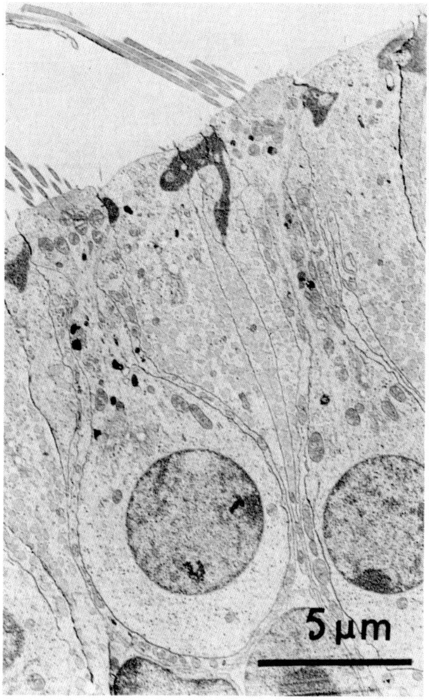

Figure 13-11. Type I sensory cells from normal crista ampullaris, containing a few lysosomes.

cell (Fig. 13-11). This cell is shaped like an amphora, with a rounded base and thin neck widening toward an apical portion that is covered by a cuticle from which a number of sensory hairs protrude. The sensory hairs on the vestibular hair cells (Fig. 13-12) are considerably longer than those on the sensory cells of the organ of Corti. They protrude into a covering layer that forms the cupula over the crista ampullaris and the gelatinous substance supporting the otoconia of the utricular and saccular maculae. The nucleus of the type I sensory cell is found in the lower portion of the cell. The type II sensory cell is cylindrical and is innervated by small nerve endings that touch the bottom of the cell. The location of the nucleus varies somewhat depending on the location of the cell in the sensory epithelium. All sensory cells contain a number of mitochondria, lysosomes, a Golgi apparatus in the supranuclear region, and ribosome-studded membranes of the so-called rough endoplasmic reticulum. In the type I sensory cells, these membranes often form a region below the nucleus with very thin parallel spaces surrounded by membranes which, in turn, are covered by ribosomes. These structural units resemble the Nissl substances in the ganglion cells. Between the sensory cells there are supporting cells of characteristic structure with a basally located nucleus. All supporting cells reach upward from the basement membrane to the cuticular surface. The supporting cells contain comparatively densely packed granules, presumably secretory, in the supranuclear portion of the cell.

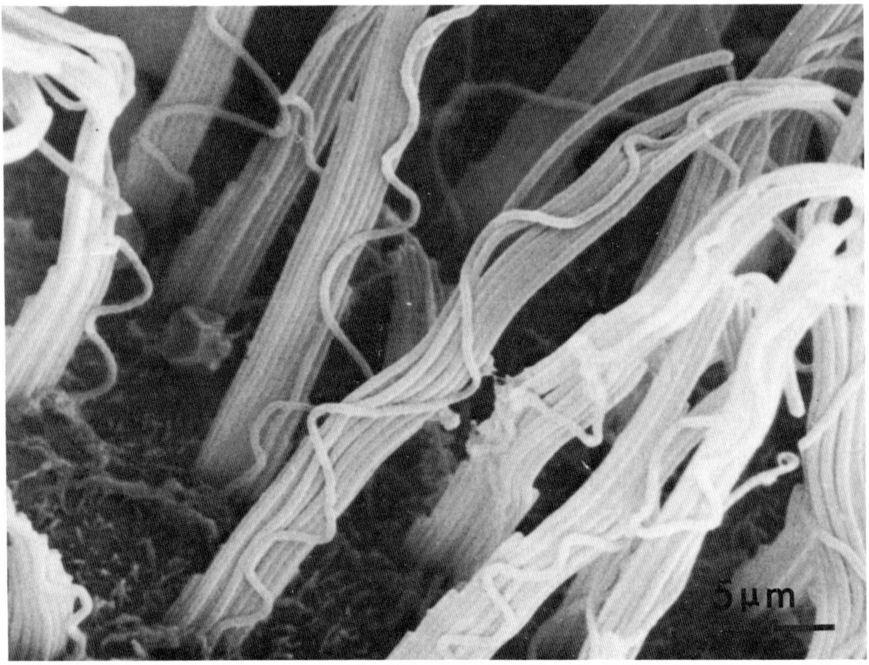

Figure 13-12. Normal sensory hair bundles on the crista ampullaris; guinea pig.

The sensory areas in the vestibular part of the labyrinth are surrounded by the so-called dark cells, specially differentiated cells that presumably take part in the fluid and ion exchange of the endolymph in the vestibular system.

The pattern of degeneration in the vestibular part of the labyrinth seems to vary, depending on the antibiotic used, the dose schedule, the total dose given, and the route of administration. Thus, concentrated solutions of streptomycin or gentamicin (25–50%) applied directly to the round window cause nuclear pyknosis and rapid disintegration of the sensory cells. A different type of damage is found when a drop of a solution containing 3 to 5 mg/ml of streptomycin or gentamicin is applied once a day during 5 to 7 days to the round window of guinea pigs. The pattern of degeneration of the sensory hairs in that case very closely follows that of the structural changes found after parenteral antibiotic treatment with comparatively low doses for 3 to 5 weeks.

Under these conditions, sensory hair fusion might be observed. Bridges are formed between neighboring sensory hairs, and progressive fusion between the sensory hairs takes place. If this fusion becomes complete, the surface plasma membrane forms a large, balloon-shaped protrusion from the sensory cell surface (Fig. 13-13). Within this protrusion the organelles of the sensory cell are found. In some cases, the whole cell may disappear into the endolymph, including the nucleus and cell organelles. In other cases, the major part of the cell remains within the sensory epithelium, where it disintegrates.

Other early signs of degeneration are formation of the same type of dark

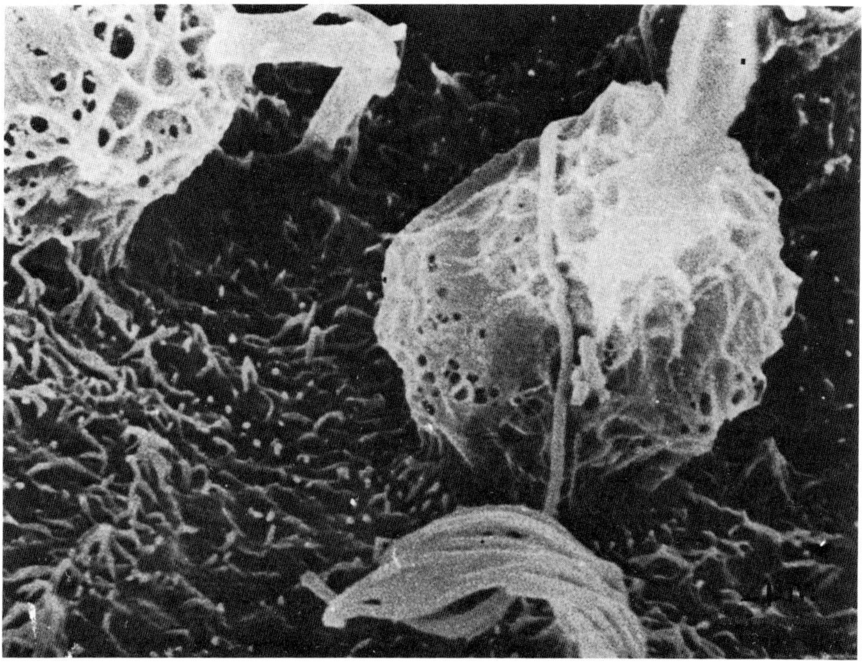

Figure 13-13. Balloon-shaped protrusions formed by sensory hair fusion after gentamicin treatment. Local application in the middle ear for 7 days. Concentration 0.3%; 0.2 ml once a day.

lamellated bodies described in the sensory cells of the organ of Corti. Some of these dark bodies are lysosomes that seem to increase in number (Figs. 13-11 and 13-14). Others are degenerated mitochondria or more or less regularly arranged accumulations of membranes, probably formed by accumulation of phospholipids from degenerated mitochondria and other cell organelles. In some cases the nucleus swells, but in most cells the density of the nucleus increases, and the nuclear pyknosis is followed by nuclear disintegration. During later stages of degeneration, vesicles form within the cytoplasm. The plasma membrane breaks down, and cellular debris is either pushed out into the endolymph between the supporting cells or taken up by the phagocytic activity of the neighboring cells. Type I sensory cells are more sensitive to degeneration than type II sensory cells. The afferent nerve endings degenerate in parallel with the sensory cells, whereas the efferent nerve fibers may remain between the supporting cells in the epithelium for some time, even after most of the sensory cells have disappeared.

The supporting cells remain intact long after the degeneration of most of the sensory cells. When the sensory cells and the nerve endings degenerate, the supporting cells take their place. Considerable flattening of the epithelium sets in; it seems, however, that the supporting cell nuclei stay intact even in very severely damaged epithelia.

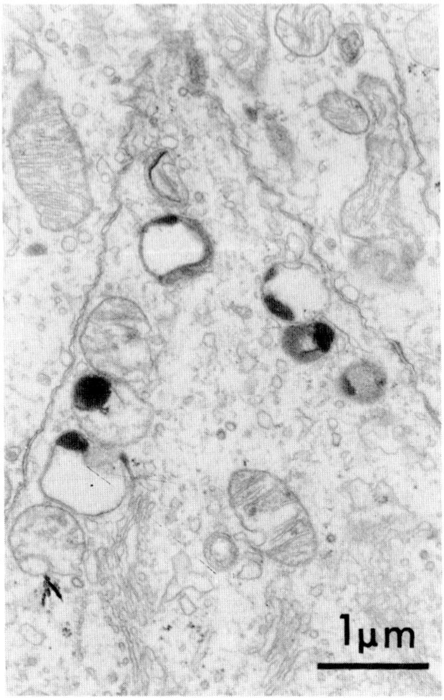

Figure 13-14. Vesiculated membrane containing bodies with dark inclusions in type I hair cells. Crista ampullaris, guinea pig. Netilmicin, 100 mg/kg for 18 days.

The nerve fibers remain in the epithelium for several weeks, even after sensory cell degeneration, but then they degenerate successively in a retrograde manner. We have not yet performed a consistent study of vestibular ganglion cells. Signs of degeneration in the ganglion cells appear during the late stages of degeneration of the vestibular sensory cells, but we do not yet know the percentage of degenerating cells after total destruction of the vestibular epithelia.

The degeneration of the vestibular sensory cells follows a regular pattern [17]. The type I sensory cells are more sensitive than the type II sensory cells in the crista ampullaris. The degeneration begins in the central part of the crista and spreads peripherally within the crista. Degeneration of the crista ampullaris precedes that of the utricle and saccule. In the utricle, the area around the striola, which contains more type I sensory cells, appears to be the most sensitive part of the utricle; the same is true for the macula sacculi.

Comments

A large number of morphologic and physiologic studies of the degeneration pattern of cochlear and vestibular sensory cells after treatment with ototoxic antibiotics are in agreement on major points. Thus, it is clearly established that some aminoglycoside antibiotics, for example, streptomycin, primarily affect the vestibular organs, whereas neomycin, kanamycin, and amikacin are more ototoxic for the cochlear sensory cells. Gentamicin may cause both vestibular and cochlear damage. It also seems to be clearly established that the toxic action is specific for the sensory cells, and that structural degeneration of sensory cells begins before any major damage is observed in the supporting cells.

There is some disagreement, however, as to whether the stria vascularis in the cochlear duct and the dark cells or other cells related to the secretion of fluid and ions in the vestibular system might be damaged at an early stage of ototoxicity. Thus far, there is no convincing evidence to indicate that damage of the secretory-reabsorptive system regulating the circulation of endolymph precedes the toxic effect of antibiotics on the sensory cells. The direct action on the sensory cells is also clearly demonstrated by the rapid and partly reversible action on lateral line organ receptor potentials by antibiotics applied locally [22].

The increase in the number of lysosomes, phagolysosomes, and irregular bodies containing debris and membranes indicates a high enzymatic degradative activity in the supranuclear portion of the cells during the early phases of ototoxic damage. This coincides with an increased activity of acid phosphatase in this area [14, 17], which demonstrates a considerable capacity of the sensory cells to digest the degenerating cell structures during an early phase of ototoxic action [20, 21].

The sensory hair fusion in the vestibular system indicates that an early action of aminoglycosides on the sensory cells affects the plasma membrane. Whether the fusion is a sign of incorporation of antibiotic into the sensory cell plasma membrane or a sign of metabolic changes in the cell cannot be proved with morphologic methods. Demonstration of interactions of neomycin with molecular films of polyphosphoinositides and other lipids indicates, however, that aminoglycoside antibiotics can interfere with phospholipid function in the plasma membrane, and possibly in other organelles in the cells, such as the membranes of the mitochondria and the endoplasmic reticulum [18].

This survey of the present knowledge of the morphologic signs of ototoxic action of the aminoglycoside antibiotics on the inner ear sensory cells supports a theory originally proposed by Duvall and Wersäll in 1964 [7]. The damage to the sensory cells can be explained primarily as an effect on the plasma membrane of the cell and on the membrane components of the mitochondria and other cell organelles, including damage to the permeability barrier. The morphologic demonstration that ribosomes disappear from many sensory cells prior to rupture of the plasma membrane [19], together with an early decrease in the RNA content of sensory cells and ganglion cells in the hearing organ of the lizard during gentamicin treatment [15], demonstrates that RNA metabolism might be affected by the antibiotics.

The degeneration of the ganglion cells and of the nerve fibers innervating the cochlear and vestibular sensory cells is due mainly to retrograde degeneration from the periphery toward the ganglion cells. This was clearly demonstrated in the study of very large numbers of guinea pigs treated with antibiotics and analyzed with regard to nerve fiber and ganglion cell population at various times after the treatment [26]. Evidence that sensory cell degeneration does not depend mainly on a primary effect on the stria vascularis or other cells of the endolymph-circulating system is provided by the fact that the pattern of damage of sensory cells is very irregular in the organ of Corti at early stages of degeneration. It seems unlikely that early damage to the endolymph-circulating system would affect only scattered sensory cells along the cochlear partition. Variations in cell metabolism and acoustic stimulation, previous treatment with aminoglycoside antibiotics, or other types of early damage to the sensory cells might increase the local effects of the antibiotics on the sensory cells. The fact that the sensory cells are much more sensitive to the drug than are the supporting cells also indicates that the composition and permeability of the plasma membrane of the sensory cells differ from those of the supporting cells. Weiner and Schacht (Chap. 7) have suggested that one of the main effects of aminoglycoside antibiotics is displacement of calcium from the reactive sites of the plasma membrane. It appears very likely that the plasma membrane of the sensory cell contains a larger number of reactive sites than do the supporting cells. This is indicated by the demonstration of the importance of calcium in transmission at receptor synapses [4]. Wersäll and Flock [22] have shown that the effect of 10 to 100 μg/ml of streptomycin on microphonic potentials of lateral line organs was reversed by exposure to a potassium-enriched medium. This finding was later confirmed with gentamicin. In these later studies, it was demonstrated that gentamicin applied locally to the surface of the lateral line organ also affects the action potentials of the innervating nerve, and that this effect also is reversible if the area is rinsed with potassium-enriched medium [24]. This relationship between potassium and calcium has to be studied further.

The present findings would suggest the following action of aminoglycoside antibiotics on the sensory cells:

1. Reversible attachment to the surface of the plasma membrane
2. Irreversible incorporation into the plasma membrane, with damage to the permeability barrier of the cell
3. Invasion of the cell by the antibiotic
4. Action of the antibiotic on the phospholipids inside the cell, including phospholipids in the mitochondria and endoplasmic reticulum, causing defects in cell metabolism
5. An effect on ribosome metabolism.

References

1. Berg, K. The toxic effect of streptomycin on eighth cranial nerve; histological investigations; a preliminary report. *Ann. Otol. Rhinol. Laryngol.* 58:448, 1949.

2. Berg, K. The toxic effect of streptomycin on the vestibular and cochlear apparatus. An experimental study on cats. *Acta Otolaryngol. (Stockh.)* [*Suppl.* 97], 1951.
3. Beck, C., and Krahl, P. Experimentelle und feingewebliche Untersuchungen über die Ototoxizität von Kanamycin. *Arch. Ohr.-Nas.- u. Kehlk.-Heilk.* 179:594, 1962.
4. Bennet, M. V. L. Transmission at Receptor Synapses. In T. Desiraju (Ed.), *Mechanisms in Transmission of Signals for Conscious Behavior.* Amsterdam: Elsevier, 1976.
5. Caussé, R. Action toxique vestibulaire et cochléaire de la streptomycine au point de vue expérimental. *Ann. Otolaryngol. (Paris)* 66:518, 1949.
6. Christensen, E., Hertz, H., Riskaer, N., and Vraa-Jensen, G. Histological investigations in chronic streptomycin poisoning in guinea pigs. *Ann. Otol. Rhinol. Laryngol.* 60:343, 1951.
7. Duvall, A. J., and Wersäll, J. Site of action of streptomycin upon inner ear sensory cells. *Acta Otolaryngol. (Stockh.)* 57:581, 1964.
8. Federspil, P. Zur Ototoxizität der Aminoglykosid-Antibiotika. *Infection* 4:239, 1976.
9. Federspil, P., Schätzle, W., and Tiesler, E. Pharmakokinetische, histologische und histochemische Untersuchungen zur Ototoxizität des Gentamicins, Tobramycins und Amikacins. *Arch. Otorhinolaryngol.* 217:147, 1977.
10. Hawkins, J. E., Jr. The ototoxicity of kanamycin. *Ann. Otol. Rhinol. Laryngol.* 68:698, 1959.
11. Hawkins, J. E., Jr., and Engström, H. Effect of kanamycin on cochlear cytoarchitecture. *Acta Otolaryngol. (Stockh.)* [*Suppl.* 188]:100, 1964.
12. Hawkins, J. E., Jr., and Lurie, M. H. The ototoxicity of streptomycin. *Ann. Otol. Rhinol. Laryngol.* 61:789, 1952.
13. Hawkins, J. E., Jr., and Lurie, M. H. The ototoxicity of dihydrostreptomycin and neomycin in the cat. *Ann. Otol. Rhinol. Laryngol.* 62:1128, 1953.
14. Ishii, T., Ishii, D., and Balogh, K., Jr. Lysosomal enzymes in the inner ears of kanamycin-treated guinea pigs. *Acta Otolaryngol. (Stockh.)* 65:449, 1967.
15. Jarlstedt, J., and Bagger-Sjöbäck, D. Gentamicin-induced changes in RNA content in sensory and ganglionic cells in the hearing organ of the lizard *Calotes versicolor. Acta Otolaryngol. (Stockh.)* 84:361, 1977.
16. Kohonen, A. Effect of some ototoxic drugs upon the pattern and innervation of cochlear sensory cells in the guinea pig. *Acta Otolaryngol. (Stockh.)* [*Suppl.* 208], 1965.
17. Lindeman, H. H. Regional differences in sensitivity of the vestibular sensory epithelia to ototoxic antibiotics. *Acta Otolaryngol. (Stockh.)* 67:177, 1969.
18. Lodhi, S., Weiner, N. D., and Schacht, J. Interactions of neomycin with monomolecular films of polyphosphoinositides and other lipids. *Biochim. Biophys. Acta* 557:1, 1979.
19. Lundquist, P. G., and Wersäll, J. The Ototoxic Effect of Gentamicin—an Electron Microscopical Study. In *Gentamicin, First International Symposium.* Basel: Schwabe, 1967. Pp. 26.
20. Wersäll, J. Studies on the structure and innervation of the sensory epithelium of the cristae ampullares in the guinea pig. *Acta Otolaryngol. (Stockh.)* [*Suppl.* 126], 1956.
21. Wersäll, J., Björkroth, B., Flock, A., and Lundquist, P. G. Sensory hair fusion in vestibular sensory cells after gentamycin exposure. *Arch. klin. exp. Ohr.-Nas.- u. Kehlk.–Heilk.* 200:1, 1971.
22. Wersäll, J., and Flock, A. Suppression and restoration of the microphonic output from lateral line organ after local application of streptomycin. *Life Sci.* 3:1151, 1964.
23. Wersäll, J., and Hawkins, J. E., Jr. The vestibular sensory epithelia in the cat labyrinth and their reactions in chronic streptomycin intoxication. *Acta Otolaryngol. (Stockh.)* 54:243, 1962.
24. Wersäll, J., and Flock, A. Unpublished observations.

25. Ylikoski, J. Guinea-pig hair cell pathology from ototoxic antibiotics. *Acta Otolaryngol. (Stockh.)* [*Suppl.* 326]:5, 1974.
26. Ylikoski, J., Wersäll, J., and Björkroth, B. Degeneration of neural elements in the cochlea of the guinea pig after damage to the organ of Corti by ototoxic antibiotics. *Acta Otolaryngol. (Stockh.)* [*Suppl.* 326]:23, 1974.

14. Effects of Gentamicin on the Development of the Embryonic Inner Ear in Organ Culture

Matti Anniko

Culture of the inner ear in vitro provides a controlled system for the study of environmental influences on its morphogenesis. Development of the avian otocyst in vitro was described many years ago [10], but culture of the mammalian inner ear was not reported until the 1970s [6, 16].

The embryologic development of the crista ampullaris of the otocyst in the CBA/CBA mouse is similar in vivo and in vitro [7]. The corresponding maturation of the cochlear part of the labyrinth, which occurs mainly postpartum in vivo, is not reproduced so well in vitro. In the latter situation, one finds aberrant coiling and cytodifferentiation of both the organ of Corti and the stria vascularis [5].

The specific structure of hair cells is not preserved after explantation of the inner ears of newborn or mature animals [3], but the secretory epithelia of these inner ears largely maintain their ultrastructure during the first week in vitro [4]. Recently, Anniko and Wroblewski [9] reported that the maturation of endolymph did not occur until 4 to 8 days postpartum in the CBA/CBA mouse. Differentiation of the crista ampullaris continues in vitro, whereas the cochlea cannot achieve corresponding maturity in culture. Both the maturation of the inner ear ultrastructure and the development of the specific composition of endolymph precede the functional capacity of the labyrinth.

In the present pilot study, I have investigated the morphologic features of murine inner ear hair cells exposed in vitro to an ototoxic aminoglycoside, gentamicin. Inner ear anlagen were explanted for incubation in gentamicin either on the thirteenth gestational day (otocyst stage) or on the sixteenth gestational day, when organogenesis is almost completed and cytodifferentiation has begun.

Supported by grants from the Karolinska Institute and funds from Tysta Skolan and the Swedish Medical Research Council (12X-720).

Materials and Methods

Animals

The CBA/CBA mouse was used in all experiments. Gestational age was determined by the vaginal-plug technique [17].

Removal of the Embryonic Inner Ear

THIRTEENTH GESTATIONAL DAY

On the thirteenth gestational day (Fig. 14-1), the otocyst has just begun to form a cochlear end by elongation of the otocyst and is developing a minimal "hook" (Fig. 14-2). During dissection, this hook may easily be damaged, allowing incubation medium to enter the inner part of the otocyst. The hook area later develops into the cochlear part of the inner ear. Damage to this structure does not interfere with the embryonic development and maturation of the vestibular part of the labyrinth, but results in either malformation or

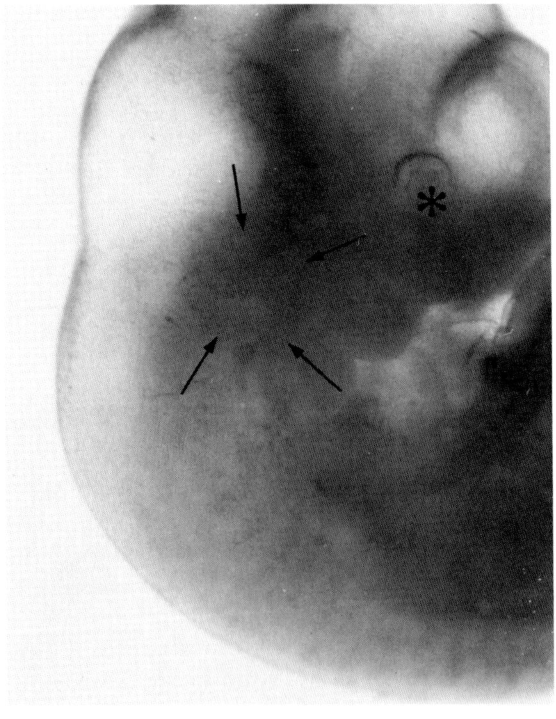

Figure 14-1. Light micrograph of a normal CBA/CBA mouse embryo on the thirteenth gestational day (×8). The otocyst region is marked by arrows. The eye is indicated by an asterisk.

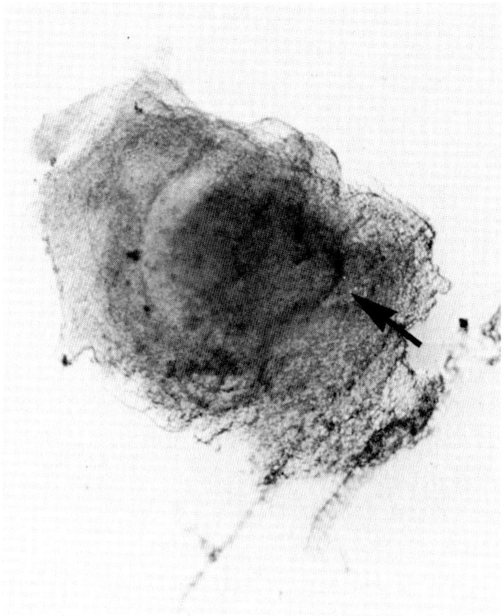

Figure 14-2. Light micrograph of a normal otocyst explant in vitro (×24). The inner ear anlage has a slight elongation indicating development of the cochlea (arrow).

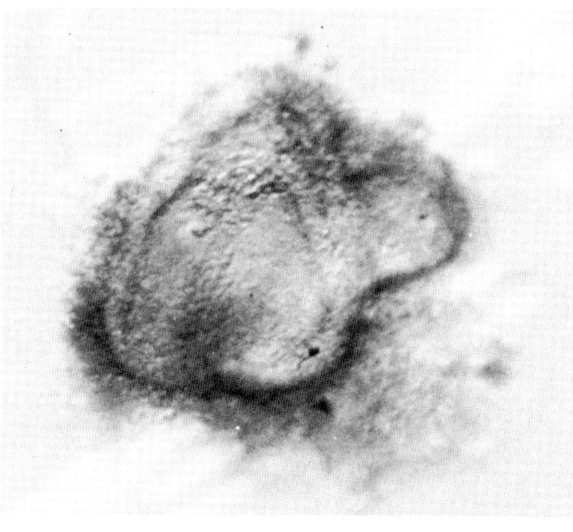

Figure 14-3. Light micrograph of an inner ear explant (thirteenth gestational day) that has been cultured in vitro for 2 days (×30). The outgrowth from the otocyst will form the cochlear portion of the labyrinth, but the semicircular canals are not yet present. This inner ear anlage was explanted without sufficient mesenchyme surrounding the otocyst. (Cf. Fig. 14-5.)

aplasia of the cochlea. In the dissection, it is important to preserve a part of the mesenchyme surrounding the otocyst because this tissue gives support for further development of the inner ear structures. In the absence of such tissue, poor development of the inner ear anlage can be misinterpreted as an exogenously induced toxic effect, e.g., as being caused by drugs in the culture medium (Fig. 14-3). Furthermore, the inner ear anlage must be allowed to attach to the bottom of the culture dish. Otherwise, embryonic development does not start or does not occur in parallel with the development in vivo.

SIXTEENTH GESTATIONAL DAY

The gross morphology of the labyrinth has developed by the sixteenth day (Fig. 14-4). It is technically easy to dissect the inner ear from the surrounding temporal bone, and damage during preparation is rare. A cartilaginous capsule now surrounds the labyrinth. At this stage, several inner ears were divided between the cochlear and vestibular portions of the labyrinth, as indicated in Fig. 14-4. This provided standardized conditions by allowing influx of medium containing gentamicin.

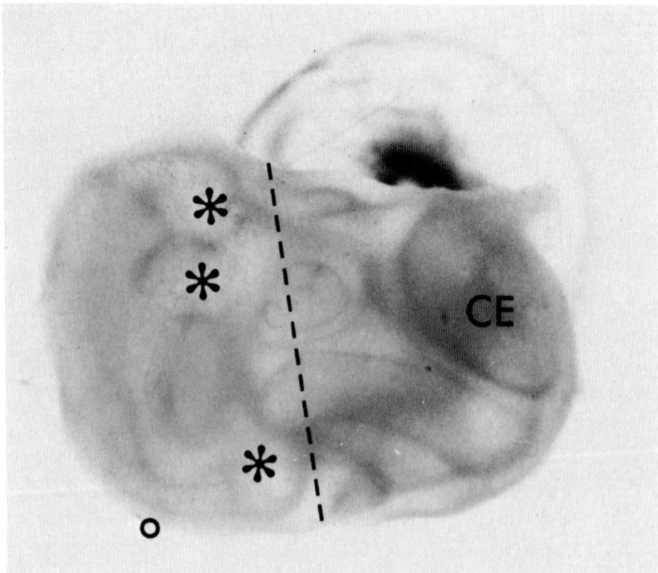

Figure 14-4. Light micrograph of an inner ear explant (sixteenth gestational day) (×20). The gross morphology reveals a nearly mature configuration. (* = cristae ampullares; CE = cochlear end [2½ coils]; ----- = the region where the vestibular and cochlear parts should be separated by microdissection.)

ORGAN CULTURE TECHNIQUE
The culture technique used has been described in detail by Van De Water [16] and Anniko et al. [6]. All experiments were performed at least in triplicate. The controls were three or more inner ears at each of the two stages of development. Each inner ear was photographed daily for study of the influence of gentamicin on the development of the gross structure.

INCUBATION WITH GENTAMICIN
Gentamicin sulfate powder was supplied by the Schering Corporation. Inner ear explants were cultured in Neuman and Tytell's serumless medium, supplemented with 10 to 15% fetal calf serum and 1% L-glutamine. Gentamicin was dissolved in the culture medium at final concentrations of 10, 100, and 1,000 μg/ml, according to the base. The nutrient solution of the organ cultures was renewed every second day.

MORPHOLOGIC PROCEDURES
Groups of otocysts explanted on the thirteenth gestational day were prepared for morphologic investigation after 1 to 5 days of incubation in gentamicin at various concentrations. A similar procedure was used for inner ears explanted on the sixteenth gestational day and incubated in gentamicin for 1 to 6 days. Fixation was performed in 3% glutaraldehyde in 0.133 M sodium phosphate buffer, after which the specimens were postfixed in 2% osmic tetroxide. After dehydration in alcohol, the specimens were embedded in epon mixture. Light-microscopic sections were stained with toluidine blue. Ultrathin sections were stained with uranyl acetate and lead citrate and examined in a Philips 400 electron microscope. A limited number of specimens were sectioned serially, and alternate sections were examined by light and electron microscopy.

Results

Effects of Gentamicin on Organogenesis

Damage to the cochlear hook during dissection affected the sensitivity to gentamicin of inner ear anlagen explanted on the thirteenth gestational day. In specimens with an intact otocyst, without direct communication between the otocyst lumen and the surrounding gentamicin-containing culture medium, gross morphologic changes were less severe.

The organogenesis of the inner ear explants from the thirteenth gestational day differed considerably between the gentamicin-treated specimens and the controls. In both groups, the regions of the cristae ampullares and the two maculae were generally identified after a few days of embryologic development in vitro. The formation of semicircular canals, however, was less distinct in the gentamicin-treated specimens, and in many cases the cristae ampullares were not distinctly separated (Figs. 14-5 and 14-6).

The sixteenth-gestational-day explants had already passed through most of their organogenesis and did not undergo gross morphologic changes after exposure to gentamicin.

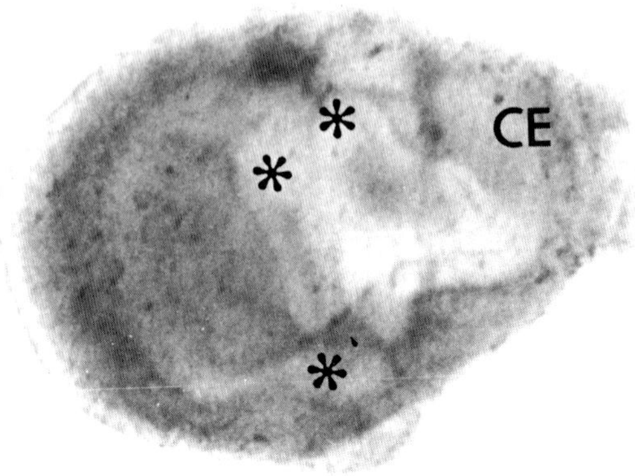

Figure 14-5. Light micrograph of an inner ear anlage (thirteenth gestational day) cultured in vitro for 1½ days without gentamicin (×20). The semicircular canals are recognizable (*), and the region containing the cristae ampullares can be identified. The cochlear end (CE) has begun to coil.

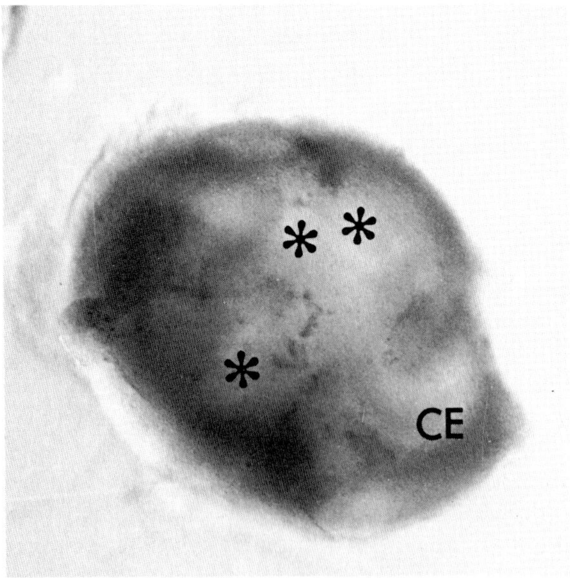

Figure 14-6. Light micrograph of an otocyst (thirteenth gestational day) exposed to 100 μg/ml of gentamicin for 2 days (×26). (* = regions of the cristae ampullares; CE = cochlear end.) An obvious malformation has occurred during organogenesis. Prior to incubation, the otocyst had been well preserved, without damage to the hook area.

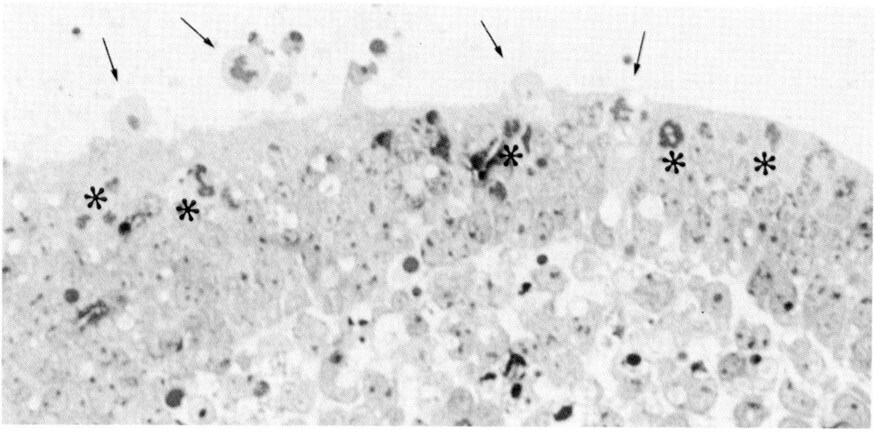

Figure 14-7. Light micrograph of an inner ear explant (thirteenth gestational day) cultured in vitro for 1 day in the presence of gentamicin, 10 μg/ml (×900). The epithelial region is forming the crista ampullaris and the utricle. Cells undergoing their terminal mitosis near the otocyst lumen differentiate into hair cells. In this specimen, several cells in mitosis are being expelled into the otocyst lumen (arrows). Many other cells in mitosis are still present in the upper part of the otocyst epithelium (*).

Effects of Gentamicin on Hair Cells

THIRTEENTH GESTATIONAL DAY INNER EAR EXPLANTS (OTOCYSTS)

In intact otocysts, specific ultrastructural changes such as sensory hair fusion, fusion of microvilli, or intracellular myelin figures restricted to sensory cells were not observed. Dose-related effects of gentamicin were seen in otocysts whose cochlear end had been damaged during dissection, allowing direct fluid flow between the otocyst lumen and the surrounding gentamicin-containing culture medium. On the thirteenth and fourteenth gestational days, however, it is not possible to differentiate with certainty between developing vestibular hair cells and supporting cells. Corresponding cochlear structures have not developed at this stage, either in the gentamicin-exposed group or in normal inner ear anlagen.

After only one day of exposure, 10 μg/ml of gentamicin caused extrusion of cells into the otocyst lumen and changes in the fine structure of cells adjacent to the lumen (Fig. 14-7). Cells undergoing mitosis appeared to be especially vulnerable. In some expelled cells, mitochondria were clumped together, but formation of myelin figures occurred only occasionally. Many cells lining the otocyst lumen lacked such findings; these were interpreted to be supporting cells. The corresponding control specimens had a normal morphology.

When the inner ear explant had been kept intact with a sufficient layer of mesenchyme surrounding the otocyst, a gentamicin concentration even as high as 100 μg/ml in the culture medium did not cause structural changes visible at the light-microscopic level. Cytologic alterations were evident in many cells under electron microscopy, however.

With increasing incubation time (3 days or more), it became easier to separate hair cells from supporting tissue. At this time, organogenesis had ended and all parts of the cristae had formed. Intact otocysts surrounded by mesenchyme at explantation showed only minor hair cell changes even when the culture period was extended to 5 days in the presence of 10 μg/ml of gentamicin.

SIXTEENTH GESTATIONAL DAY INNER EAR EXPLANTS

When this stage of embryonic development was reached, a large number of vestibular hair cells had already been formed. The lowest concentration of gentamicin (10 μg/ml) caused morphologic changes in vestibular hair cells after 2 days. Many of the hair cells appeared swollen (Fig. 14-8), and myelin figures were noted in these cells (Figs. 14-9 and 14-10). Severe hair cell degeneration appeared only occasionally during 5-day culture of these explants in 10 μg/ml of gentamicin. At higher gentamicin concentrations, 100 to 1,000 μg/ml, much more severe hair cell damage was seen after the same time interval (Fig. 14-11).

Ototoxic damage to the cochlear portion of the inner ear was also evaluated. After exposure of explants to gentamicin at 100 to 1,000 μg/ml for 3 to 4 days, no severely degenerating hair cells were seen under light microscopy. After similar treatment in only 10 μg/ml of gentamicin, however, mitochondrial disintegration in cochlear hair cells and protrusion of the apical part of the hair cells were evident under electron microscopy (Fig. 14-12). These changes were not observed in controls (Fig. 14-13).

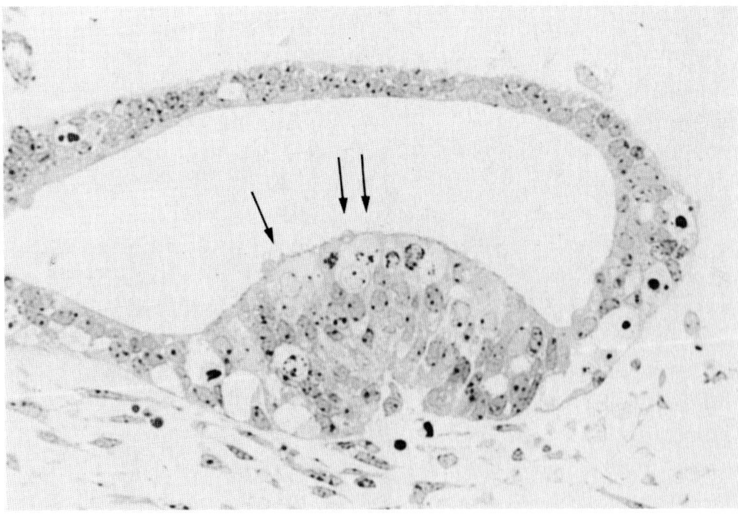

Figure 14-8. Light micrograph of crista ampullaris (×310). Inner ear explant (sixteenth gestational day) exposed to 10 μg/ml of gentamicin for 4 days. Swollen hair cells are indicated by arrows.

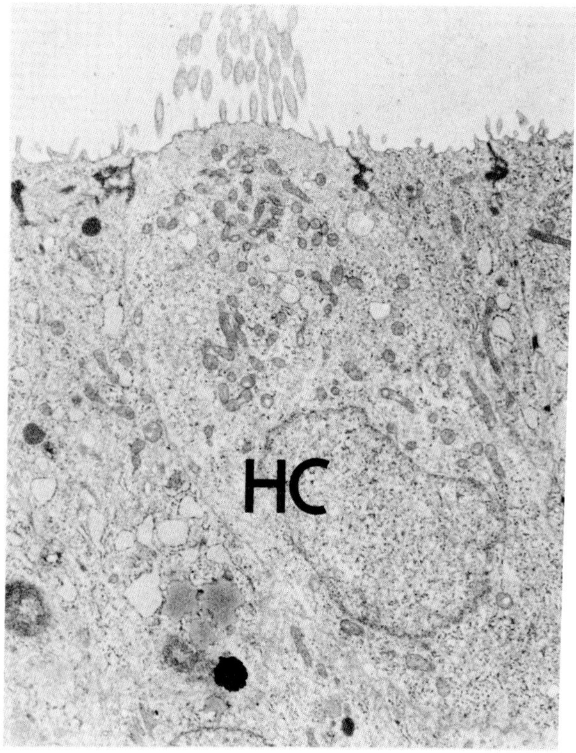

Figure 14-9. Electron micrograph of an inner ear explant (sixteenth gestational day) cultured for 2 days (×4,500). Normal hair cell (HC) from the crista ampullaris.

Comments

The present investigation reveals that embryonic mammalian hair cells in culture are vulnerable to the ototoxic effect of aminoglycoside antibiotics. This vulnerability was present during both early and late gestational ages, although the effect was less specific at the otocyst stage.

With the in vitro technique, I have attempted to obtain a model system for the study of ototoxicity by exposing inner ear hair cells to ototoxic agents at concentrations achieved in vivo. The vestibular portion of the inner ear reaches maturation before birth, except for the final innervation of vestibular hair cells [14]. Therefore, this portion of the inner ear constitutes a suitable model for ototoxicity studies in vitro, as has been suggested by Anniko, Van De Water, and Nordemar [8]. This model may also be useful if one wishes to examine the possibility of intrauterine ototoxicity.

In the in vitro system, the hair cells are exposed to gentamicin at a constant concentration. In the maternal circulation, however, the serum level of the antibiotic may vary considerably between peaks and troughs, when the drug is

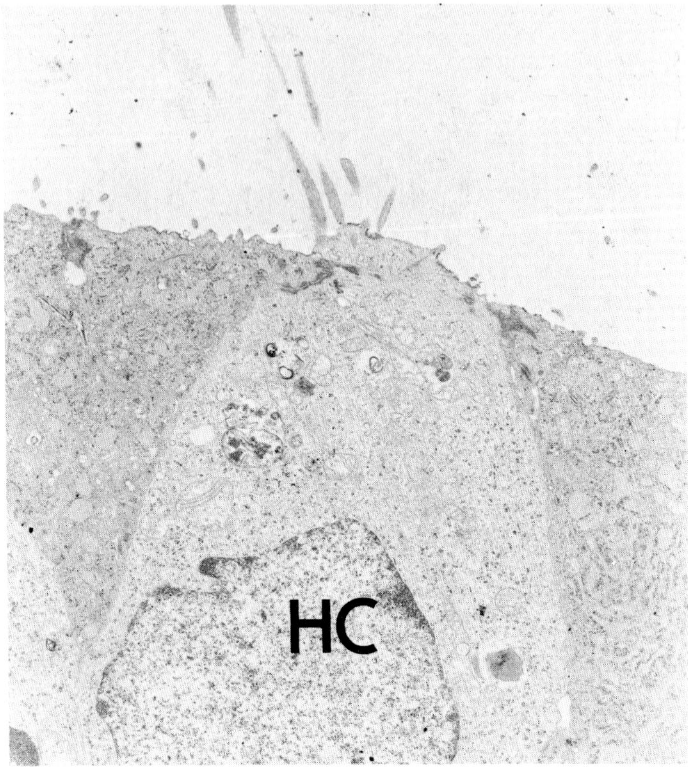

Figure 14-10. Electron micrograph of explant similar to that shown in Fig. 14-9, except that culture was performed in medium containing 10 μg/ml gentamicin (×6,000). Myelin figures are present in the hair cell (HC) cytoplasm, but no sensory hair fusion is visible.

Figure 14-11. Light micrograph of crista ampullaris (×360). Inner ear explant (sixteenth gestational day) exposed to 100 μg/ml of gentamicin for 4 days. Degenerating hair cells can be identified at the light-microscopic level (arrows).

Figure 14-12. Electron micrograph of outer hair cells (OHC) in the basal coil of the cochlea (×3,700). Inner ear explant (sixteenth gestational day) cultured for 6 days in the presence of 10 μg/ml gentamicin. The hair cells reveal mitochondrial disintegration (arrows). The apical part of one hair cell protrudes into the endolymphatic space (*). Hair fusion has not occurred.

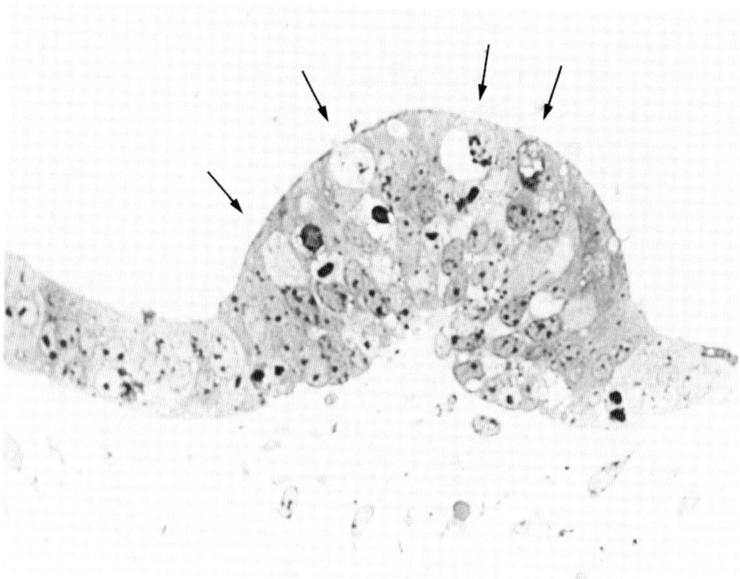

14-11

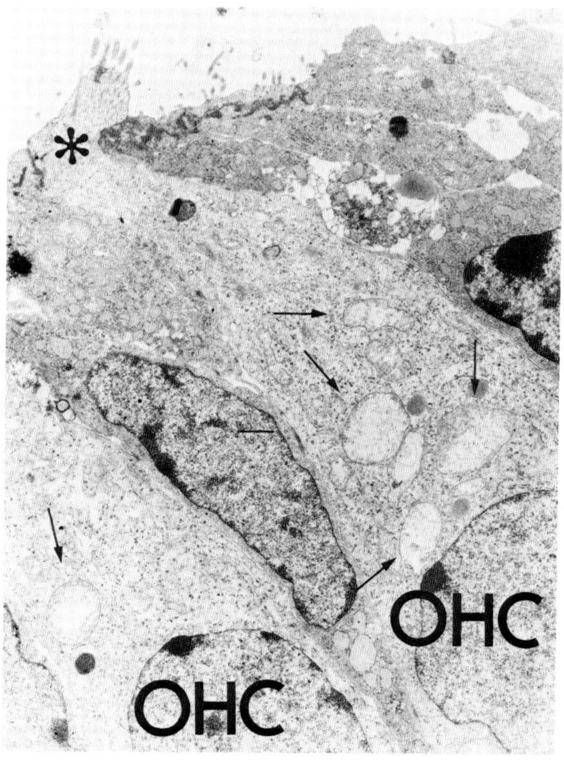

14-12

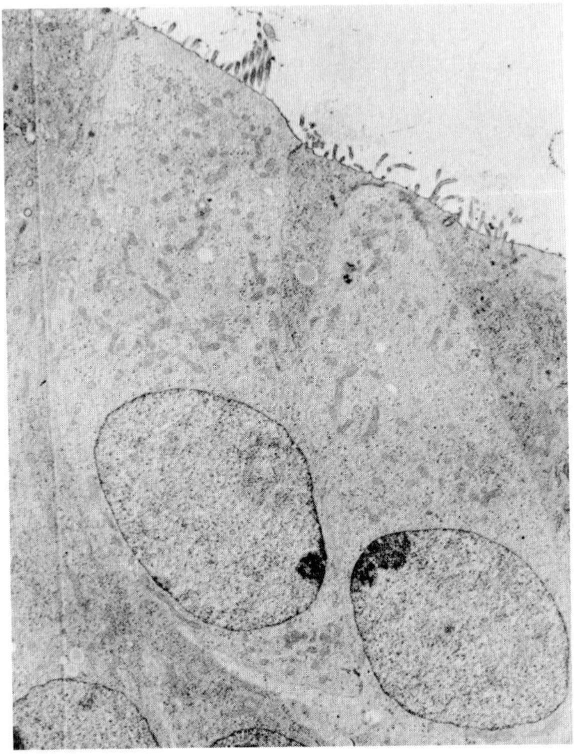

Figure 14-13. Electron micrograph of outer hair cells (×2,700). Control specimen. Experimental conditions were the same as in Fig. 14-12, but gentamicin was omitted. The cell organelles have normal morphology. No protrusion of outer hair cells was observed.

administered in the usual regimen of intermittent infusion or injection. There is little information on the rate of transplacental passage of aminoglycosides in man and animals. In one study, Andersen and Pedersen [2] treated guinea pigs in the terminal stages of pregnancy with frequently repeated doses of kanamycin so that the level of kanamycin in the serum reached at 2 hours was maintained fairly constantly. Kanamycin was detected in fetal serum within 1 hour, and by 6 hours the level was in equilibrium with that of the maternal serum. The equilibrium level in fetal serum was approximately 7 percent of that in maternal serum over a ten-fold range of doses and maternal serum levels.

Mirkin [13] concluded that the general pattern of drug distribution in the fetus frequently resembles that in the mother. The distribution of drugs in the fetus may, however, be influenced by differences in permeability of specialized membranes, binding to specific proteins, selective distribution of the fetal circulation, and active secretion of drugs by the yolk sac.

Intrauterine ototoxicity is seldom reported in man [12]. It may be difficult to separate aminoglycoside-induced effects from those of other noxious agents. In animals, ototoxicity of aminoglycoside antibiotics has been noted during intrauterine development [15]. Akiyoshi et al. [1] showed damage to both outer and inner hair cells in the basal coil of the fetal cochlea after treatment of pregnant guinea pigs with dideoxykanamycin B.

Hair cell damage by aminoglycosides in vitro has previously been reported only by Friedmann and Bird [11]. In their study of the fowl embryo otocyst, incubation was performed at extremely high concentrations. The present model for in vitro culture is likely to be better suited for screening of potentially ototoxic drugs, since the developing inner ear of a mammal is treated with clinically achievable concentrations of aminoglycosides.

References

1. Akiyoshi, M., Sato, K., Shoji, T., Sugahiro, K., Tajima, T., Koeda, T., Odaki, M., and Yokota, M. Ototoxic effects of 3,4-dideoxykanamycin B on the inner ear in the intrauterine guinea-pigs. *J. Antibiot. (Tokyo)* 27:735, 1974.
2. Andersen, J. B., and Pedersen, C. B. A method for the determination of transplacental transmission of drugs. *Acta Pathol. Microbiol. Scand. [B]* 79:204, 1971.
3. Anniko, M. Extracorporeal preservation—organ culture of the post-natal mammalian inner ear. *Acta Otolaryngol. (Stockh.)* 88:211, 1979.
4. Anniko, M. The postnatal mammalian labyrinthine secretory epithelium *in vitro*. *Acta Otolaryngol. (Stockh.)* 90:237, 1980.
5. Anniko, M. Unpublished observations.
6. Anniko, M., Nordemar, H., and Van De Water, T. R. Embryogenesis of the inner ear. I. Development and differentiation of the mammalian crista ampullaris *in vivo* and *in vitro*. *Arch. Otorhinolaryngol.* 224:285, 1979.
7. Anniko, M., Nordemar, H., and Wersäll, J. Comparative embryologic development *in vivo* and *in vitro* of mammalian hair cells of the crista ampullaris. *Proc. Bárány Society* (3rd Ordinary Meeting in Uppsala):4, 1978.
8. Anniko, M., Van De Water, T. R., and Nordemar, H. Organ culture of the 16th gestational day mouse labyrinth. *Acta Otolaryngol. (Stockh.)* 86:52, 1978.
9. Anniko, M., Wroblewski, R., and Wersäll, J. Development of endolymph during maturation of the mammalian inner ear. *Arch. Otorhinolaryngol.* 225:161, 1979.
10. Friedmann, I. The Ear. In E. N. Willner (Ed.), *Cells and Tissues in Culture.* New York, London: Academic, 1965. Vol. 2, pp. 521–547.
11. Friedmann, I., and Bird, E. S. The effect of ototoxic antibiotics and of penicillin on the sensory areas of the isolated fowl embryo otocyst in organ cultures: An electron-microscope study. *J. Pathol. Bacteriol.* 81:81, 1961.
12. Jones, H. C. Intrauterine ototoxicity. *J. Natl. Med. Assoc.* 65:201, 1973.
13. Mirkin, B. L. Maternal and fetal distribution of drugs in pregnancy. *Clin. Pharmacol. Ther.* 14:643, 1973.
14. Nordemar, H., and Anniko, M. Postnatal maturation of vestibular hair cells. Congress abstract. 16th Workshop on Inner Ear Biology, Bern, Switzerland, 1979.
15. Uziel, A., Romand, R., and Marst, M. Electrophysiological study of the ototoxicity of kanamycin during development in guinea-pigs. *Acta Otolaryngol. (Stockh.)* In press.
16. Van De Water, T. R. Effects of removal of the statoacoustic ganglion complex upon the growing otocyst. *Ann. Otol. Rhinol. Laryngol. [Suppl.* 33]:2, 1976.
17. Van De Water, T., and Ruben, R. J. Organ culture of the mammalian inner ear: A tool to study inner ear deafness. *Laryngoscope* 84:738, 1974.

Discussion of Chapters 12, 13, and 14

Dr. L. Nordström (Malmö General Hospital, Malmö, Sweden): Dr. Hawkins, do you notice presbycusis in your "old" animals? If so, do you also see age-related changes in the vestibular system?

Dr. Hawkins: Changes in the vestibular system with aging are certainly very real, and I should have pointed out that those rather deplorable-looking otoconia that I showed at the end of my talk are almost identical to those that Lars Johnsson and Muriel Ross and others have described in aging human subjects.

Dr. Wersäll: Long-term studies in an animal such as the guinea pig are difficult because we have, as Dr. Hawkins and Dr. Engström have shown, presbycusis or presbyastasia in the aging animals, and that comes after about 2 years of life.

Dr. Nadol: Dr. Wersäll, are the ototoxic changes that you see in hair cells in either the vestibular or auditory system, where there is protrusion into the endolymphatic space, caused by changes in the intercellular junctional complex that plays a role in dividing endolymph from perilymph? Also, what are the ultrastructural correlates of the first-order neuronal changes that Dr. Hawkins showed especially with neomycin?

Dr. Wersäll: We have not satisfactorily studied the membranes with very high ultrastructural resolution. As far as the ganglion cells are concerned, which Dr. Ylikoski studied in our laboratory, it was quite clear that there were early changes in both the ganglion cells and the nerve fibers. It was possible to follow the degeneration. After 12 months, those ganglion cells that are preserved will have a very normal appearance.

Dr. Matz: Dr. Anniko, have you seen any changes in your embryo model with doses less than 10 μg/ml?

Dr. Anniko: I have not used those doses yet.

Dr. Schacht: Dr. Wersäll, you alluded to the sequence of events when a particular type of cell is damaged. There seems to be some discrepancy in the literature as to whether there are certain very sensitive tissues that are damaged prior to other tissues in the inner ear.

Dr. Wersäll: In my opinion, dark-cell damage, for example, comes rather late. You can have damaged sensory cells and still have most of the supporting cells in the vestibular system intact. This might also depend on the concentration or the duration of drug treatment. The pattern of degeneration in the various parts of the ear will vary depending not only on the route of administration, but also on the dose rate, both in the cochlea and in the vestibular system.

Dr. Hawkins: I once proposed the working hypothesis that ototoxicity depends on a derangement of the microhomeostasis of the cochlea, and the suggestion that perhaps the earliest events occur in the spiral ligament and stria vascularis, which presumably are charged with the maintenance of this microhomeostasis. I feel now that the changes in the hair cells probably come first.

Dr. J. Ylikoski (University of Helsinki, Helsinki, Finland): One of the examples of the sequence of degeneration in the end organ due to aminoglycosides, or in other types of end-organ lesions, is a retrograde degeneration of the cochlear nerve.

Dr. Brummett: One of the things we have noticed in our studies on the interaction between the aminoglycosides and the loop diuretics is that, as a late effect, changes are seen in the cochlear hair cells similar to changes observed with the aminoglycosides alone. The mitochondria are damaged, and the nucleus shows chromatin clumping. The hair cells are distorted, and all of the cilia are fused together. One of the two earliest changes is an alteration in the plasma membrane in localized areas. The other change is the nuclear chromatin clumping of the hair cells, which is very obvious and is not seen in any other cell. The supporting cells directly beneath the hair cells look very nice and neat. At least in our system, we have been able to observe these changes; but whether they apply to the aminoglycosides alone, we don't know.

Dr. Wersäll: One problem is that we are working with several systems in the cells. Morphologically, the fenestrated membranes are actually shaped by the plasma membrane, and you showed this morning that there are small half-pinocytotic vesicles on the surface. These vesicles are found in the normal cell, and I think this represents a continuity between the surface and the fenestrated membranes.

Your picture showed that an important part of the ototoxicity may be due to the passage of fluid into the hair cells. This might indicate that the direct action of the diuretic is on the hair cells. Dr. Hawkins pointed out that one of the factors in toxicity may be enzyme activity on the cell surface membrane. We may have here a very complicated combination of two types of toxicity.

Dr. Federspil: Previously, the destruction of the outer hair cells was described as proceeding from the base to the apex, and the destruction of the inner hair cells began in the apical part of the cochlea. These studies were done mainly with neomycin and kanamycin. Studies with the newer aminoglycosides, such as gentamicin, tobramycin, and amikacin, show that lesions begin at the basal turn in both outer and inner hair cells. How do you explain these differences?

Dr. Hawkins: I think it is certainly true that in the guinea pig one tends to see loss of inner hair cells at the apical end and loss of outer hair cells at the basal end initially; this may be due to a characteristic of the animal. There is something very peculiar about the apical portion of the organ of Corti in the guinea pig: even in perfectly normal control animals, the outer hair cells are often swollen. This may be an artifact of preparation, but it suggests to me that perhaps these cells can be abnormal even without aminoglycoside treatment.

Dr. Wersäll: One interesting comment was made by Dr. Ernstson, who studied the waltzing guinea pig and found consistently that degeneration of the organ of Corti starts in the upper part of the basal coil, at the point where the differentiation starts in the embryo. This would indicate that the basal turn is susceptible to later degeneration by aminoglycosides.

In some of the material, the hook area, which is the most distal portion of the basal coil, plus the upper part of the basal coil are the two sites where early changes are found. Thus, changes do not always start in the most apical portion. I think you yourself demonstrated that about 20 percent of your specimens had degeneration in other parts of the cochlea. So, it seems to be a rule with many exceptions.

Dr. Igarashi: Dr. Wersäll, would you kindly explain why type I vestibular hair cells are more sensitive to aminoglycosides than type II? Also, I would like to hear about your findings on the efferent nerve endings for the hair cells. Dr. Anniko, would you explain what you found out about the cupula, otoconial membrane, and tectorial membrane in your specimens?

Dr. Wersäll: It seems impossible right now to decide why one cell type is more sensitive than the other; but I think it is quite clear that the metabolism and the function of the type I and type II cells are different.

We know now that, in the waltzing guinea pig, the pathologic actin rod which goes through the whole cell is found only in the type I cells and never in type II cells. Recently, we demonstrated exactly the same thing in the Shaker 2 mouse; the type I sensory cell has one actin rod and the type II cell doesn't. So, there is something different in the metabolism that might cause a difference in sensitivity to toxicity.

Dr. Anniko: Concerning the otoconial membrane, you very seldom get development of otoconia in vitro. I don't know on what this depends; probably there is not enough calcium in the nutrient solution. As to the tectorial membrane, I am analyzing it and don't have enough material. I have not seen any great changes in the cupula, but the number of animals or specimens is too small (less than 40).

II. Studies in Human Subjects

Testing Inner Ear Function

The earliest reports on streptomycin ototoxicity described patients with symptoms of vestibular and auditory disorders. Audiometry has long been available for precise recording of hearing loss. By means of monitoring procedures with standardized audiometric tests, as described by Patricia Thompson and Jerry Northern and by Harris J. Mowry et al., one can detect toxic effects of aminoglycosides and thereby facilitate the rehabilitation of patients who suffer hearing loss. Analysis of the cochlear microphonic and eighth nerve action potential has been applied by Richard Ramsden to patients undergoing aminoglycoside therapy. With these techniques, the early electrophysiologic effects of these drugs can be detected objectively. In tests for auditory toxicity in very young children, particularly in neonates, nonbehavioral methods such as the measurement of auditory brainstem response have been used. Terese Finitzo-Hieber shows that, in neonates, such testing can be as effective as impedance audiometry and auditory behavioral methods in identifying hearing loss caused by ototoxicity.

Techniques for evaluation of human vestibular function that match the precision of audiometric methods are not yet well established. Recently, a battery of vestibular tests has been devised by Leonard Proctor and his co-workers for prospective studies of aminoglycoside toxicity. Precise vestibular tests like theirs will have to be applied to large numbers of aminoglycoside-treated patients to provide data on the actual incidence of vestibular toxicity. We have included a study by James Roeder et al. on the intrasubject variability of serial vestibular caloric tests in adults, in which the authors attempted to evaluate the reliability of these tests as indicators of vestibular toxicity. Like auditory tests, vestibular tests are difficult to perform and interpret in very young children. Lydia and Abraham Eviatar achieve effective evaluation of vestibular dysfunction in children by combining postural tests, measurement of developmental reflexes, and electronystagmography.

15. Audiometric Monitoring of Patients Treated with Ototoxic Drugs

Patricia L. Thompson and Jerry L. Northern

Numerous clinical reports on aminoglycoside ototoxicity have been published since 1945. Ototoxicity has been described in children and adults receiving streptomycin therapy for tuberculosis [24, 44]. Ototoxic effects of neomycin were reported in neonates [24] and in patients receiving the drug by a variety of routes, including oral [32, 52], intermittent lavage of a surgical cavity [33], topical aerosol [1, 31], and application with porcine skin xenografts for burns [47]. Several studies describe vestibular and auditory toxicity caused by gentamicin used systemically and topically [8, 11, 12, 18, 26, 36]. The severe deafness that occurred in some patients after treatment with neomycin or kanamycin was not a serious problem during early clinical trials with gentamicin. Ototoxicity with gentamicin seemed to be less frequent and less severe than with its predecessors [22].

Since the introduction of gentamicin, tobramycin, and amikacin, the use of aminoglycosides has increased markedly, possibly accompanied by an increase in the overall number of patients with ototoxicity. The use of repeated courses in many patients has also increased the likelihood of toxic effects. The introduction and widespread use of other ototoxic drugs, especially the loop diuretics, have further complicated the risks of therapy. For example, in one case, a mother and infant were severely deafened after treatment of the mother with kanamycin and ethacrynic acid during pregnancy [25].

The use of aminoglycosides is limited by the relatively low toxic-therapeutic ratio. Not all the clinical and pharmacologic factors that contribute to toxicity are clearly defined. Because of this uncertainty, and because of the relatively limited amount of information available about the manifestations and detection of subtle, early toxicity, there is no firm agreement as to which parameters or procedures should be used for monitoring of ototoxicity.

Audiometry has become generally recognized as an important source of statistical data on new aminoglycosides during clinical trials. Audiometric and vestibular testing for identification and quantification of toxic reactions according to well-defined and standardized criteria will help to provide information on the incidence of drug toxicity and on the correlation of toxicity with drug doses, serum levels, and renal function. In recent prospective and comparative clinical studies on the toxicity of gentamicin, tobramycin, amikacin, and netilmicin, objective testing has been used to a greater extent than previously [3, 15, 21, 27, 28, 30, 34, 39, 43, 46, 48, 54].

Audiometric monitoring may help to provide early evidence of decreased hearing, so that a drug can be discontinued in an effort to prevent further hearing loss. The practical usefulness of such monitoring has been questioned, since continued drug treatment is often indicated despite the appearance of ototoxicity, and since ototoxicity may progress or even appear after aminoglycoside therapy is discontinued. Some clinicians believe that symptoms of vestibular or auditory toxicity are readily apparent to the physician or patient, and that it is not necessary to rely on audiometry [4, 49]. Routine use of audiometry for monitoring has also been considered too costly, time-consuming, and not feasible for the seriously ill patient. Others feel that audiometry is potentially a useful procedure for monitoring of toxicity, at least in some patients [3, 5, 9, 15, 20, 29, 34, 35]. Yet audiometry is used inconsistently, without guidelines as to which patients should be monitored, what procedures should be used, and how the resulting information should be applied.

Audiometry serves two potential functions for patients undergoing aminoglycoside therapy: (1) prevention and reduction of the severity of ototoxicity and (2) identification of drug-induced hearing loss for immediate and appropriate rehabilitative management. Although the controversy about the use of audiometry centers mainly on its utility in prevention, we feel that this is secondary to its main contribution in identifying incurred hearing loss.

If audiometry detects minimal changes in auditory thresholds and the offending drug can be stopped, the hearing loss might stabilize sooner and at a less severe level, or might even return toward the baseline level. It has been amply demonstrated that behavioral observation of symptoms is not a reliable detector of early hearing loss [3, 24, 33, 38, 44, 54]. A mild to moderate hearing loss can go unnoticed by a patient who is not in his natural listening environment and may be in a generally depressed state brought on by serious illness.

In infants and prelanguage children, early identification of hearing loss is vitally important, but hearing loss is also more difficult to detect. Mild hearing loss of only 15 to 25 dB has been shown to have an adverse effect on language development and academic achievement [40]. The importance of early detection of hearing loss for immediate and long-term management is therefore of concern to physicians treating young children with ototoxic drugs.

Adults treated with ototoxic drugs may also be handicapped by resulting hearing loss. The critical degree of hearing loss is less obvious in adults than in children and varies among individuals, depending on their communication needs and adaptability. We know that many individuals with mild hearing decrease, such as 20 to 25 dB in the speech frequencies, often voluntarily seek

Table 15-1. University of Colorado Criteria for Selection of High-Risk Patients for Audiometric Monitoring During Therapy with Ototoxic Drugs

1. Ototoxic drug administered in the presence of decreased renal function
2. Ototoxic drug administered in increased daily doses or for an extended period
3. Assay showing high peak or trough level of ototoxic drug
4. Multiple ototoxic drugs administered concurrently or in consecutive courses (within 1 week)
5. Special patient conditions such as preexisting hearing loss or severe visual impairment or blindness
6. Ear symptoms reported by patient: tinnitus, hearing loss, dizziness

help for their communication problems. The American Medical Association recently accepted the recommendation of the American Academy of Ophthalmology and Otolaryngology that defines a beginning hearing handicap as 25 dB for the averaged frequencies of 0.5, 1.0, 2.0, and 3.0 kHz [19]. Of course, hearing at frequencies $\leq$ 3.0 kHz is generally affected later by aminoglycoside toxicity than is hearing at higher frequencies.

The audiometric monitoring program we have developed for use at our institution is applied only to patients receiving aminoglycosides who are considered to be at high risk for hearing loss. The procedure takes a short time, yields only essential information, involves the smallest possible number of hospital personnel, is minimally demanding of the seriously ill patient, and is done at reasonable cost. The program utilizes bedside testing with a portable audiometer; this is least demanding of the patient and other supportive personnel. Ambient noise in the hospital room usually does not significantly interfere with adequate pure-tone threshold measurements, since it affects only the lower frequencies (usually up to a maximum intensity of 20 dB hearing level) and not the higher test frequencies (2–8 kHz), which are of greatest interest in monitoring of ototoxicity. Testing can generally be completed in 10 minutes and is not costly. The fee in our hospital for an initial or follow-up bedside hearing test is less than that for a single serum creatinine value, creatinine clearance test, or serum drug assay.

We have encountered very few patients in whom audiometric testing with the techniques to be described could not be accomplished. Success in obtaining reliable test results is largely dependent on the skill of the person performing the test in eliciting good responses from patients who may be quite ill. In patients who are to receive sedatives, audiometric testing is scheduled prior to administration of such drugs, while they are optimally attentive. Patients who are so ill that their alertness is very depressed cannot respond reliably to psychoacoustic testing.

Table 15-1 indicates the risk factors we use in the selection of patients for audiometric monitoring. A patient meeting any one of the six criteria is monitored during drug therapy.

Testing is recommended for patients with decreased renal function, whether

Table 15-2. University of Colorado Protocol for Audiometric Monitoring of Patients on Ototoxic Drug Therapy

1. Baseline hearing level is established as soon as possible
2. Obtain air conduction thresholds bilaterally at 0.5, 1.0, 2.0, 4.0, and 8.0 kHz
3. If hearing loss is noted, bone conduction thresholds are obtained, and referral for additional audiologic and otologic work-up is considered
4. Patient is questioned about ear symptoms: tinnitus, hearing loss, dizziness. Dizzy patient is referred for electronystagmography
5. Results are recorded in patient's hospital chart
6. Criterion for change: $\leq$ 15 dB at any test frequency

or not adjustments in the dose of the ototoxic drug have been made. This includes patients with chronic or acute renal failure and patients who develop altered renal function during a course of therapy with nephrotoxic antibiotics.

Table 15-2 outlines our protocol for bedside testing. Air conduction thresholds at the indicated frequencies are obtained during each test in the course of drug therapy. Tests are repeated every 2 to 7 days, depending on the degree of risk of ototoxicity for the patient. Patients with a demonstrated decline in hearing or high serum levels are followed especially closely.

At present, there is no objective method, based on electronystagmographic techniques, that can be used at the bedside for routine monitoring of vestibular function. Therefore, we refer patients who develop symptoms of vestibular damage during the course of audiometric monitoring for whatever electronystagmographic evaluation can be undertaken. The development of a sensitive and reliable test of vestibular function to be utilized as a screening procedure would be a significant contribution, since patients with early vestibular damage are not always symptomatic. Vestibular damage has traditionally been viewed less seriously than hearing loss because of the compensatory mechanisms that may permit good subjective recovery from vestibular dysfunction. A number of patients, however, have suffered permanent debility due to ototoxic vestibular impairment [8, 9, 18, 53].

An audiometric record is maintained in the patient's hospital chart. A brief interpretive comment is included in the daily progress notes of the chart. Our criterion for a possible change in hearing is a decrease in sensitivity of at least 15 dB at any test frequency. The physician is notified, and the testing schedule is altered as follows: (1) If the physician indicates that there is a possibility of altering drug therapy, daily audiometric testing is continued to confirm the change in hearing or a possible progression of hearing loss. (2) If the physician indicates that there is no possibility of altering drug therapy, testing is continued every 3 days.

Our follow-up procedures are summarized in Table 15-3. Emphasis in our audiometric monitoring program is on identification of drug-induced hearing loss for appropriate management. In some cases, the first follow-up test, at 1 week after drug therapy, can be accomplished while the patient is still hos-

Table 15-3. Follow-up Protocol Used for Audiometric Monitoring of Patients Treated with Ototoxic Drugs

1. Bedside testing continued to the end of drug therapy
2. After drug therapy, audiometric tests done at 1 week, 1 month, and 3 months after therapy; additional periodic testing until the toxicity has stabilized
3. Follow-up of infants may be necessary up to age 3 to 4 years
4. Counseling, rehabilitation assistance provided as necessary

pitalized. Before the patient is discharged, the audiologist schedules a return appointment for the next follow-up hearing test in the clinic. The testing protocol described in Table 15-2 is used for follow-up tests given in the audiology clinic, as well as for outpatients who are monitored in the clinic during drug therapy.

We use the criteria described in Table 15-3 for selection of "high-risk" pediatric patients on ototoxic drugs who are to receive routine audiometric tests. The testing techniques described, however, must obviously be altered for infants and preschool children. Testing techniques for children from birth through the preschool years have been described in detail [41]. The main difficulty is adequate follow-up, as it may be necessary to follow children up to the age of 3 to 4 years, when standard audiometric testing can be completed. The primary physician can be helpful in this regard in supporting and encouraging follow-up tests.

The clinical measurement of high-frequency hearing (8 kHz to 18 kHz) has been investigated as a means of early detection of drug ototoxicity. In the late 1960s, following the development of the Rudmose clinical suprahigh-frequency audiometer [16, 37], a number of studies were published suggesting various clinical applications of high-frequency audiometry [10, 50, 51]. High-frequency hearing was evaluated in patients with meningitis [17], noise-induced hearing loss [6], and coronary heart disease [45], and also in patients receiving ototoxic drugs [23]. In the last study, the authors tested seven kanamycin-treated patients on a weekly basis by using the Rudmose audiometer. Each patient's initial audiogram was used as a control; 4 patients revealed marked high-frequency changes which were identified 41 to 76 days prior to detection of a hearing change in the conventional frequency range.

By 1972, interim threshold reference levels at frequencies between 8 kHz and 18 kHz were recommended [42]. The Rudmose high-frequency audiometer fell into disrepute because of equipment problems, however. Therefore, a number of clinicians have developed their own instrument systems for studying the significance of high-frequency hearing loss in certain diseases [2, 7].

Stephen Fausti and others in the Auditory Research Laboratory at the Portland Veterans Administration Medical Center have been active in high-frequency audiometric evaluations since 1975, particularly in relation to ototoxicity [14]. They have developed a new testing system reported to amplify high-frequency signals with high fidelity through an earphone with a ceramic diaphragm (Koss, Model HV/IA), one which can be calibrated similarly to conventional audiometers. They have accumulated normative data and, apparently, a satisfactory testing technique [14]. Fausti has conducted studies on high-frequency hearing during the administration of known and potentially ototoxic drugs. He reports that, with high-frequency audiometry, he detects ototoxicity earlier than with conventional audiometric testing, although the time between drug therapy and hearing loss varies considerably among patients.

High-frequency audiometry has not yet reached the stage of routine clinical application. Well-standardized data on threshold norms and test-retest reliability must be obtained. Reliable portable equipment to be used at the bedside is not yet available. In our experience with the Rudmose high-frequency audiometer, patients often stated that the high-frequency signals were much more difficult to listen to than pure-tone signals in the standard audiometric range.

Undoubtedly, some of the limitations of high-frequency audiometry will be overcome as more research data are gathered, but whether high-frequency audiometry should replace standard-frequency audiometry as a clinical technique for monitoring of the effects of ototoxic drug therapy is still subject to debate. If the primary role of a monitoring program is to identify hearing loss incurred as a result of therapy with ototoxic drugs, the method of choice is still conventional audiometry. If, however, monitoring audiometry is viewed as an aid in the prevention of ototoxic effects, the high-frequency technique may be preferable.

Whether conventional or high-frequency audiometry is preferred for monitoring, a threshold technique should be utilized rather than screening at some suprathreshold level. A screening method would not have the sensitivity of a threshold technique in detecting early and minimal changes in hearing sensitivity.

The basis of a practical audiometric monitoring program is the selection of patients to be tested rather than which audiometric technique is to be used, since it is neither feasible nor justifiable to test all patients treated with ototoxic drugs.

Comments

We have described an audiometric monitoring program in which the primary purpose is to identify patients with hearing loss caused by therapy with ototoxic drugs, so that such patients can receive immediate and appropriate rehabilitative guidance. Such a monitoring program may also be of help in the prevention of ototoxicity. Specific criteria are listed according to which our patients at high risk for ototoxic hearing loss are tested. We have described specific audiometric procedures which we use in a monitoring program. Clinical application has shown the procedures discussed here to be time- and cost-efficient and feasible for most patients. The testing program needs to be applied more rigorously to greater numbers of patients, so that its sensitivity can be determined and guidelines established for various risk factors and testing schedules.

References

1. Bamford, M. F., and Jones, L. F. Deafness and biochemical imbalance after burns treatment with topical antibiotics in young children: Report of 6 cases. *Arch. Dis. Child.* 53:326, 1978.
2. Berlin, C. I., Wexler, K. F., Jerger, J. F., Halperin, H. R., and Smith, S. Superior ultra-audiometric hearing: A new type of hearing loss which correlates highly with unusually good speech in the "profoundly deaf." *Otolaryngology* 86:ORL-111, 1978.
3. Black, R. E., Lau, W., Weinstein, R. J., Young, L. S., and Hewitt, W. L. Ototoxicity of amikacin. *Antimicrob. Agents Chemother.* 9:956, 1976.
4. Bodey, G. P. Discussion following session on review of clinical trials with amikacin. Ninth International Congress of Chemotherapy. *J. Infect. Dis.* 134 [*Suppl.*]:S447, 1976.
5. Carey, J. T., and Wichter, M. D. Testing for ototoxicity: Amikacin and gentamicin (Letter to the editor). *N. Engl. J. Med.* 296:1124, 1977.
6. Corliss, L. M., Doster, M. E., Simonton, J., et al. High frequency and regular audiometry among selected groups of high school students. *J. Sch. Health* 40:400, 1970.
7. Cunningham, D. R., and Goetzinger, C. P. Extra-high frequency hearing loss and hyperlipidemia. *Audiology* 13:470, 1974.
8. Dayal, V. S., Chait, G. E., and Fenton, S. S. Gentamicin vestibulotoxicity: Long term disability. *Ann. Otol. Rhinol. Laryngol.* 88:36, 1979.
9. Dayal, V. S., Smith, E. L., and McCain, W. G. Cochlear and vestibular gentamicin toxicity. A clinical study of systemic and topical usage. *Arch. Otolaryngol.* 100:338, 1974.
10. Downs, M. P., Hemenway, W. G., and Doster, M. E. Sensory overload. *Hear. Speech News* 37:10, 1969.
11. Echeverria, P., Fina, D., Norton, S., and Smith, A. L. Ototoxicity of gentamicin: Clinical experience in a children's hospital. *Chemotherapy* 24:267, 1978.
12. Elfving, J., Pettay, O., and Raivio, M. A follow-up study on the cochlear, vestibular and renal function in children treated with gentamicin in the newborn period. *Chemotherapy* 18:141, 1973.
13. Fausti, S. A., Frey, R. H., Rappaport, B. Z., and Erickson, D. A. An investigation of the effect of bumetanide on high frequency (8–20 KHz) hearing in humans. *J. Aud. Res.* 19:243, 1979.
14. Fausti, S. A., Frey, R. H., Erickson, D. A., Rappaport, B. Z., and Cleary, E. J. A system for evaluating auditory function from 8000–20,000 Hz. *J. Acoust. Soc. Am.* 66:1713, 1979.
15. Fee, W. E., Jr., Vierra, V., and Lathrop, G. R. Clinical evaluation of aminoglycoside toxicity: Tobramycin versus gentamicin, a preliminary report. *J. Antimicrob. Chemother.* [A] 4:31, 1978.
16. Fletcher, J. L. Reliability of high-frequency thresholds. *J. Aud. Res.* 5:133, 1965.
17. Fletcher, J. L., Cairns, A. B., Collins, F. G., and Endicott, J. High frequency hearing following meningitis. *J. Aud. Res.* 7:223, 1967.
18. Gailiunas, P., Jr., Dominguez-Moreno, M., Lazarus, M., Lowrie, E. G., Gottlieb, M. N., and Merrill, J. P. Vestibular toxicity of gentamicin. Incidence in patients receiving long-term hemodialysis therapy. *Arch. Intern. Med.* 138:1621, 1978.
19. Guide for the evaluation of hearing handicap. American Academy of Otolaryngol-

ogy Committee on Hearing and Equilibrium, and American Council of Otolaryngology Committee on the Medical Aspects of Noise. *J.A.M.A.* 241:2055, 1979.
20. Gydé, M. C. When the weeping stopped: An otologist views otorrhea and gentamicin. *Arch. Otolaryngol.* 102:542, 1976.
21. Huizing, E. H., and Carrière, E. G. J. Hearing loss due to gentamicin therapy. *ORL* 37:359, 1975.
22. Jackson, G. G., and Arcieri, G. Ototoxicity of gentamicin in man. A survey and controlled analysis of clinical experience in the United States. *J. Infect. Dis.* 24[*Suppl.*]:S130, 1971.
23. Jacobson, E. J., Downs, M. P., and Fletcher, J. L. Clinical findings in high-frequency thresholds during known ototoxic drug usage. *J. Aud. Res.* 9:379, 1969.
24. Johnsonbaugh, R. E., Drexler, H. G., Light, I. J., and Sutherland, J. M. Familial occurrence of drug-induced hearing loss. *Am. J. Dis. Child.* 127:245, 1974.
25. Jones, H. C. Intrauterine ototoxicity. A case report and review of literature. *J. Natl. Med. Assoc.* 65:201, 1973.
26. Kricsfeld, B., and Ware, F. Gentamicin neurotoxicity: A case report. *Nebr. Med. J.* 61:291, 1976.
27. Lane, A. Z., Wright, G. E., and Blair, D. C. Ototoxicity and nephrotoxicity of amikacin: An overview of phase II and phase III experience in the United States. *Am. J. Med.* 62:911, 1977.
28. Lau, W. K., Young, L. S., Black, R. E., et al. Comparative efficacy and toxicity of amikacin/carbenicillin versus gentamicin/carbenicillin in leukopenic patients: A randomized prospective trial. *Am. J. Med.* 62:959, 1977.
29. Lerner, S. A., and Matz, G. J. Suggestions for monitoring patients during treatment with aminoglycoside antibiotics. *Otolaryngol. Head Neck Surg.* 87:222, 1979.
30. Lerner, S. A., Seligsohn, R., and Matz, G. J. Comparative clinical studies of ototoxicity and nephrotoxicity of amikacin and gentamicin. *Am. J. Med.* 62:919, 1977.
31. Little, P. J., and Lynn, K. L. Letter: Neomycin toxicity. *N.Z. Med. J.* 81:445, 1975.
32. Lowry, L. D., May, M., and Pastore, P. Acute histopathologic inner ear changes in deafness due to neomycin: A case report. *Ann. Otol. Rhinol. Laryngol.* 82:876, 1973.
33. Masur, H., Whelton, P. K., and Whelton, A. Neomycin toxicity revisited. *Arch. Surg.* 111:822, 1976.
34. Meyer, R. D., Lewis, R. P., Carmalt, E. D., et al. Amikacin therapy for serious gram-negative bacillary infections. *Ann. Intern. Med.* 83:790, 1975.
35. Mittelman, H. Ototoxicity of "ototopical" antibiotics: Past, present and future. *Trans. Am. Acad. Ophthalmol. Otolaryngol.* 76:1432, 1972.
36. Moffat, D. A., and Ramsden, R. T. Profound bilateral sensorineural hearing loss during gentamicin therapy. *J. Laryngol. Otol.* 91:511, 1977.
37. Myers, C. K., and Harris, J. D. Comparison of seven systems for air conduction audiometry from 8-20 KC-S. United States Navy Submarine Medical Center Laboratory, Report No. 567, 1969.
38. Noone, P., Pattison, J. R., and Davies, D. G. The effective use of gentamicin in life-threatening sepsis. *Postgrad. Med. J.* 50[Suppl. 7]:9, 1974.
39. Nordström, L., Banck, G., Belfrage, S., Juhlin, I., Tjernström, Ö., and Toremalm, N. G. Prospective study of the ototoxicity of gentamicin. *Acta Pathol. Microbiol. Scand.* [*B*] [*Suppl.* 241]:58, 1973.
40. Northern, J. L., and Downs, M. P. In *Hearing in Children* (2nd ed.). Baltimore: Williams & Wilkins, 1979. Pp. 1–15.
41. Northern, J. L., and Downs, M. P. In *Hearing in Children* (2nd ed.). Baltimore: Williams & Wilkins, 1979. Pp. 113–147.
42. Northern, J. L., Downs, M. P., Rudmose, W., Glorig, A., and Fletcher, J. L. Recommended high-frequency audiometric threshold levels (8000 to 18000 Hz). *J. Acous. Soc. Am.* 52:585, 1972.

43. Panwalker, A. P., et al. Netilmicin: Clinical efficacy, tolerance and toxicity. *Antimicrob. Agents Chemother.* 13:170, 1978.
44. Pražić, M., and Salaj, B. Ototoxicity with children caused by streptomycin. *Audiology* 14:173, 1975.
45. Rosen, S., and Olin, P. Hearing loss and coronary heart disease. *Arch. Otolaryngol.* 82:236, 1965.
46. Smith, C. R., Baughman, K. L., Edwards, C. Q., Rogers, J. F., and Lietman, P. S. Controlled comparison of amikacin and gentamicin. *N. Engl. J. Med.* 296:349, 1977.
47. Sugarbaker, P. H., Sabath, L. D., and Morgan, A. P. Neomycin toxicity from porcine skin xenografts. *Ann. Surg.* 179:183, 1974.
48. Tjernström, Ö., Banck, G., Belfrage, S., Juhlin, I., Nordström, L., and Toremalm, N. G. The ototoxicity of gentamicin. *Acta Pathol. Microbiol. Scand.* [*B*] [*Suppl.* 241]:73, 1973.
49. Torok, N. Discussion following session on pharmacology and toxicity. International Symposium on Gentamicin. *J. Infect. Dis.* 119:442, 1969.
50. Vassallo, L., Sataloff, J., and Menduke, H. Air conduction thresholds for high frequencies. *J. Occup. Med.* 9:353, 1967.
51. Vassallo, L., Sataloff, J., and Menduke, H. Very high frequency audiometric technique. *Arch. Otolaryngol.* 88:251, 1968.
52. Ward, K. M., and Rounthwaite, F. J. Neomycin ototoxicity. *Ann. Otol. Rhinol. Laryngol.* 87:211, 1978.
53. Wilmot, T. J. Vestibular analysis in streptomycin ototoxicity. *J. Laryngol. Otol.* 87:235, 1973.
54. Winkel, O., Hansen, M. M., Kaaber, K., and Rozarth, K. A prospective study of gentamicin ototoxicity. *Acta Otolaryngol.* 86:212, 1978.

Discussion of Chapter 15

Dr. Matz: What is your definition of baseline audiometry at your institution? Would you consider obtaining a baseline audiogram within the first 48 to 72 hours, or does it have to be before drug therapy?

Mrs. Thompson: Naturally, you want to test the patient before drug therapy, but it is just not practical; so, if you can test within 24 to 48 hours, I think that is reasonable, and it is possible in many cases. I think it is a misconception that auditory symptoms will be apparent to either the physician or the patient; this is not always the case in patients with ototoxic hearing loss. It has been amply demonstrated that even moderate hearing loss can go unnoticed by the patient who is not in a natural listening environment and may be seriously ill. Therefore, clinical observation of symptoms is an inadequate way of monitoring hearing loss.

If a physician refers a patient to me who has been on gentamicin for 2 weeks and is already complaining of symptoms, I won't say I can't test the patient because baseline audiometry is lacking. Audiometric testing is important if you find hearing loss at that time. You merely have to be careful about the judgment you make as to the cause of the hearing loss in this instance, but the information can be used for management of the patient.

Dr. Smith: In some of our patients, we have wondered how to interpret a single-frequency change at 500 Hz of 15 dB or more in the audiometric threshold. How would you interpret that kind of clinical information, and what would you do about it in terms of the aminoglycoside treatment of the patient?

Mrs. Thompson: Ambient noise is a problem at 500 Hz. In a noisy hospital room where there is supportive equipment, a normal low-frequency threshold can be depressed by as much as 30 dB. I like to include testing at 500 Hz, because some of the ototoxic diuretics have resulted in changes at lower frequencies and in a trough- or flat-type audiogram rather than a high-frequency loss. I think a minimal change in the audiogram indicates the need to step up your testing schedule and to follow the patient to see if there is progression of hearing loss.

Dr. Smith: So you would disregard low-frequency change as possibly being related to aminoglycoside toxicity?

Mrs. Thompson: No. If the noise in the hospital room remains the same, a change in the audiogram would indicate possible ototoxicity.

Dr. Federspil: I think it is important to question patients treated with gentamicin and tobramycin about dizziness, and to test vestibular function.

Mrs. Thompson: I agree. I excluded vestibular testing from my paper, since it is a topic left up to other people in this symposium.

16. Auditory and Vestibular Assessment of Patients Receiving Aminoglycosides

Harris J. Mowry, James W. Roeder, Gregory J. Matz, and Stephen A. Lerner

The reported incidence of auditory and vestibular toxicity brought on by aminoglycoside therapy has been highly variable, ranging from less than 1 percent to more than 20 percent (Chap. 23). This variability can be attributed in part to a lack of uniform, consistent procedures for audiometric and vestibular evaluation.

We have found it impractical to monitor the hearing and vestibular function of all patients receiving aminoglycosides. There are several categories of high-risk patients, however, who may benefit from periodic audiometric and vestibular evaluations if their clinical condition permits it. These patients include (1) individuals receiving a prolonged course of aminoglycoside therapy, (2) patients with a previous history of ototoxicity, and (3) those with occupations in which even mild auditory or vestibular toxicity could prove catastrophic. It is especially important to monitor auditory and vestibular function in these patients, because toxicity that is subclinical initially may not become apparent until they return to work.

Audiometric Evaluation

All audiometric studies in our clinic are performed by a qualified audiologist. Additionally, all patients to be evaluated with audiometry and electronystagmography are examined by an otolaryngologist who can determine whether there is any condition, e.g., impacted cerumen or a perforated tympanic membrane, that would preclude testing or could seriously affect the reliability of the test results.

For uniformity of audiometric test results, the procedures and audiometric symbols in ANSI Standard S3.21-1978 [1], Methods for Manual Pure-Tone Threshold Audiometry, are used for all patients.

When an audiometric protocol is established for monitoring of patients receiving aminoglycosides, it will not always be possible to meet the background noise criteria specified in ANSI Standard S3.1-1977 [2], especially for patients whose clinical condition requires that they be tested at the bedside. In many typical hospital rooms, the background noise level at 0.25 to 0.75 kHz is too great to permit reliable threshold measurements. Although it is desirable to obtain thresholds at these low frequencies, thresholds obtained above 1.0 kHz are more critical for monitoring of effects of aminoglycoside ototoxicity. In our clinical practice, we obtain pure-tone thresholds at 1.0, 2.0, 3.0, 4.0, 6.0, and 8.0 kHz; 0.25 and 0.5 kHz are included only when the examiner feels that the thresholds obtained are accurate. The threshold at 6 kHz is included to corroborate a deficit at 8 kHz, which is often difficult to assess, especially if the patient complains of high-pitched tinnitus. In some instances, variability in the patient's high-frequency thresholds resulting from confusion of the test tone with high-frequency tinnitus can be overcome if a pulsed rather than a continuous tone is used. If the baseline audiogram is obtained with pulsed tones, all subsequent audiograms are obtained with pulsed tones. A second reason for testing at 6 kHz is to assist in differentiating ototoxicity from hearing loss secondary to a standing wave in the ear canal at 8 kHz.*

As an alternative to audiometric testing outside a sound-isolated room, several manufacturers have introduced audiometric receiver enclosures intended to reduce the ambient noise level. We do not use these routinely because of difficulties encountered in calibration of the headphones mounted in the enclosures. Furthermore, some of these noise-excluding headsets have been designed with headbands that apply excessive pressure. With this increased pressure, the incidence of hearing loss caused by collapsible ear canals increases significantly.

For patients receiving aminoglycoside therapy, we consider it acceptable to perform baseline audiometric studies within the first 72 hours after initiation of therapy. Justification of this baseline period is derived from other studies in man and animals indicating that ototoxicity generally does not appear earlier than 5 days after the initiation of aminoglycoside treatment [16]. If the results of the baseline study are abnormal, additional tests of speech discrimination, tone decay, alternate binaural loudness balance, and impedance audiometry may be indicated. After the baseline studies, we perform audiometric evaluations at weekly intervals. A deterioration from the baseline values of at least 15 dB at two or more frequencies in both the air and bone conduction thresholds for either ear is considered possible evidence of ototoxicity. The patient's physician is then informed of the result. We obtain a second audiogram within 48 hours to verify such a finding.

Despite evidence of auditory toxicity, a patient's medical condition may necessitate the use of an aminoglycoside for effective treatment of infection.

*A standing wave is created whenever a pure tone is introduced into a closed system having the same length as the wavelength of the tone. The tone reflected from the closed end of the system cancels the original one because the two tones are 180 degrees out of phase. This cancellation effect is frequently seen at 8 kHz, where the wavelength of the tone and the distance from the diaphragm of an audiometric headphone to the eardrum are often equal (about 1½ inches).

Any individual in whom ototoxicity has been identified is then evaluated twice weekly. After treatment has been discontinued, the patient is reevaluated 1 week and, if possible, 3 months after the last dose of the drug.

High-Frequency Audiometry

Experiments in animals have shown that aminoglycoside ototoxicity is detectable initially at ultrahigh frequencies, and the effects on auditory function are then seen at progressively decreasing frequencies [7, 12, 14]. Jacobson et al. [15] noted that high-frequency audiometry (above 8 kHz) was effective in monitoring of ototoxicity in patients receiving either kanamycin or streptomycin therapy for tuberculosis. Decreased high-frequency auditory sensitivity was apparent prior to reports of tinnitus and before the onset of hearing loss as detected by conventional pure-tone audiometry.

Investigations are under way at several institutions on refinement of the instrumentation for high-frequency audiometry and on high-frequency hearing in patients receiving a variety of potentially ototoxic drugs.

Auditory Brainstem Responses (ABR)

Auditory brainstem responses are both cochlear and central auditory responses to sound. The recording of ABR has the advantages of being noninvasive and can be used in patients whose medical condition precludes administration of conventional audiometric tests. Several investigators [3, 10, 17, 18] have been able to measure ABR thresholds at 1, 2, and 4 kHz to within 15 to 25 dB of thresholds obtained with standard pure-tone audiometry. Before ABR can be used in the evaluation of ototoxicity, however, studies concerning the test-retest variability of ABR thresholds in both normal and hearing-impaired individuals must be performed. At this time, we are not certain how much of a shift from the baseline ABR threshold can be considered evidence of ototoxicity.

Vestibular Testing

In addition to impairing cochlear function, aminoglycosides may be toxic to the vestibular system. Patients who develop symptoms including vertigo, nausea, instability of gait, and difficulties with ocular fixation during their treatment course may be experiencing vestibular toxicity. In many instances, however, it is extremely difficult to differentiate between balance disorders resulting from vestibular toxicity and those resulting from deterioration in the patient's condition, central nervous system disorders, or concomitant drug therapy. The majority of patients in whom we have identified vestibular toxicity were asymptomatic during their hospitalization.

The standard test employed in the evaluation of vestibular function is the Fitzgerald-Hallpike Bithermal Caloric Test with electronystagmographic recording of the response [13]. As a screening test of vestibular function, some clinicians utilize caloric stimulation and observe the nystagmus through Frenzel glasses. This technique is not satisfactory for monitoring the effects of ototoxic drugs on the vestibular system because the only nystagmus parameter which can be evaluated is duration. Several investigators [13] (see also Chap. 22) have concluded that duration is the most variable of nystagmus parameters, and they discourage the use of this measure. Another severe limitation of this screening caloric test is that there is no objective means of comparing one test with another. We strongly advocate graphic recording of the nystagmus, especially in patients for whom serial examinations of vestibular function are indicated. A number of recorders specifically designed for recording of eye movements are commercially available. We use nystagmographs capable of recording in both AC and DC modes. For a more detailed discussion of nystagmographs, the reader is referred to papers by Barber et al. [4] and Coats [8].

In our clinics, any patient receiving an aminoglycoside and requiring monitoring of the vestibular system during therapy is given an otologic examination to ascertain that the tympanic membranes are visible and intact and that there are no conditions that would preclude caloric irrigation. Electrodes are attached in the conventional configuration [4, 8], while the patient is lying on the examination table with the back elevated to 30 degrees. Considerable care is taken in attaching of the electrodes, since poor skin contact will result in poor recordings of eye movement. Once the electrodes have been attached and the electrode leads connected to the recorder, the patient is asked to gaze straight ahead. The tracing obtained should appear clear and unwavering.

If the tracing is satisfactory, the examiner checks the polarity of the electrodes by having the patient look alternately to the right and left, then up and down. In electronystagmography, movement of the eyes to the right should (by convention) yield an upward deflection of the pen; movement of the eyes to the left should yield a downward deflection. If a second recording channel is used, upward and downward eye movements yield corresponding deflections.

Calibration is accomplished by having the patient look alternately between two dots (lights) separated by a distance yielding a 20-degree movement of the eyes. The recorder is adjusted so that 20 degrees of eye movement yields a 20-mm pen deflection. A similar procedure is used in the calibration of the recorder for vertical eye movements.

In tests of vestibular function on patients receiving aminoglycoside therapy, calibration of the nystagmograph, examination for preexisting nystagmus, and bithermal caloric testing are carried out. One may also record spontaneous, optokinetic, gaze, and positional nystagmus. It is necessary to examine the patient for preexisting nystagmus while he is in the caloric test position, so that a correction can be applied to nystagmus induced by caloric stimulation. In this position, the lateral semicircular canal is oriented in a vertical plane and thus maximally stimulated with caloric irrigations. The test is carried out with the eyes closed, in a dimly lit room. The recorder is allowed to run for at least 15 seconds prior to the irrigation, and the patient is given mental alerting tasks to perform. We irrigate each ear canal for 30 seconds with water at 30°C and at 44°C. The temperature of the water at the irrigator tip is carefully regulated to within 0.5°C. The irrigations are carried out in the following sequence: 30°C left, 30°C right, 44°C left, and 44°C right, with rest periods of at least 8 minutes between irrigations.

In analyzing the record for nystagmus induced by caloric irrigation, the examiner may note that some patients with normal vestibular function have only a marginal response. In many of these cases, the response becomes more pronounced if the examiner gently holds the patient's eyelids. The most common causes of a weak or absent response are a break or short circuit in an electrode lead or in the electrode input cable, inadequate irrigation, inability to keep the patient mentally alert, and recent administration of a central nervous system depressant. To assure valid and reliable test results, the cause for an unexpected weak or absent caloric response must be identified and corrected. This may necessitate having the patient return for vestibular testing at a later date.

In patients with perforated tympanic membranes, caloric irrigations with water are contraindicated. In these instances, caloric studies may be performed with air [5, 9], in a closed-loop system [6], or with a protective latex fingercot inserted into the external auditory canal [11]. Before these alternative techniques are applied in the clinical evaluation of vestibular toxicity, however, test-retest data on subjects with normal vestibular function are needed. It should be noted that data obtained with these techniques cannot be compared directly to data obtained with conventional caloric testing. In our opinion, this is not a serious shortcoming in the evaluation of vestibular toxicity, since, for any given patient, one is most concerned with changes from baseline values.

We perform baseline vestibular studies, like audiometric studies, within 72 hours after the start of treatment. After the baseline study, vestibular tests are carried out at weekly intervals. The maximum average slow-phase velocity for each ear is determined during irrigation with water at 30°C and at 44°C. The two velocities for a given ear are averaged. A decrease in one of these mean values of 50 percent or more from baseline is regarded as possible evidence of vestibular toxicity in the corresponding ear. We perform a second vestibular study within 48 hours to verify this finding. If the repeat electronystagmogram still indicates ototoxicity, the patient's physician is so informed.

Comments

Audiometric testing, in general, is easier to perform than vestibular testing on ill patients, since examinations with portable audiometric equipment can be carried out at the bedside. Inter- and intrasubject variability is less for audiometric than for vestibular examinations. For these reasons, in most large series of aminoglycoside-treated patients, vestibular tests have been performed only sparingly (see Chap. 23). High-frequency audiometry promises to be a predictor of subclinical ototoxicity, provided that normative and test-retest standards can be developed along with a reliable bedside portable high-frequency audiometer.

The problem encountered most frequently in the assessment of vestibular function in patients receiving aminoglycosides is that the serious medical condition of many of these patients at the outset of therapy, or after deterioration during the course of therapy, precludes valid and reliable caloric testing. Most patients undergoing caloric studies experience minimal or no side effects.

Some patients, however, become extremely nauseated and vertiginous during caloric testing. Such patients usually refuse to participate in any future vestibular tests.

It is likely that many of the disadvantages encountered in vestibular testing can be eliminated, or at least greatly reduced, with precisely controlled testing in a rotating chair [19]. Although we have not applied rotational testing in monitoring vestibular function of patients receiving ototoxic drugs, data obtained on patients with normal vestibular function, and on patients with a variety of peripheral and central vestibular lesions, indicate that the technique may be highly promising for evaluation of vestibular toxicity.

References

1. American National Standards Institute. Standard S3.21-1978. Methods for manual pure-tone threshold audiometry.
2. American National Standards Institute. Standard S3.1-1977. Criteria for permissible ambient noise during audiometric testing.
3. Anthony, P. F., Durrett, R., Pulec, J. L., and Hartstone, J. L. A new parameter in brainstem evoked response: Component wave areas. *Laryngoscope* 89:1569, 1979.
4. Barber, H. O., and Stockwell, C. W. *Manual of Electronystagmography.* St. Louis: Mosby, 1976.
5. Barber, H. O., Harmand, W. M., and Money, K. E. Air caloric stimulation with tympanic membrane perforation. *Laryngoscope* 88:1117, 1978.
6. Brookler, K. H., Baker, A. H., and Grams, G. Closed loop water irrigation system. *Otolaryngol. Head Neck Surg.* 87:364, 1979.
7. Brummett, R. E. Drug-induced ototoxicity. *Drugs* 19:412, 1980.
8. Coats, A. C. *Manual of Electronystagmographic Technique.* Houston: L. T. Instruments, 1971.
9. Coats, A. C., Hebert, F., and Atwood, G. The air caloric test, a parametric study. *Arch. Otolaryngol.* 102:343, 1976.
10. Davis, H., and Hirsch, S. K. The audiometric utility of brain-stem responses to low frequency sounds. *Audiology* 15:181, 1976.
11. Eviatar, A., and Goodhill, V. A dry calorization method for vestibular function studies. *Laryngoscope* 78:1746, 1968.
12. Fausti, S. A., Frey, R. H., Erickson, D. A., Rappaport, B. Z., Cleary, E. J., and Brummett, R. E. A system for evaluating auditory function from 8000 to 20,000 hertz. *J. Acoust. Soc. Am.* 66:1713, 1979.
13. Fitzgerald, G., and Hallpike, C. S. Observations on the directional preponderance of caloric nystagmus resulting from cerebral lesions. *Brain* 65:115, 1942.
14. Hawkins, J. E., Stebbins, W. C., Johnsson, L-G., Moody, B. D., and Muraski, A. The patas monkey as a model for dihydrostreptomycin ototoxicity. *Acta Otolaryngol.* 83:123, 1977.
15. Jacobson, E. J., Downs, M. T., and Fletcher, J. L. Clinical findings in high frequency thresholds during known ototoxic drug usage. *J. Aud. Res.* 9:379, 1969.
16. Lerner, S. A., and Matz, G. J. Aminoglycoside ototoxicity. *Am. J. Otolaryngol.* 1:169, 1980.
17. Picton, T. W., Ouellett, J., Hamal, G., and Smith, A. D. Brainstem evoked potentials to tone pips and notch noise. *J. Otolaryngol.* 8:289, 1979.
18. Suzuki, T., Hirai, Y., and Horiuchi, K. Auditory brainstem responses to pure tone stimuli. *Scand. Audiol.* 6:51, 1977.
19. Van Egmond, A. A. J., Groen, J. J., and Jongkees, L. B. W. The turning test with small regulable stimuli. I. Method of examination: Cupulometria. *J. Laryngol. Otol.* 2:63, 1948.

17. Transtympanic Electrocochleographic Monitoring of the Immediate Effects of Tobramycin and Gentamicin

Richard T. Ramsden

Our understanding of the electrical events occurring in the inner ear and in its central connections following acoustic stimulation has increased greatly since the identification, in the 1930s, of the cochlear microphonic (CM) and the eighth nerve action potential (AP) by Wever and Bray [17] and by Saul and Davis [13]. The development of relatively inexpensive and compact electronic averaging equipment has allowed physicians to use for clinical purposes many of the observations hitherto noted in the animal laboratory, thus opening up the field of clinical electric response audiometry (ERA).

The occurrence of these electrical phenomena in the peripheral receptor, the eighth nerve, the brainstem with its various relay stations, the higher centers, and the cerebral cortex can be monitored on the oscilloscope screen. The responses are identified by means of their latency, magnitude, polarity, and waveform. Their detection is of great value in the objective assessment of auditory threshold, and alteration in one or more of their characteristic features may, in many instances, assist in localizing pathologic changes within the auditory pathway. At present, the two most useful techniques in clinical practice are brainstem evoked response audiometry (BERA) and electrocochleography (ECoG).

Electrocochleography assesses the earliest electric responses to a sound stimulus—those occurring in the cochlea itself and in the eighth nerve. In a normal ear, at high stimulus intensity, these events are over within 2 msec of the stimulus, and their magnitude is in the range of 1 to 50 μV. Identification of such small responses is facilitated by the positioning of the recording electrode as near as possible to their sites of origin. Although it is possible to

My co-workers in this study were Dr. Peter Wilson and Dr. W. P. R. Gibson of the Departments of Microbiology and Otolaryngology, The London Hospital, E.1.

I am grateful to the editor of the *Journal of Laryngology and Otology* for permission to publish the illustrations, and to the Department of Medical Illustration, Manchester Royal Infirmary, Manchester, for their preparation.

obtain adequate recordings from an electrode placed in the external auditory meatus, close to the drum, much larger and clearer waveforms are obtained from the promontory overlying the basal turn of the cochlea. Early workers in clinical electrocochleography attempted to place the recording electrode onto the round window membrane. Although they were often successful in recording potentials if the electrode was well positioned, the obliquity of the round window niche made placement of the electrode very difficult; furthermore, the potentials obtained were often very small and difficult to identify. The introduction of the electronic technique of time-domain averaging revolutionized electrocochleography by enabling the desired response to be enhanced and the unwanted random background electrical activity to be suppressed. Thus, good recordings could be obtained from electrode positions somewhat remote from the round window: the external meatus [19], the earlobe [15] and mastoid process [16], and the nasopharynx [7]. The clearest potentials, however, are obtained from a transtympanic needle electrode situated on the promontory. This technique has been widely employed in France by Portmann and his co-workers [10] and by most investigators in the United Kingdom [3, 12].

Materials and Method

With the patient lying relaxed on a couch, a fine sterile stainless steel electrode of approximately 0.3-mm diameter is passed under microscopic control through the posteroinferior quadrant of the tympanic membrane, midway between the umbo and the annulus, and is advanced until it comes to rest on the medial wall of the middle ear. The tip of the needle is placed on the promontory, which overlies the basal coil of the cochlea, close to the round window. Anesthesia of the tympanic membrane is achieved by iontophoresis of a solution of 2% lidocaine and 1:2,000 adrenalin [11]. A current of 0.5 mA is passed through this solution for 10 minutes, and the drum is totally anesthetized for up to 2 hours. The only discomfort occasionally experienced may occur when the tip of the needle makes contact with the promontory, which is not affected by the iontophoresis, causing mild temporary irritation in the throat by referred pain through the glossopharyngeal nerve. Of several hundred transtympanic ECoGs performed by the author, fewer than a dozen have had to be abandoned because of discomfort. Those patients who had both ECoG and caloric tests of labyrinthine function usually stated a preference for ECoG. No permanent perforations have occurred. Indeed, it is often impossible, even immediately after the needle has been removed, to detect the point of perforation. No otitis media has followed ECoG in our experience.

The active (transtympanic), reference (ear lobe), and ground (forehead) electrodes are connected via a preamplifier to the averaging and display device (Medelec Amplaid Mark III system). Acoustic stimuli, produced by a research audiometer, are introduced to the ear through a shielded metal earphone attached magnetically to a headband which also supports the needle electrode. The most commonly used stimuli have been a 100-μsec electrical click of a wide-frequency spectrum, with the maximum energy at 3 kHz, and pure-tone bursts of 2 to 6 sine waves at specific audiometric frequencies.

The electrical activity recorded by transtympanic ECoG is a complex mixture of several components. The three most important of these are the cochlear microphonic (CM), compound eighth nerve action potential (AP), and summating potential (SP).

The CM is thought to be dependent on the presence of intact cochlear hair cells in the organ of Corti. Mechanical displacement of the basilar membrane by the traveling wave causes distortion of the hairs embedded in the tectorial membrane. It has been suggested that this distortion produces the CM by a piezoelectric mechanism. The magnitude of the CM is proportional to the degree of displacement of the basilar membrane, and in a normal ear it reproduces faithfully in an electrical form the waveform of the acoustic signal. Whether the CM is a prerequisite for the generation of the AP, or merely a coincidental phenomenon, is not clear.

The AP represents the combined, relatively synchronous firing of a large number of individual fibers in the eighth nerve. This synchrony is greatest in the fibers supplying the basal turn of the cochlea, i.e., the part that is sensitive to the highest frequencies. For that reason as well as others, basal turn activity predominates in the compound AP. The typical AP waveform has a brief latent period, a negative deflection (N1), a positive limb, and often a second, much smaller negative deflection (N2). It has been suggested by Aran and Darrouzet [1] that the N1 wave, which dominates the normal AP, reflects activity in nerve fibers serving the basal turn of the cochlea, whereas N2, which is smaller and of longer latency, originates in the more remote apical regions.

The SP is a drift in the baseline of the CM, occurring as a DC shift, usually in a negative direction, at high stimulus intensities and reflecting nonlinearities or asymmetry of movement of the basilar membrane.

The ECoG was originally applied for objective estimation of the auditory threshold in subjects difficult to test by conventional means, for example, in infants. Many workers, including the author, also find the technique of great value in the differential diagnosis of peripheral hearing disorders, notably Menière's disorder and acoustic neuroma. The transtympanic ECoG also provides the investigator with a unique opportunity to study the short-term effects of certain drugs on human peripheral auditory function, notably the dehydrating effect of glycerol [8] and the action of vasodilators [4] and of the aminoglycoside antibiotics [18].

A group of patients receiving either tobramycin or gentamicin has been studied with ECoG. All were inpatients in the London Hospital, and all were ill with gram-negative infections, including septicemia, bronchopneumonia, or wound infections. Each patient had normal tympanic membranes, and hearing was either normal or close to normal. Renal function was normal in each patient. Once it had been decided to institute therapy with one of the aminoglycoside antibiotics, arrangements were made for continuous electrocochleographic monitoring before and for up to 2 hours after the intravenous administration of the first dose. Because most of the patients given aminoglycosides were too ill to cooperate in such a study, only three patients receiving tobramycin and five receiving gentamicin have been studied in detail. Blood samples were taken before infusion and then at 10-minute intervals until the end of the experiment. The serum antibiotic levels were measured by microbiologic plate assay methods.

Results

Tobramycin-Treated Patients

The findings were very similar in all three patients tested; one will be described in detail as being typical of the group. This 69-year-old woman underwent an abdominoperineal resection for an adenocarcinoma of the rectum in November 1975. Her postoperative recovery was complicated by a wound dehiscence and infection with *Pseudomonas aeruginosa*, for which treatment with tobramycin was begun. The patient gave no history of any previous ear disease, and no abnormality of the tympanic membrane was found on examination. Her renal function, as assessed by plasma urea and creatinine studies, was normal. A pure-tone audiogram before tobramycin administration (Fig. 17-1A) revealed a slight degree of sensorineural impairment, accountable for by her age. A transtympanic ECoG was then carried out on the right ear; this confirmed the pure-tone subjective threshold and revealed normal-shaped AP and CM both to clicks and to a 4-kHz 2-sine-wave tone burst. Next, a bolus of 120 mg of tobramycin was given intravenously over 30 seconds into the opposite arm, and further ECoG tracings were then made 60 and 85 minutes after the infusion. Blood samples for serum tobramycin were taken between the ECoG recordings. By the end of the 85-minute period, the AP response to the 100-dB click stimulus had decreased to approximately 70 percent of the preinfusion magnitude, and the waveform showed apparent widening caused by a relative increase in the size of the N2 component. A comparable decrease in the magnitude of the CM was observed. One week later, the patient was

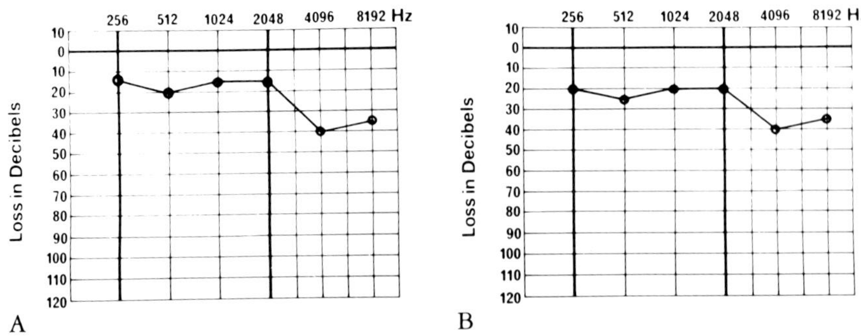

Figure 17-1. Pure-tone audiograms of test ear of the first patient treated with tobramycin. A. Pretreatment audiogram. B. Posttreatment audiogram.

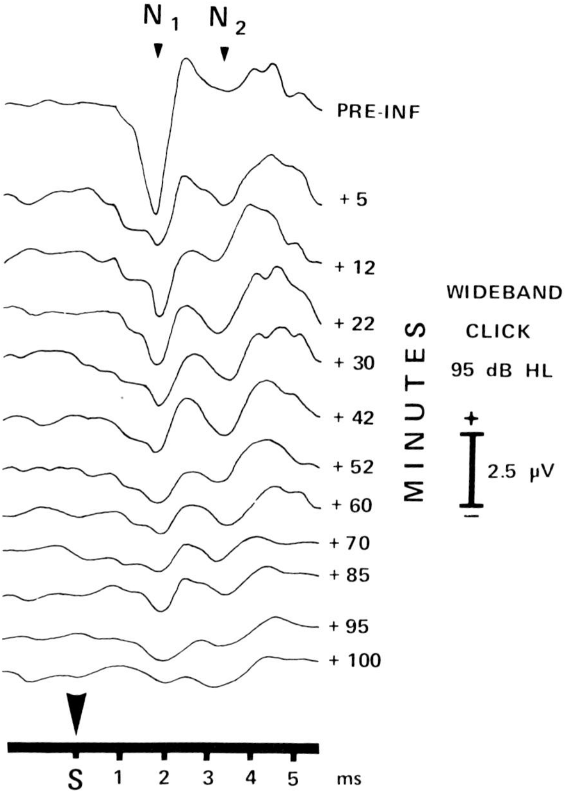

Figure 17-2. Changes in compound eighth nerve action potential following IV infusion of 80 mg of tobramycin. N_1 decreased rapidly in magnitude and N_2 remained relatively prominent, thus producing a dissociated waveform. (S = stimulus.)

tested again. In the interim, she had been receiving 80 mg of tobramycin every 8 hours by intramuscular injection. She did not complain of deafness or tinnitus. The ECoG was timed to coincide with a scheduled dose of tobramycin so that serum levels of the antibiotic were at a "trough" level. The preinfusion ECoG again showed normal-shaped AP and CM. After the bolus infusion of 80 mg of tobramycin, a remarkable and immediate change was observed in the click-induced waveforms. Within 5 minutes of the infusion, a diminution in the magnitude of the N1 response and a relative increase in the size of N2 occurred (Fig. 17-2). The overall decrease in the size of the AP progressed up to the end of the test at 100 minutes, by which time N1 was very small and N2 had become the main component of the waveform. No sign of recovery was apparent at this stage. Similarly, the CM decreased rapidly, so that, within 15 minutes of the infusion, it had diminished to 44 percent of the preinfusion level. It continued to decrease gradually up to 100 minutes, by which time it was 22 percent of the preinfusion level (Fig. 17-3). There was no evidence of

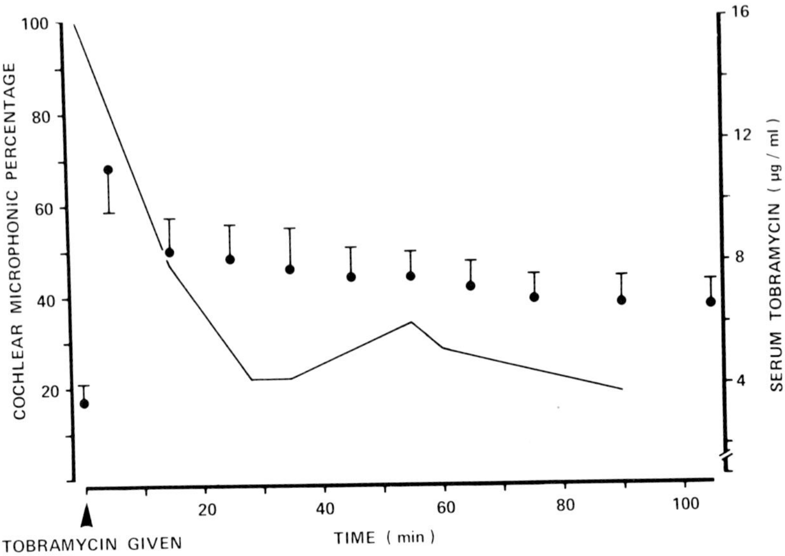

Figure 17-3. Changes in magnitude of cochlear microphonic (CM) and serum level following IV infusion of 80 mg of tobramycin. Same patient as in Fig. 17-2. (—— = magnitude of CM; ⫯ = serum levels with one standard deviation.)

recovery at this time. The AP response to the 4-kHz 2-sine-wave tone burst showed a progressive decrease in amplitude up to 95 minutes, by which time it was 30 percent of the original magnitude; but there was no significant change in the shape of the complex. The peak serum tobramycin level within 5 minutes of the infusion was 11.2 μg/ml. Levels exceeding 8 μg/ml were maintained for 30 minutes. Treatment with tobramycin was continued in the same dosage for 6 more days. Five days after discontinuation, a final ECoG was performed which showed that the AP and CM had reverted to a normal form. At no time during the treatment did the patient complain of tinnitus or deafness. Pure-tone audiograms obtained both midway through and after treatment (Fig. 17-1B) were virtually identical to that recorded before the first dose of tobramycin.

Figure 17-4 illustrates similar changes occurring in the second patient tested. On this occasion, following a bolus of 120 mg of tobramycin, an immediate diminution in the magnitude of AP and CM ensued, and the AP assumed the dissociated waveform. Serum levels reached a peak of 15.6 μg/ml, and levels exceeding 8 μg/ml were maintained for 60 minutes. No pure-tone audiograms were available for comparison, but the patient complained at no time of any change in auditory acuity or of tinnitus.

The third patient was monitored on two occasions, once at the beginning of treatment (Fig. 17-5A) and once during the course of therapy. During both tests there was an immediate decrease in the size of both AP and CM, to approximately 70 percent of the preinfusion level on the first occasion and 50

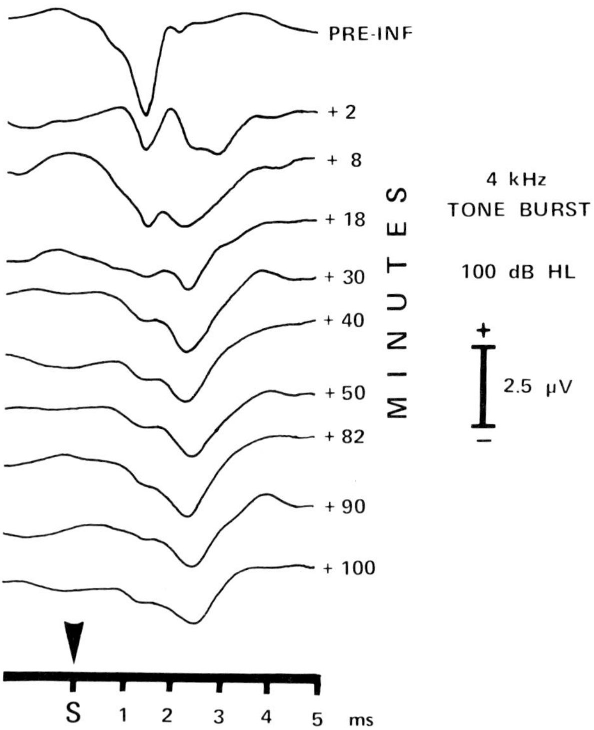

Figure 17-4. Changes in action potential following IV infusion of 120 mg of tobramycin. The dissociated waveform is particularly obvious. (S = stimulus.)

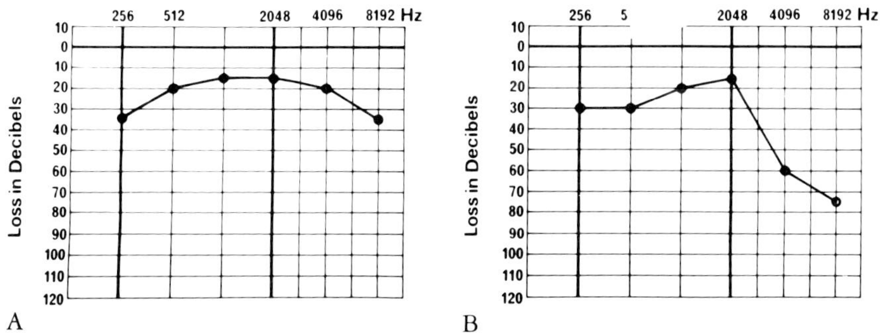

Figure 17-5. Pure-tone audiograms of test ear of the third patient treated with tobramycin. A. Pretreatment audiogram. B. Midtreatment audiogram.

percent on the second. The tendency to a dissociated waveform was less marked in this patient. The serum levels of tobramycin never exceeded 7 to 8 μg/ml during either test. Throughout the period of tobramycin therapy, the patient did not complain of deafness or tinnitus, but a 60-dB sensory deafness at 8 kHz and 4 kHz developed during the week's therapy (Fig. 17-5B).

Gentamicin-Treated Patients

Five patients receiving gentamicin were tested during their initial dose, according to the procedure described for tobramycin-treated patients. The doses ranged from 60 to 160 mg, and the peak blood levels were between 8 μg/ml and 17 μg/ml. In no case was there any change either in the magnitude of the AP or CM or in the shape of the AP waveform. Three of the five patients were retested during therapy, and again no changes in AP or CM were observed. All five patients retained normal pure-tone audiograms throughout the course of treatment (Figs. 17-6 and 17-7).

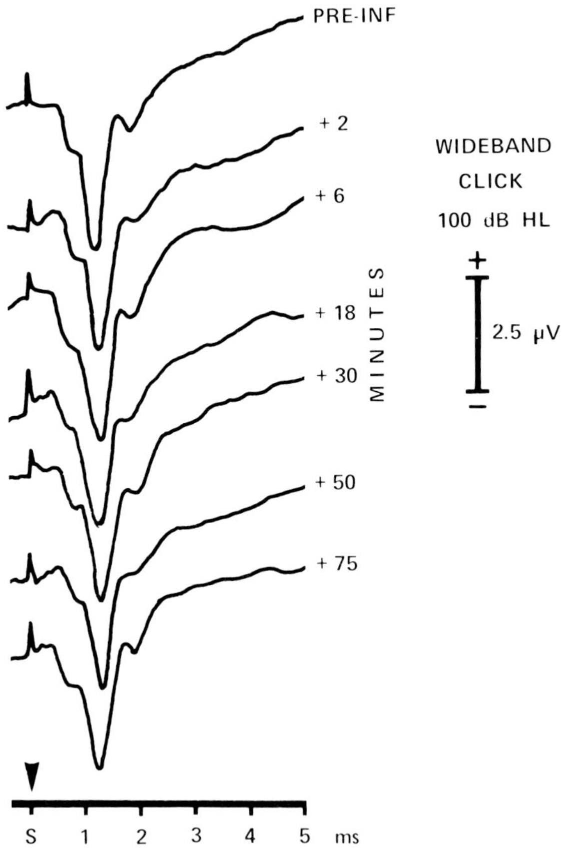

Figure 17-6. Action potential following IV infusion of 160 mg of gentamicin. There is no change in the magnitude or waveform of the complex. (S = stimulus.)

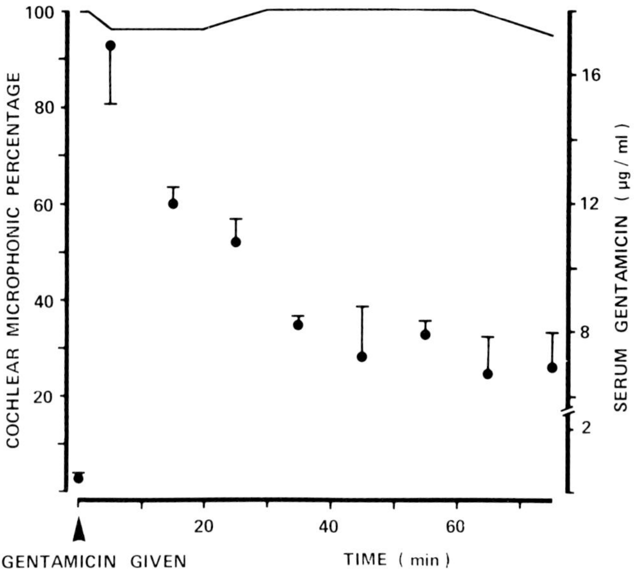

Figure 17-7. Cochlear microphonic (CM) following IV infusion of 160 mg of gentamicin. There is no change in the magnitude of the waveform. (—— = magnitude of CM; ⫱ = serum levels with one standard deviation.)

Comments

An immediate diminution in cochlear output was observed in three patients, each monitored on five occasions after single intravenous doses of tobramycin. Reductions in the magnitude of the cochlear microphonic and the compound eighth nerve action potential occurred within minutes of the achievement of peak antibiotic levels in the blood. Furthermore, there was a tendency for the first negative peak (N1) of the AP to become smaller and for the second negative peak (N2) to dominate the waveform. This is the so-called dissociated waveform. These changes progressed up to at least 90 minutes after the injection of tobramycin. They were not associated with any subjective complaint of hearing loss or of tinnitus. Although one patient developed a hearing loss at 4 and 8 kHz that was demonstrable audiometrically, a second patient retained audiometrically normal hearing at least up to 8 kHz during the entire course of treatment.

These results agree closely with the observations of Logan and his colleagues [6], who demonstrated in guinea pigs a dose-related decrease in both AP and CM within 5 minutes of tobramycin infusion. Furthermore, they were able to record from an intracochlear electrode an immediate and profound decrease in the magnitude of the endolymphatic potential. The rapidity of onset of the changes observed both in the guinea pig and in man suggests a metabolic block at one or more sites in the cochlea, possibly the organ of Corti or the stria vascularis. Blocking of cation transport [2], interruption of cell respiration, and interference with phosphoinositide metabolism [14] are the most probable modes of action of the drug.

The dissociated waveform has been described by Aran and Darrouzet [1] in guinea pigs that have received prolonged treatment with kanamycin. They feel that this waveform reflects damage to the basal coil of the cochlea. The N1 wave, which dominates the normal AP and arises mainly in the basal turn of the cochlea, decreases in magnitude and allows N2, which arises in the more apical turns of the cochlea, to emerge as the predominant component. The absence of any subjective complaint of deafness suggests that any temporary hearing loss may be occurring at frequencies well above the normal speech range, although one patient in this study did suffer a loss at 4 kHz without being aware of it. Further studies involving closer correlation with pure-tone audiometry would be of great interest in clearing up this point.

Five patients treated with gentamicin and tested in a similar manner on a total of eight occasions failed to exhibit any of the changes observed with tobramycin, despite comparable blood levels of the drugs. Vestibular function was not assessed in these patients, but the differences in the observed effects of the two antibiotics may reflect the fact that gentamicin has been found in some series to exert a greater toxic effect on the vestibular system than on hearing [5, 9].

References

1. Aran, J-M., and Darrouzet, J. Observation of click-evoked compound VIII nerve responses before, during, and over seven months after kanamycin treatment in the guinea pig. *Acta Otolaryngol.* 79:24, 1975.
2. Crawford, L. M., and Bowen, J. M. Calcium binding as a property of kanamycin. *Am. J. Vet. Res.* 32:357, 1971.
3. Gibson, W. P., and Beagley, H. A. Trans-tympanic electrocochleography in the investigation of retro-cochlear disorders. *Rev. Laryngol. Otol. Rhinol.* [*Suppl.*] 97:507, 1976.
4. Gibson, W. P., Ramsden, R. T., and Moffat, D. A. The immediate effects of naftidrofuryl on the human electrocochleogram in Menière's disorder—preliminary findings. *J. Laryngol. Otol.* 91:679, 1977.
5. Jackson, G. G., and Arcieri, G. Ototoxicity of gentamicin in man: A survey and controlled analysis of clinical experience in the United States. *J. Infect. Dis.* 124 [*Suppl.*]:S130, 1971.
6. Logan, T. B., Prazma, J., Thomas, W. G., and Fischer, N. D. Tobramycin ototoxicity. *Arch. Otolaryngol.* 99:190, 1974.
7. Martin, J. L., and Coats, A. C. Short-latency auditory evoked responses recorded from human nasopharynx. *Brain Res.* 60:496, 1973.
8. Moffat, D. A., Gibson, W. P., Ramsden, R. T., Morrison, A. W., and Booth, J. B. Transtympanic electrocochleography during glycerol dehydration. *Acta Otolaryngol.* 85:158, 1978.
9. Nordström, L., Banck, G., Belfrage, S., Juhlin, I., Tjernström, Ö., and Toremalm, N. G. The prospective study of the ototoxicity of gentamicin. *Acta Pathol. Microbiol. Scand.* [*B*] 241:58, 1973.
10. Portmann, M., LeBert, G., and Aran, J-M. Potentiels cochléaires obtenus chez l'homme en dehors de toute intervention chirurgicale. *Rev. Laryngol.* 88:157, 1967.
11. Ramsden, R. T., Gibson, W. P., and Moffat, D. A. Anaesthesia of the tympanic membrane using iontophoresis. *J. Laryngol. Otol.* 91:779, 1977.

12. Ramsden, R. T., Moffat, D. A., and Gibson, W. P. Transtympanic electrocochleography in patients with syphilis and hearing loss. *Ann. Otol. Rhinol. Laryngol.* 86:827, 1977.
13. Saul, L. J., and Davis, H. A. Action currents in the central nervous system. 1. Action currents of the auditory tracts. *Arch. Neurol. Psychiatry* 28:1104, 1932.
14. Schacht, J. Interaction of neomycin with phosphoinositide metabolism in guinea pig inner ear and brain tissues. *Ann. Otol. Rhinol. Laryngol.* 83:613, 1974.
15. Sohmer, H., and Feinmesser, M. Cochlear action potentials recorded from the external ear in man. *Ann. Otol. Rhinol. Laryngol.* 76:427, 1967.
16. Spreng, M., and Keidel, W. D. Separierung von Cerebroaudiogramm (CAG), Neuroaudiogramm (NAG) und Otoaudiogramm (OAG) in der objektiven Audiometrie. *Arch. klin. exp. Ohr.-, Nas.- u. Kehlk.-Heilk.* 189:225, 1967.
17. Wever, E. G., and Bray, C. W. Action currents in the auditory nerve in response to acoustic stimulation. *Proc. Natl. Acad. Sci. USA* 16:344, 1930.
18. Wilson, P., and Ramsden, R. T. Immediate effects of tobramycin on human cochlea and correlation with serum tobramycin levels. *Br. Med. J.* 1:259, 1977.
19. Yoshie, N., Ohashi, T., and Suzuki, T. Non-surgical recordings of auditory nerve action potentials in man. *Laryngoscope* 77:76, 1967.

Discussion of Chapter 17

Dr. Brummett: Dr. Ramsden, did you give saline as a control to any patients who received tobramycin?

Dr. Ramsden: Saline was given in the opposite arm, and no changes in the cochlear electrical potentials were seen.

Dr. Brummett: Dr. Prazma's work indicated that doses of 200 mg/kg given IV over a 5-minute period result in a reduction of the cochlear potential, which corresponds to a reduction in the blood pressure.

Dr. Ramsden: There was no evidence that my patients were becoming hypotensive. We did not measure blood pressure every 5 minutes; however, these patients had normal blood pressure prior to and after therapy.

Dr. Lietman: How was the gentamicin given? Was it given as a very quick bolus intravenously or was it given intramuscularly? Might early cochlear changes be related to the neuromuscular paralysis that is seen when you get transient high levels?

Dr. Ramsden: We gave the antibiotic intravenously over about 1 minute.

Dr. Brummett: Then I assume you would get very transient high levels which may lead to neuromuscular paralysis, causing a defect in neuronal transmission.

Dr. P. A. Bernard (Laval University, Quebec): Do you think there are differences in ototoxicity between gentamicin and tobramycin? We see that tobramycin appeared to be less ototoxic than gentamicin in many experiments.

Dr. Ramsden: We see more gentamicin ototoxicity than tobramycin ototoxicity in man. Gentamicin ototoxicity in man tends to be vestibular. Patients tend to get dizzy rather than deaf, although, in a previous report, we described a case of profound deafness with gentamicin.* There is a species

*D. A. Moffat and R. T. Ramsden. Profound bilateral sensorineural hearing loss during gentamicin therapy. *J. Laryngol. Otol.* 91:511, 1977.

difference, of course. In the guinea pig, gentamicin is more cochleotoxic than tobramycin.

Dr. Proctor: In view of Dr. Lietman's question, I wonder what the effect of gentamicin was on the cochlear microphonic. This may settle the question whether there was a neural transmission paralysis.

Dr. Ramsden: In patients treated with gentamicin, there was no alteration in the magnitude of either the cochlear microphonic or the action potential. In those treated with tobramycin, the cochlear microphonic decreased in magnitude in parallel with the action potential.

Dr. Proctor: It was parallel in time and in magnitude?

Dr. Ramsden: Yes.

Dr. Hawkins: I wonder if you have had occasion to repeat this type of experiment with patients receiving a bolus of furosemide or other diuretics.

Dr. Ramsden: We plan to start a trial with furosemide.

Dr. Brummett: Because of the known calcium-binding capacity of aminoglycosides, we also looked at Versine, given to guinea pigs in equal molar amounts, and we noted that the cochlear microphonic was the same when we gave Versine as when we gave tobramycin. We also observed a decrease in blood pressure.

Dr. Ramsden: Peter Bull, who was working in Bristol at the time, performed experiments similar to these, using gentamicin and amikacin, and, as far as I know, he obtained results similar to those we obtained with tobramycin.

Dr. Brummett: I wonder if anybody knows whether there is a difference in calcium-binding capacity between tobramycin and gentamicin.

Dr. Ramsden: Nobody knows.

18. Auditory Brainstem Response in Assessment of Infants Treated with Aminoglycoside Antibiotics

Terese Finitzo-Hieber

Neonates with dysfunction of multiple organ systems are frequently treated with aminoglycoside antibiotics. Because of the suspected ototoxicity of these drugs, such infants have required extensive audiologic follow-up, as described by Finitzo-Hieber et al. [5]. The auditory sensitivity of some multiply handicapped children in that study could be described only in qualitative terms, even after 4 years of ongoing evaluation.

Such limitations in the audiologic evaluation of high-risk infants need no longer occur, however. The auditory brainstem response (ABR) described by Jewett and Williston [10] yields unequivocal information about the peripheral auditory system and the brainstem nuclei and tracts in adults, neonates, and even premature infants whose gestational age is only 26 to 28 weeks. The ABR provides a valuable aid in identifying etiologic agents that are significant causes of childhood deafness. The ABR can be used prospectively for monitoring the auditory sensitivity of premature, high-risk infants. We are currently using this method in a study of infants treated with two potentially ototoxic antibiotics; their responses are being compared with those of a non-treated control group matched according to gestational age, weight, and sex.

The ABR is recorded in the first 10 msec following a click stimulus. A schematic diagram of the apparatus used is shown in Fig. 18-1. The EEG is recorded continuously from surface electrodes attached to the vertex and mastoid process. The response is amplified, filtered, and computer averaged for ease of identification. The electrical click stimulus is a 0.1-msec square wave presented at 2 hearing levels (60 dB hearing level and 30 dB hearing level relative to the click threshold of a normal adult) through a shielded earphone.

The author wishes to thank Karen Clinton Brown and Linda Parker for their dedication and their meticulous data collection, Trudy Coleman for her artwork, and Deborah R. Price for collating the data on premature babies. Special thanks go to Dr. George McCracken for his continuing support, encouragement, and friendship.

This chapter was completed as part of a study funded by the Schering Corporation.

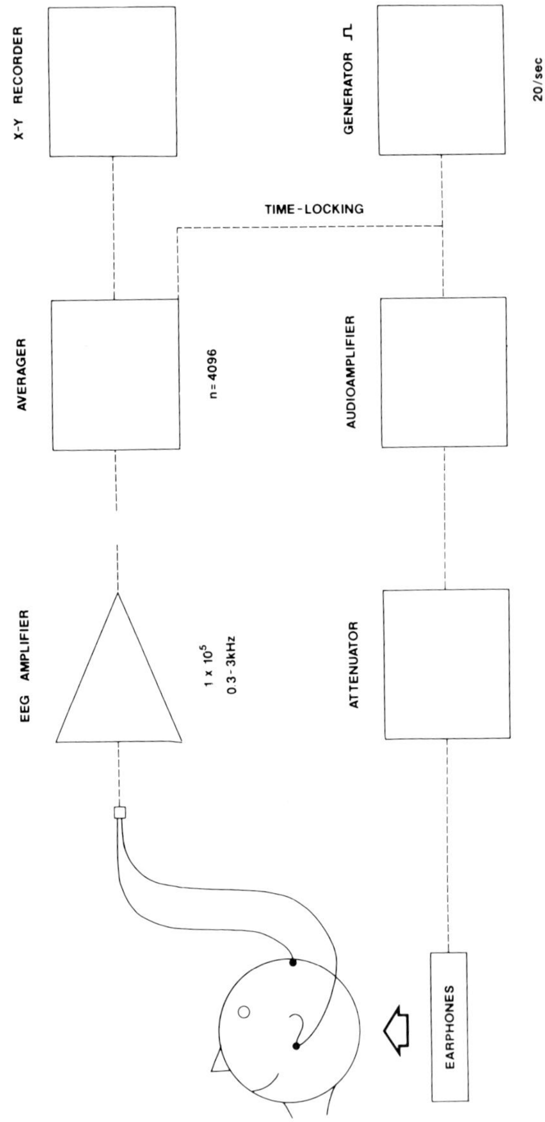

Figure 18-1. Instrumentation used for recording of ABR.

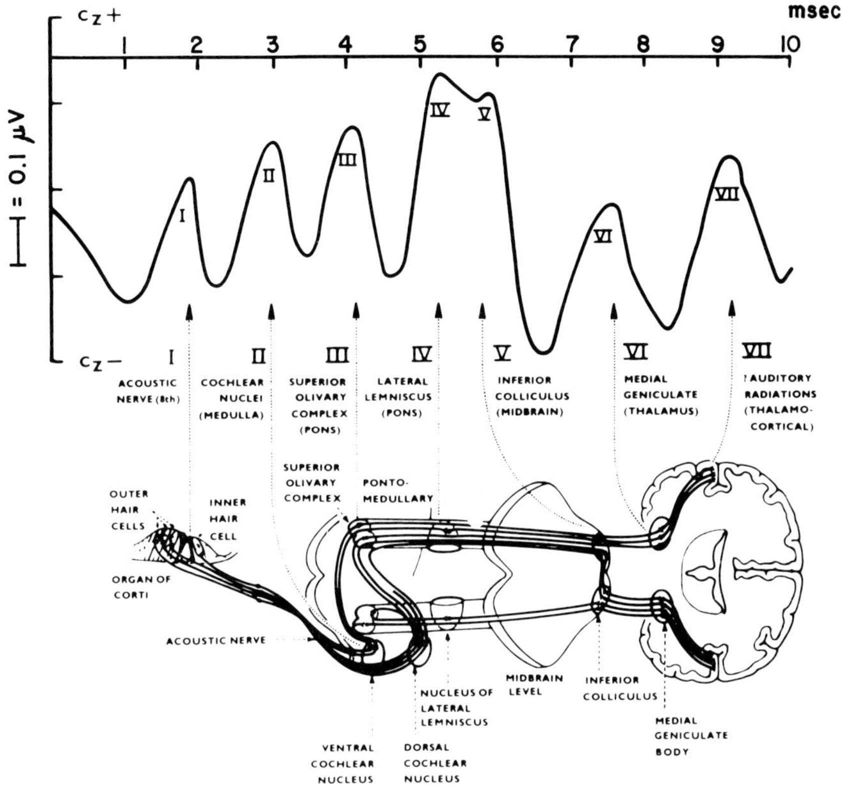

Figure 18-2. Normal ABR (waves I–VII) at a rate of 10 clicks per second. Suggested sites for the origin of the components are marked. In this and all subsequent figures, positivity at the vertex is up. (From J. J. Stockard, J. E. Stockard, and F. W. Sharbrough, Detection and localization of occult lesions with brainstem auditory responses. *Mayo Clin. Proc.* 52:761, 1977. Reprinted by permission.)

A repetition rate of 20 clicks per second is routinely used in our laboratory. Use of more rapid repetition rates results in a loss of the early components of the ABR.

The ABR consists of five to seven components, which are shown in the simplified diagram in Fig. 18-2. Wave I represents the activity of first-order neurons in the eighth cranial nerve (the action potential seen in electrocochleography recordings); wave II arises from the cochlear nucleus; wave III may arise from the superior olivary nucleus, and the IV-V complex may be from the region of the lateral lemniscus and inferior colliculus. Waves VI and VII may represent midbrain and thalamic contributions.

Developmental Norms

Prior to beginning the current study of premature and full-term infants, we considered it critical to quantify variations in waveform latency, amplitude, and threshold occurring at different gestational ages, particularly in infants with no risk factors other than prematurity. Accurate assessment of hearing loss in this population requires age-specific norms that may change from week to week [2]. In a premature infant of 34 weeks, for example, our initial judgment as to whether auditory development was on schedule or was affected by some external factor would be based on deviations from these norms. Maturation of auditory function proceeds at the same rate in both intrauterine and extrauterine environments [3, 16]. Therefore, a baby born at 30 weeks' gestational age and tested at 2 weeks of life would demonstrate maturation similar to that of a baby of 32 weeks' gestational age tested at 1 day of life. Our norms for the latency of wave V are shown in Fig. 18-3.

Wave V, the strongest component of the ABR, is clearly visible, although with extended latency, by a gestational age of 30 weeks. The latency gradually decreases with increasing gestational age; in addition, the response is present at lower stimulus intensities. Figure 18-3 shows that wave V latency decreases by almost 2 msec between 30 and 42 weeks' gestational age, compared to the less than 0.5-msec change that occurs in infants between 6 months and 12 months. Adult ABR norms are achieved between 12 and 18 months of age. For the structural and functional basis of these evoked-potential characteristics, the reader is referred to a discussion by Hecox [7].

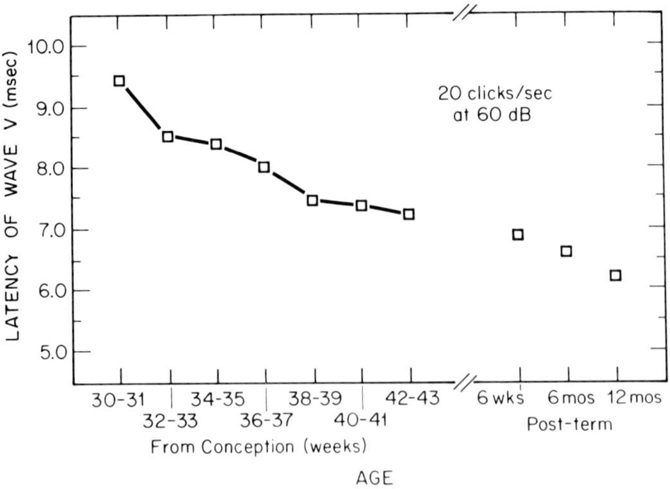

Figure 18-3. Maturation of wave V latency in premature infants at 60 dB HL, 20 clicks per second.

Clinical Utility

We analyzed the complex ABR waveform to determine which of its characteristics are valuable in the clinical evaluation of the auditory system. Based on data by Hecox and Galambos [9], Cone et al. [2], and Starr and Achor [15], we are using the absolute latency of waves I and V, the latency-intensity function, the response threshold, the interwave interval (conduction time in msec from wave I to wave V), and the wave V to wave I amplitude ratio to identify hearing impairment and to distinguish it from neurologic disorders.

The latency of wave V is clinically the most useful parameter for determination of the presence or absence of hearing loss [1, 2, 4, 9]. Because the latency is sensitive to stimulus intensity, changes in the latency of the response with changes in intensity provide information about the type and degree of auditory impairment. The latency-intensity function portrays the latency shift that occurs with change in stimulus intensity. The shaded area of the graph in Fig. 18-4 illustrates the normal latency-intensity function for adults and the values for one of our "normal" premature infants tested at 35, 38, and 46 weeks from conception and again at 6 months postterm. This graph illustrates the inverse relationship of latency to intensity and age. In general, we consider an increase of between 30 and 60 μsec for each decibel decrease in intensity to be within normal limits in our 6-week-old and older infants.

Figures 18-5 and 18-6 demonstrate how absolute latency and latency-intensity functions aid in defining the degree and type of auditory impairment. Figure 18-5 shows absolute latencies for a 6-week-old infant with normal

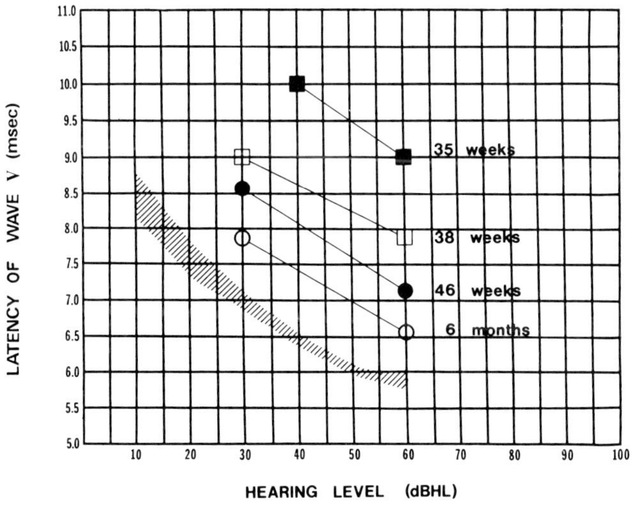

Figure 18-4. Developmental changes in the latency-intensity function for 1 premature infant treated with gentamicin, tested at 35, 38, and 46 weeks from conception and at 6 months postterm.

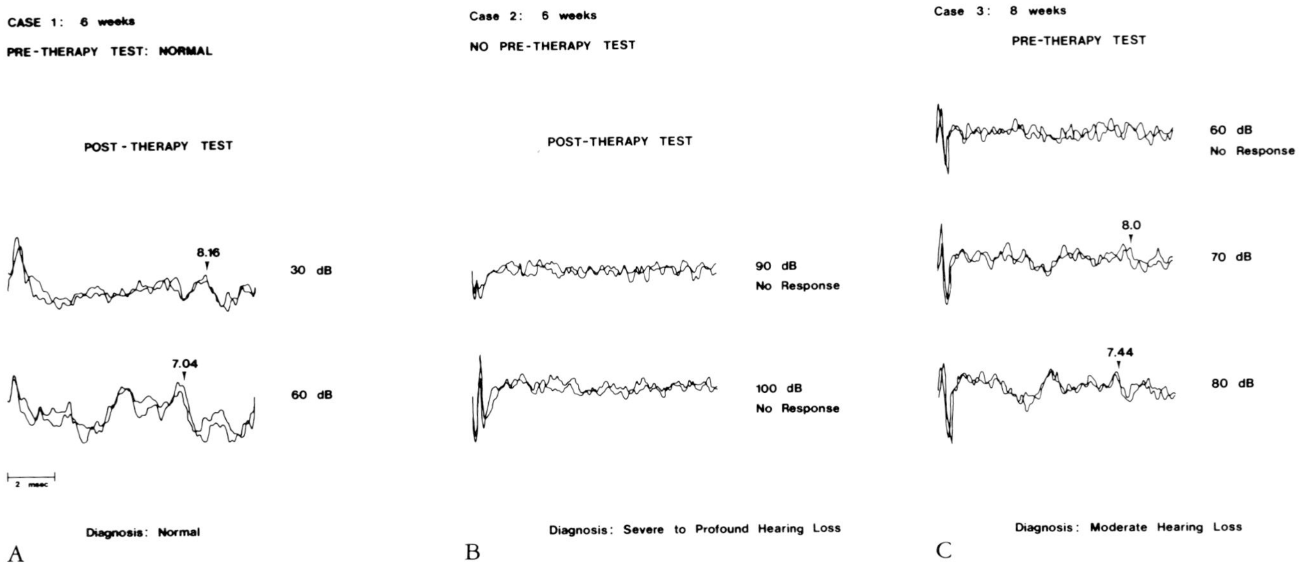

Figure 18-5. Scalp-recorded ABRs in 2 infants at 46 weeks postconception and 1 infant at 48 weeks postconception (6 and 8 weeks postterm). Each trace is the computer average of 2,048 responses. A. Normal response of aminoglycoside-treated infant without inner ear damage. B. Severe to profound hearing loss after aminoglycoside treatment. C. Moderate hearing loss present before aminoglycoside therapy. These results highlight the importance of predrug ABR assessment in the evaluation of premature infants with dysfunction of multiple organ systems. (▼ = Wave V response.)

responses after gentamicin treatment, and those for two 6-week-olds with highly abnormal responses after treatment with two other aminoglycosides. In the normal baby, wave V in response to a 60 dB hearing level (HL) is present at 7.04 msec, and to 30 dB HL at 8.16 msec, for a latency-intensity function of 37 μsec per dB.

In the second infant, despite signal intensities up to 100 dB HL, no response was obtained in either ear. No pretherapy test had been obtained on this infant. Subsequent evaluations confirmed the presence of a severe to profound sensorineural hearing loss.

The third infant had multiple risk factors, including staphylococcal pneumonia and hydrocephalus. At the pretherapy assessment there was no response at 60 dB or below. At 70 dB, the wave V response latency was similar to the normal infant's response at 30 dB. The degree of hearing impairment in this case was moderate prior to aminoglycoside therapy.

These three examples illustrate the need for pretherapy assessment. Without such evaluation, as in the second infant, it is impossible to determine whether a particular drug regimen may be implicated in hearing impairment.

Latency-intensity functions for three infants are presented in Fig. 18-6 as general examples of different types of auditory impairment, with the normal function shown for comparison. The upper graph is a latency function of a neonate with a right atresia, i.e., a conductive impairment, and with a normal left ear. The latencies for the atretic ear are displaced to the right of the normal neonatal function; however, the curve is parallel to the normal function. In this case, prolonged latency in the ear with conductive loss is the result of the decreased signal intensity reaching the cochlea [4].

The middle graph illustrates a recruiting sensory impairment in an 18-month-old with a history of low birth weight, perinatal asphyxia, and hyperbilirubinemia. The latencies in both ears are prolonged at low hearing levels, near the patient's threshold, but they attain near-normal values as the intensity increases. Thus, there is an abnormally rapid decline in wave V latency with increasing intensity, with the function changing at a rate greater than 60 μsec per dB. These findings are consistent with previous studies on adults with sensory impairment characterized by recruitment. Galambos and Hecox [6] report that between 5 and 20 dB are required for convergence of the normal and abnormal functions in their adult patients with Menière's disease, very similar to the results for this infant.

In some cases of severe high-frequency hearing loss, very little latency change occurs as the intensity increases. An example of the resulting curve, shown in the lower graph of Fig. 18-6, may be interpreted as illustrating that, for latency to decrease, the participation of fibers from the basal end of the basilar membrane is necessary [6]. In this case, the usual decrease in latency with increased intensity does not occur, presumably because the hair cells at the basal end of the basilar membrane have been destroyed or are missing. When an audiogram on this child could be obtained, it confirmed a marked loss above 1,000 Hz, with moderate impairment at the middle frequencies.

Thus, the absolute latency, the latency-intensity function, and the response

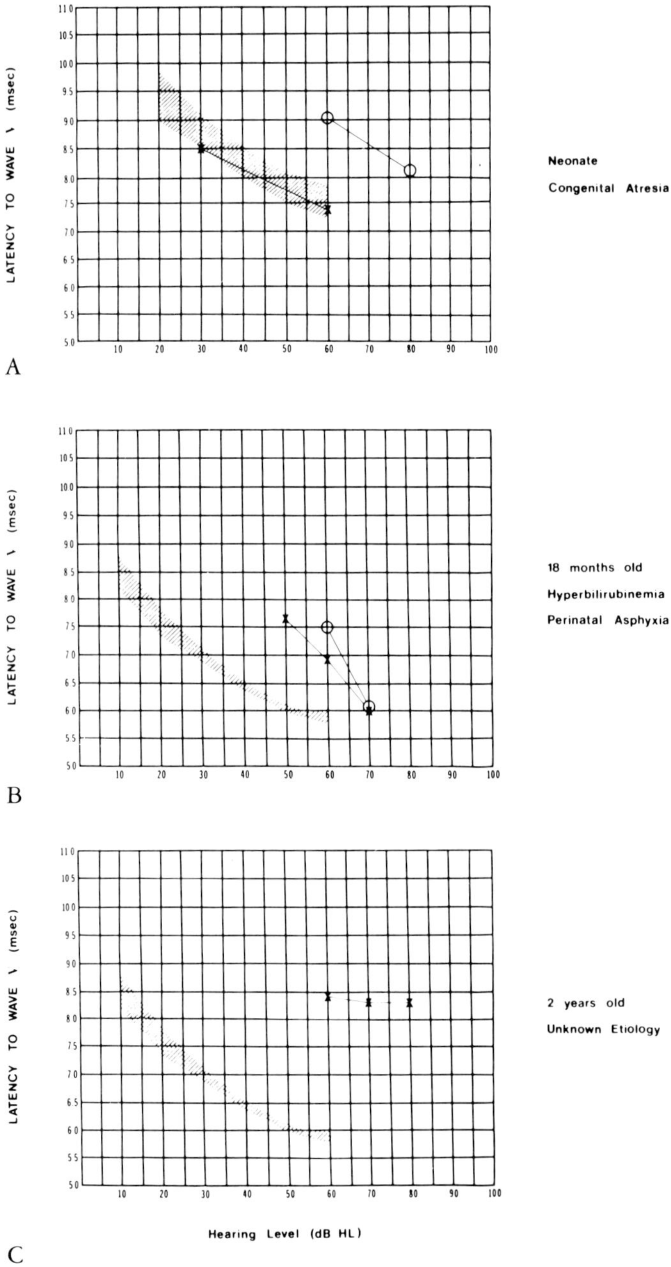

Figure 18-6. Wave V latency-intensity functions for three infants. A. Neonate with congenital atresia of the right outer ear (○) and normal left ear (×). The unilateral impairment, with a normal slope of the curve, was subsequently confirmed to be conductive in nature and of moderate degree. B. Infant with bilateral moderate sensory impairment. The steep slope of the curve for both ears is indicative of recruitment. C. Infant with a left high-frequency impairment and a shallow slope of the latency-intensity curve.

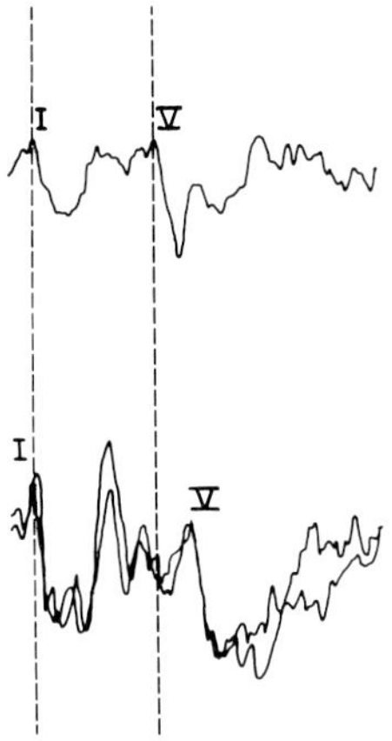

Figure 18-7. Interwave interval abnormality in an 8-month-old baby with postanoxic encephalopathy (lower trace), compared to a response from a normal 8-month-old (upper trace). (From K. Hecox, B. Cone, and M. Blau, Application of brainstem evoked potentials to pediatric neurology. *Arch. Neurology,* in press. Reprinted by permission.)

threshold are used together in the assessment and quantitation of cochlear function. The ABR, however, can also provide neurophysiologic data about the pathways of the auditory brainstem. The wave I to wave V transmission time (the interwave interval) is one criterion by which peripheral disease can be differentiated from brainstem damage. For example, Fig. 18-7 presents the waveforms from an infant with a history of hypoxic encephalopathy [8] and from a normal infant of the same age. The latency of wave V in the brain-damaged infant is prolonged compared to that of the normal 8-month-old. The latency of wave I, the eighth-nerve response, was not prolonged, however. Therefore, the abnormality is in the brainstem and not in the peripheral auditory system. Since aminoglycosides are not implicated in brainstem disease, they would not explain the auditory impairment in such a case. This example illustrates the importance of examining more than just one ABR component. In this case, the latencies of wave I as well as wave V were measured.

Finally, the relative amplitudes of waves V and I are also a useful indicator of brainstem function. Wave V typically has a greater amplitude than wave I in adults, but this is not the case in neonates. A V/I amplitude ratio of 0.5 was established for term infants [2]. In the example in Fig. 18-8, the ABR of a normal 6-week-old infant is compared with that of a 2-month-old who had multiple congenital anomalies, including microencephaly. In the latter case, a wave I response to 60 dB was present at 2.96 msec, but wave V could not be identified. At 70 dB, the amplitude of wave I was greater than that of wave V, and the I-to-V interval was prolonged. The ABR threshold was also elevated, because no response was obtained below 60 dB. Therefore, both peripheral and brainstem involvement were present.

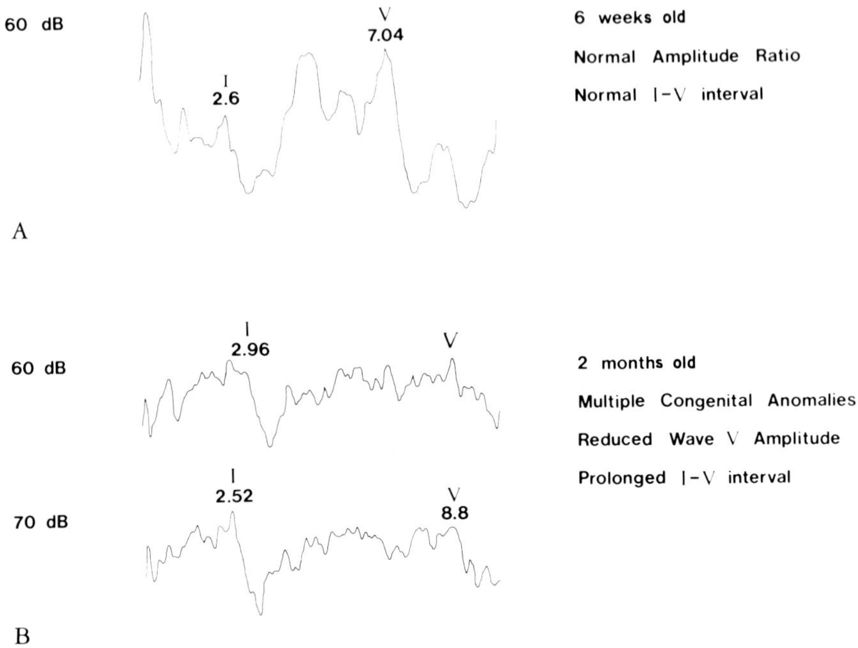

Figure 18-8. A. Normal amplitude ratio and interwave interval in a 6-week-old infant. For comparison (B), the abnormal wave V amplitude at 60 and 70 dB for a 2-month-old microencephalic infant is shown.

Comments

In the design of an ototoxicity study on neonates, it is necessary first to confirm that a laboratory's "normal" values are in agreement with those at other centers. The findings in this study of premature and full-term infants are in agreement with those of Despland and Galambos [3] and others [13, 14, 16].

In our study, appropriate bacteriologic smears and cultures are obtained before antibiotic therapy is initiated, and again at the end of therapy for patients with documented infections. Blood is drawn for assay of serum antibiotic levels during and after therapy for evaluation of the pharmacokinetics of the drugs studied. For monitoring of hematopoietic and renal function, complete blood counts, urinalyses, and serum creatinine concentrations are determined prior to and at the end of antibiotic therapy. Because of the high incidence of sensorineural losses associated with congenital cytomegalovirus infections [12], urine cultures and cord blood antibody studies for this virus are carried out.

We attempt to monitor the multiple factors that might affect an infant's auditory brainstem response. Thus, careful evaluation is essential, not only pre- and posttherapy, but also if there is a significant change in the clinical condition. Reassessment is indicated if there is a sudden variation in levels of bilirubin, glucose, or oxygen, or in acid-base balance.

Follow-up audiometric testing after an aminoglycoside-treated infant has left the hospital is also essential. Each baby is retested at 6 weeks postterm (46 weeks postconception), which is 6 to 8 weeks after administration of the aminoglycoside. If the results are favorable, an infant is not reassessed until 6 months postterm. The tests used are impedance audiometry, including tympanometry and measurement of acoustic reflexes, behavioral audiometric evaluation, and another ABR. Additional audiologic and developmental assessments are made at 12 and 18 months.

Conclusion

Auditory brainstem response is proving to be an effective tool in identifying hearing loss, with a sensitivity greater than that of other measures easily available. For example, with ABR we identify 20-dB conductive impairment caused by otitis media in 6-week-old infants who have type A tympanograms, thus supporting the evidence against the effectiveness of impedance audiometry as a clinical test in very young infants [11, 18]. During our behavioral evaluation at 6 and even 12 months, some infants with normal auditory brainstem responses have not responded sufficiently to auditory stimuli to permit determinations of hearing impairment on that basis.

The ABR has its limitations, but it is a noninvasive procedure that can be used for measurement of auditory sensitivity in high-risk infants. It can identify significant auditory impairment with greater precision than either impedance measurement or behavioral test techniques.

References

1. Cone, B. The auditory evoked potential in the human neonate. University of Texas at Dallas. Unpublished dissertation, 1979.
2. Cone, B., Hecox, K., and Finitzo-Hieber, T. The brainstem auditory evoked response in neonates: A normative study. Presented at the 1977 Annual Meeting of the American Academy of Ophthalmology and Otolaryngology, October 2–6, 1977, Dallas, Texas.
3. Despland, P., and Galambos, R. The auditory brainstem response (ABR) is a useful diagnostic tool in the infant intensive care unit. *Pediatr. Res.* 14:154, 1980.
4. Finitzo-Hieber, T., Hecox, K., and Cone, B. Brain stem auditory evoked potentials in patients with congenital atresia. *Laryngoscope* 89:1151, 1979.
5. Finitzo-Hieber, T., McCracken, G. H., Roeser, R. J., Allen, D. A., Chrane, D. F., and Morrow, J. Ototoxicity in neonates treated with gentamicin and kanamycin: Results of a four-year controlled follow-up study. *Pediatrics* 63:443, 1979.
6. Galambos, R., and Hecox, K. Clinical Applications of the Brainstem Auditory Evoked Potentials. In J. Desmedt (Ed.), *Auditory Evoked Potentials in Man. Psychopharmacology Correlates of Evoked Potentials. Progress in Clinical Nerophysiology.* Basel: Karger, 1977. Vol. 2, p. 1.
7. Hecox, K. Electrophysiological Correlates of Human Auditory Development. In L. B. Cohen and P. Salapatek (Eds.), *Infant Perception: From Sensation to Cognition.* New York: Academic, 1975. P. 151.
8. Hecox, K., Cone, B., and Blau, M. Application of brainstem evoked potentials to pediatric neurology. *Neurology.* In press.

9. Hecox, K., and Galambos, R. Brainstem auditory-evoked responses in human infants and adults. *Arch. Otolaryngol.* 99:30, 1974.
10. Jewett, D., and Williston, J. Auditory evoked far fields averaged from the scalp of humans. *Brain* 94:681, 1971.
11. Paradise, J. L., Smith, C. G., and Bluestone, C. D. Tympanometric detection of middle ear effusion in infants and young children. *Pediatrics* 58:198, 1976.
12. Reynolds, D. W., Stagno, S., Stubbs, G., Dahle, A. J., Livingston, M. M., Saxon, S. S., and Alford, C. A. Inapparent congenital cytomegalovirus infection with elevated cord IgM levels. *N. Engl. J. Med.* 290:291, 1974.
13. Salamy, A., and McKean, C. Postnatal development of human brainstem potentials during the first year of life. *Electroencephalogr. Clin. Neurophysiol.* 40:418, 1976.
14. Schulman-Galambos, C., and Galambos, R. Brainstem auditory evoked responses in premature infants. *J. Speech Hear. Res.* 18:456, 1975.
15. Starr, A., and Achor, J. Auditory brain stem responses in neurological disease. *Arch. Neurol.* 32:761, 1975.
16. Starr, A., Amlie, R. N., Martin, W. H., and Sanders, S. Development of auditory function in newborn infants by auditory brainstem potentials. *Pediatrics* 60:831, 1977.
17. Stockard, J. J., Stockard, J. E., and Sharbrough, F. W. Detection and localization of occult lesions with brainstem auditory responses. *Mayo Clin. Proc.* 52:761, 1977.
18. Zarnock, J., and Balkany, T. Tympanometric Screening of Normal and Intensive Care Unit Newborns: Validity and Reliability. In E. Harford, F. Bess, C. Bluestone, and J. Kleing (Eds.), *Impedance Screening for Middle Ear Disease in Children.* New York: Grune & Stratton, 1978. P. 69.

Discussion of Chapter 18

Dr. Weiner: I have a question about the greater susceptibility of larger babies to ototoxicity as compared to the smaller ones. Larger babies have a greater blood volume, but not necessarily a greater amount of perilymph. For example, I think it has been found that the amount of ocular fluid in small babies is very nearly the same as found in large babies; and if the dose is determined on a weight basis, this would possibly cause a higher concentration of the drug in the perilymph of the larger babies. This, of course, may make larger babies more susceptible to ototixicity.

Dr. R. Amlie (University of California, Irvine): That is certainly possible.

Dr. P. A. Bernard (Laval University, Quebec): We have considered the same problem. We found no relation between weight and ototoxicity, but we found a clear relation between the total amount of antibiotic per kilogram of a baby's body weight and ototoxicity. Secondly, we never have been able to find recovery when we saw an alteration of brainstem evoked response.

Dr. Finitzo-Hieber: We have seen recovery of auditory function when we did follow-up examinations with ABR.

Dr. Bernard: In some cases, it is very difficult to see wave V clearly. This wave is very flat, and its absence may have to be explained.

Dr. Finitzo-Hieber: Sometimes, in very young sick babies, wave V is not easily identified. However, a wave I response can be seen in these infants. The depressed brainstem function may be responsible for the absence of wave V. Wave V may have a latency of 10 or 14 msec in very young babies.

Dr. Amlie: I know that Dr. Hecox's group studied hypoxia and noted disappearance of wave V. We have not seen that. The hypoxic effect has been that of increased latency, but not a specific loss of certain waves.

Dr. R. A. Butler (University of Chicago, Chicago): I share the enthusiasm for the progress in brainstem-evoked response and how it applies to clinical medicine. But notice how it has changed our language—at least I think it has. Now we talk about hearing loss on this electrophysiologic response. I don't think I am being professionally provincial when I say that I think hearing is an overt response to sound. What I think this points up, though, is that infant audiometry is lagging far behind the technology that you people have developed.

Dr. Amlie: I think it should be made clear that we cannot say depression of brainstem evoked response is hearing loss. We are not measuring perception. We are measuring whether the auditory pathway is intact or not.

Dr. Federspil: I have studied normal neonatal guinea pigs for ototoxicity. In eight animals, I could see a significant increase of ototoxicity with tobramycin. The renal damage, which has also been described,* is greater in neonates. I would like to hear your comments on the case with netilmicin.

Dr. Finitzo-Hieber: I was using that case to illustrate the importance of a pretherapy assessment on each of these babies. The baby who received netilmicin turned out ultimately to be deaf. This was a 1½-year-old child who had severe to profound hearing loss, with no acoustic reflexes and continued absent response on ABR. This was a very sick, premature baby weighing less than 1,500 g.

Dr. Amlie: Have you seen any specific period when babies are more sensitive to aminoglycoside antibiotics? I have not observed babies in whom I could state that the effect on the abnormal ABR was due to aminoglycoside ototoxicity.

Dr. Finitzo-Hieber: Neither have I at this point.

Dr. Lerner: Have you made correlations with treatment of the mother during pregnancy to obtain information on intrauterine toxicity?

Dr. Finitzo-Hieber: We are collecting those data.

Dr. L. Eviatar: As a pediatrician, I can appreciate the difficulty and the beauty of Dr. Finitzo-Hieber's prospective study. We should have more correlation between brainstem evoked responses and audiometry and then try to compare both, because these are babies that may have several risk factors, including bilirubinemia, hypoxia, and possibly intraventricular hemorrhage. All of these are critical factors in terms of brainstem findings, and they are superimposed on the effect of aminoglycosides. Therefore, I don't think you can really draw statistical conclusions about aminoglycoside ototoxicity, because the patients selected in your study were critically ill.

Dr. Nadol: Dr. Finitzo-Hieber, could you review your criteria for distinguishing between a conductive and a sensorineural hearing loss? This is critical, because many of these children are intubated or have a serous otitis; others have unresolved mesenchyme in the middle ear space that may give you transient conductive hearing loss.

Dr. Finitzo-Hieber: In the nursery we have a pediatric resident who will make an effort to look in the ear and tell us whether or not he believes there

*P. J. Federspil, W. Schätzle, M. Kayser, K. Sack, and J. Schentag. Influence of total dose, division of daily dose, age, and pregnancy on aminoglycoside ototoxicity. *Current Chemotherapy and Infectious Disease.* In Proceedings of the 11th ICC and the 19th ICAAC, American Society of Microbiology, 1980. P. 607.

is a conductive hearing loss. We make no effort to use impedance audiometry in the nursery. I think there are enough data to suggest that impedance audiometry in the baby under 6 months is questionable in identifying conductive hearing loss. When these children are retested at 6 weeks or 6 months, they are examined by a neonatologist or a pediatrician as well as a research nurse. At this time, we also do impedance audiometry and ABR. The criterion proposed by Drs. Hecox and Galambos is that a shift in wave V, maintaining the same slope as in normals, can be considered to be compatible with a conductive loss or a flat sensorineural hearing loss. We are making an effort to differentiate transient conductive hearing loss from sensorineural loss.

Dr. Nadol: I would like to emphasize not only behavioral audiometry, but histopathology. I am not sure there is one report yet that correlates evoked response with standard light-microscopic histopathology. We have such a case, however, since we have been studying neonates in the intensive care unit. The only correlate with conductive hearing loss that we could find was the shift in wave V, which was due to unresorbed mesenchyme in the middle ear; so it seemed to be a conductive lesion. Hair cells, neurons, and the brainstem were normal.

19. A Test Battery for Detection of Vestibular Toxicity in Man

Leonard R. Proctor, Robert N. Glackin, Craig R. Smith, and Paul S. Lietman

Strategies for detection of vestibular toxicity must take into account the fact that a disturbance in the action of vestibular reflexes may be partially or even completely concealed by compensating mechanisms within the nervous system. For example, it has been pointed out that the vestibulo-ocular reflex, the usual object of clinical tests, is a self-repairing mechanism [17]: Changes in the gain of the reflex, caused by disease or injury, are adjusted promptly to normal levels, so that unwanted image motion on the retina during head movements is avoided. Thus, tests measuring performance at physiologic levels may fail to detect small degrees of damage to the system. For this reason, clinical workers have traditionally relied upon caloric or impulsive rotatory tests, in which the vestibulo-ocular reflex is deliberately driven far beyond physiologic levels so that disturbed function can more readily be observed. Another type of problem occurs when posture or gait tests are used for detection of vestibular dysfunction: Reflexes utilizing touch, pressure, and kinesthesia receptors tend to compensate for vestibular deficits, obscuring the latter from detection by such tests [13].

The caloric test is currently the most widely accepted clinical method for assessment of vestibular function. Unfortunately, test scores show a high degree of intersubject variability [1, 2, 10, 15], and therefore measurements are customarily expressed in relative terms for clinical use: Responsiveness from one labyrinth is related to responsiveness from its mate ("right-left difference" or RLD score). Similarly, nystagmus intensity to the right is related to nystagmus intensity to the left in the "directional preponderance" (DP) score. The RLD and DP scores have proved useful in detecting labyrinthine disease, especially when it is asymmetric [1, 10, 14]. On the other hand, the

This work was supported in part by USPHS Grant CMS 5 R01 13780-03 and a grant from the Schering Corporation.

RLD and DP scores are relatively insensitive to the presence of disease when both sides of the vestibular system are affected equally and simultaneously, as is often the case in antibiotic ototoxicity [4, 5, 12, 18, 21]. Therefore, when bilateral disease is suspected, absolute scores for induced nystagmus intensity are required. The variability of response scores is a well-documented phenomenon. On the other hand, variability is a somewhat lesser problem in the test-retest situation, once a baseline response level is established for a given subject [2, 15].

One factor that may be responsible for a certain degree of variability in test results is the physical stimulus itself. For control of the rotatory stimulus, a motor-driven chair and rigid head restraint are considered important [1, 9]. For caloric stimulation, control of irrigation fluid temperature and head position is essential [1, 10, 14]. A second factor contributing to the variability of vestibular test scores is the influence of the central nervous system: The nystagmic response to vestibular stimulation may undergo sudden capricious changes in intensity or orderliness, thus seriously interfering with attempts to score the test result [1, 3, 10, 11, 19]. To prevent such disruptions, the tester maintains a high level of "alertness" in the test subject through requests for mental arithmetic or other tasks [1, 3, 10, 19]. Another problem is that repeated simulation may result in a progressive decrement in response intensity, a phenomenon referred to as habituation [1, 11]. In view of the above difficulties, it must be admitted that there are certain limitations to the precision and diagnostic effectiveness of clinical vestibular testing, but the development of new methods for applying caloric stimulation [6, 15, 16] and the availability of computerized techniques for measuring the nystagmic response [9, 16, 20] have given us hope that the situation may be improved.

This report describes a battery of tests we chose to detect evidence of vestibular toxicity in normal young adult male volunteers receiving a 10-day course of aminoglycoside antibiotics in a study at the Johns Hopkins Hospital. Those candidates who pass a series of vestibular, auditory, and renal screening tests are admitted to the hospital for a period of 3 weeks. Criteria for entry into the study are shown as screening test values in Tables 19-1 and 19-2. Posture and gait criteria are slightly modified from normal values suggested by Fregly et al. [7, 8]. Criteria in Table 19-2 are based on empirical values from our laboratory. Renal and auditory tests are performed throughout the hospital stay, but are not discussed in this report. During each of the first 3 days of hospitalization, baseline vestibular tests are applied. Next, subjects receive either a placebo or a standard clinical regimen of one of the aminoglycoside antibiotics by intravenous infusion for 10 days. The vestibular test battery is repeated 3 times weekly during, and for 1 week following, the period of drug or placebo administration. Tests are then repeated weekly for 1 month and at 3 months after cessation of drug administration.

Our main purpose in the study is to determine whether differences in toxicity can be demonstrated between two types of aminoglycoside antibiotics when sensitive tests of auditory, renal, and vestibular function are used in subjects whose test performance is not disturbed by concurrent organic dis-

Table 19-1. Tests of Posture and Gait

Test		Limit Value for Screening Test*	Limit for Toxicity†
SR	(Sharpened Romberg)	154 sec	30%
SEO	(Stand, eyes open, on ¾-inch rail)	5 sec	30%
SEC	(Stand, eyes closed, on 2¼-inch rail)	5 sec	30%
SOLEC	(Stand on one leg, eyes closed)	54 sec	30%
WOFEC	(Walk on floor, eyes closed)	26 (no. of steps taken)	60%

*Limit values for screening tests are lowest acceptable scores for entry into the study.
†Limits for toxicity indicate the lower limit of performance acceptable, as a percentage of averaged baseline performance.
Source: Limit values for screening tests were modified from A. R. Fregly and A. Graybiel, An ataxia test battery not requiring rails. *Aerospace Med.* 39:277, 1968.

ease. It should be emphasized that we expect to demonstrate significant evidence of toxicity only by showing slight differences in group means at the conclusion of the study. We consider it very unlikely that any individual will show clinically evident toxic effects. If, however, clinically evident vestibular toxicity occurs in any subject during drug administration, we hope to detect it at the earliest possible moment. Toxicity criteria have been established to allow immediate termination of drug administration based on changes in test results or clinical appraisal of signs or symptoms of toxicity.

Our test battery includes an interview for symptoms, tests for spontaneous or positional nystagmus, oculomotor task performance, and posture, gait, rotational, and caloric tests. Enrollment and toxicity criteria for the tests of posture and gait (Table 19-1) take into account an expected high day-to-day variability and the large differences demonstrated by Fregly et al. [7, 8] between labyrinthine-defective and normal men. Fregly showed 71 percent to 96 percent differences in mean scores for all tests except WOFEC, in which a difference of 47 percent occurred. Criteria for rotatory, caloric, and other tests were set to accommodate the degree of variability expected among normal subjects for individual tests, while retaining the greatest possible sensitivity.

Rotational testing consists of a sudden stop after 1 minute at constant angular velocity (30 degrees per second) with eyes closed. Clockwise and counterclockwise rotations are used. Caloric stimulation is applied by means of a temperature-switching aqueous irrigation that is in routine clinical use in our laboratory. The stimulus profile shown in the upper curve of Fig. 19-1 is produced by a continuous aural irrigation at 500 ml per minute, run first at a hot temperature (43.5°C × 45 seconds), and then abruptly switched to a cold temperature (30.5°C × 23 seconds). One advantage derived from the temperature-switching test is the fact that the stimulus is promptly eliminated

Table 19-2. Screening Test and Toxicity Limits for Spontaneous and Induced Nystagmus and Oculomotor Tests

Test	Screening Test	Toxicity Limit
1. Oculomotor tests (pursuit, saccades, optokinetic nystagmus)	Any definite abnormality	Same
2. Spontaneous nystagmus	6 beats/10 sec	Baseline + 6 beats/10 sec
3. Positional nystagmus	5°/sec	Baseline + 5°/sec
4. Average of clockwise and counterclockwise post-rotatory responses	10°/sec	60% of baseline
5. Average caloric responses from right side	10°/sec	60% of baseline
6. Average caloric responses from left side	10°/sec	60% of baseline
7. Right-left difference	±15%	±30%
8. Directional preponderance	±20%	±40%

Note: Scores shown for tests 2, 3, 7, and 8 are upper limits of acceptable performance; scores for tests 4, 5, and 6 are lower limits.

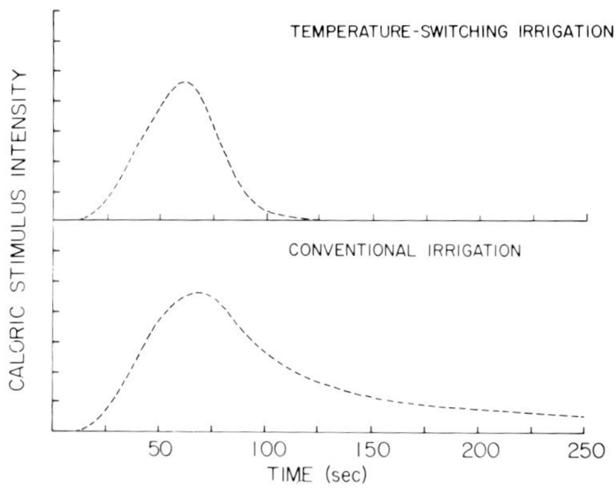

Figure 19-1. Upper curve shows time course of predicted caloric stimulus intensity produced by temperature-switching aural irrigation (43.5°C × 45 sec; 30.5°C × 23 sec). Lower curve shows time course of predicted caloric stimulus intensity from aural irrigation at 43.5°C for 30 seconds.

after the desired level is reached, in contrast to the prolonged stimulation produced by the conventional method (Fig. 19-1, lower curve). Another feature is the convenience with which the stimulus intensity can be adjusted by changes in the duration of the hot/cold pulses [6]. Our test, however, is otherwise equivalent to the four caloric stimulations (hot, left and right, and cold, left and right) produced by conventional methods [16]. In addition to the above, we apply a series of incremental stimulations in the left ear at 20 percent, 40 percent, and 120 percent of the standard intensity. The nature of the responses to be expected from these three stimuli has not been established, however, and they are not used as criteria for toxicity.

A special feature of the caloric and rotatory tests is an arrangement for dealing with the notorious problem of intrasubject variation observed with repeated testing. For example, a subject may become drowsy temporarily despite efforts to maintain alertness, and his response to stimulation may thereby be reduced markedly. When the test is repeated, normal responses may be seen. Our schedule calls for an analysis of results of the rotatory and caloric tests while the subject awaits further examination. If analysis shows that he failed any of the tests, they are repeated. Failure on reexamination is considered bona fide evidence of toxicity.

A computerized program of nystagmus analysis is of crucial importance for rapid, precise determination of slow-phase eye speed. The practicality and reliability of the technique were established in a previous study [16]. Figure 19-2 shows how the eye movement signal is registered in the computer while simultaneously being recorded on magnetic tape for storage and displayed on a strip chart recorder for immediate inspection. The tape recording preserves

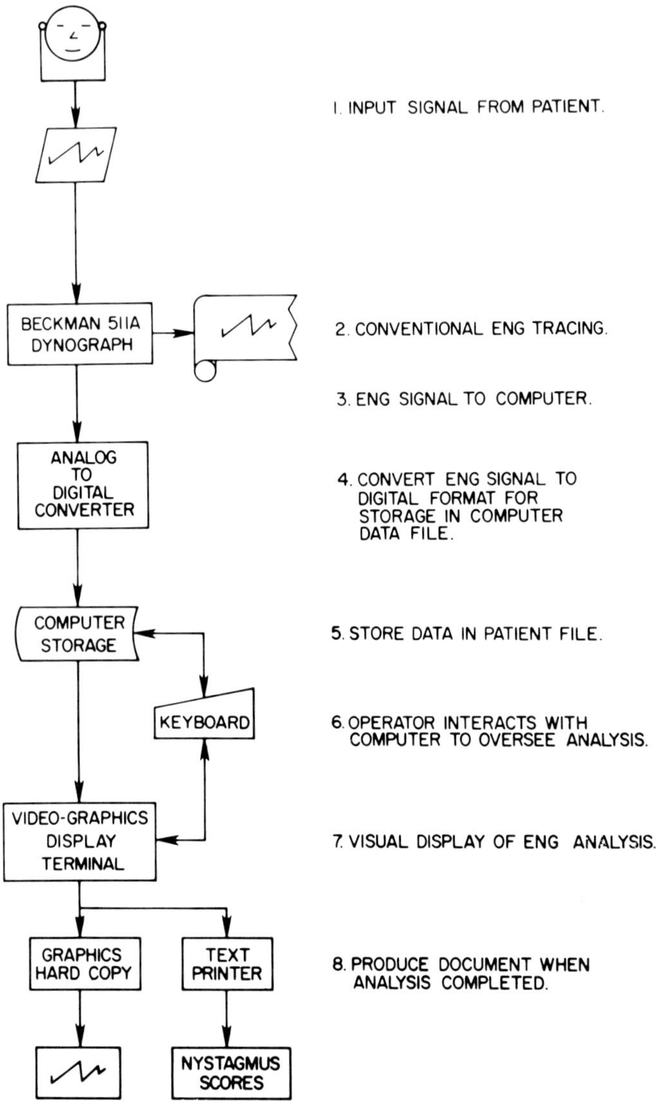

Figure 19-2. Flow diagram for computerized analysis program used to measure average slow-phase eye speed of induced nystagmus. Abnormal test scores are indicated automatically by the computer program.

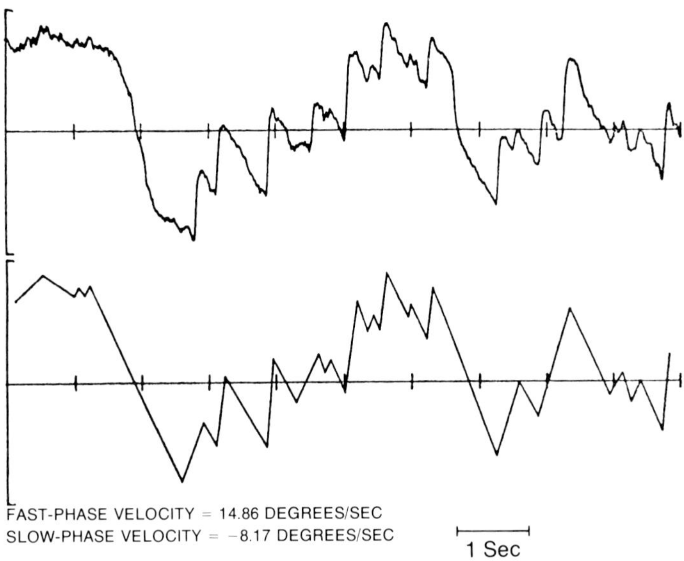

Figure 19-3. Computer-analyzed nystagmus signal (lower tracing) is reconstructed on graphics display terminal (cf. Fig. 19-2) along with original record of nystagmus (upper tracing). In this case, computerized analysis was judged to be satisfactory, and slow-phase velocity (−8.17 degrees/sec) was accepted as final score for this 10-second segment. (Ordinate: Eye position.)

the signal for reprocessing in the event of difficulties with the initial analysis. A key feature of the analysis program is the interaction between computerized processing and the human editor-overseer (Fig. 19-2). Figure 19-3 shows how the raw nystagmus signal is displayed along with a reconstruction based on the computerized analysis, so that the human editor can decide whether a proper analysis was performed on this segment of the record. The computer also calculates caloric stimulus intensity based on temperature measurements from within the irrigation nozzle during each test. Deviations from intended stimulus strength (usually less than 5 percent to 10 percent) are applied linearly to "correct" the corresponding nystagmus eye-speed score.

Because tests are scored as soon as they are completed, a definitive evaluation can be made promptly. Baseline criteria for diagnosing vestibular toxicity are determined for each test subject by averaging of scores from the three baseline test sessions (Tables 19-1 and 19-2). Toxicity is considered to be present in any individual when a test score (corroborated by immediate retesting) falls outside the limits set for the test; under such circumstances, drug administration would be discontinued immediately. Furthermore, as in any clinical research, drug administration is also discontinued if it is perceived at any time that the health of the test subject is in jeopardy.

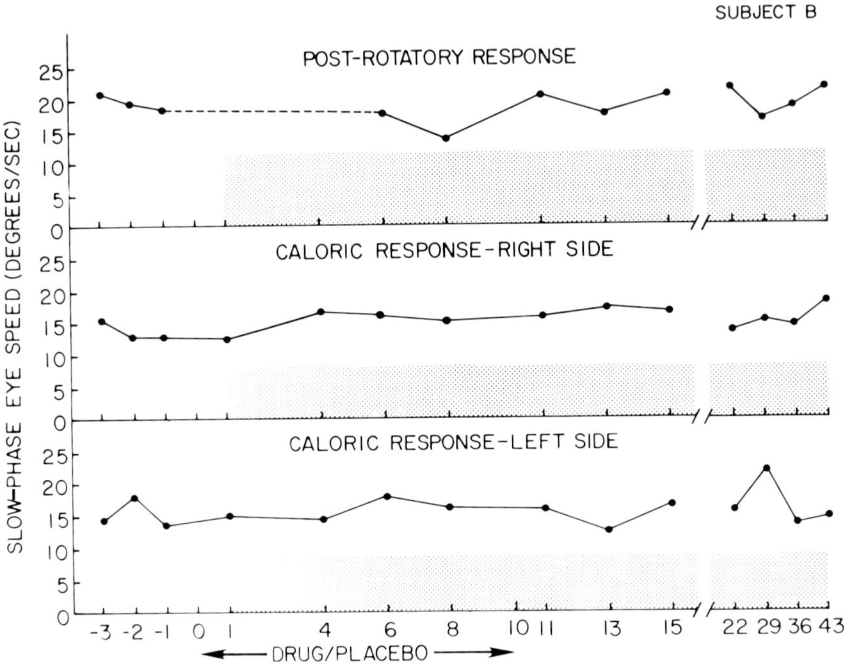

Figure 19-4. Rotatory and caloric test results on successive test days for second subject in study. Caloric test scores are the average of hot and cold responses for each ear. Gray zone indicates criterion level for toxicity (cf. Table 19-2). Technical problems prevented completion of rotatory test on days 1 and 4 (dotted line). "Habituation" is absent except during baseline sessions (prior to day 0), where a slight downward trend is suggested. (Abscissa: Time [days].)

Comments

In agreement with a previous study [15] employing the temperature-switching technique, we have observed only minor habituation effects as individual tests are repeated. The total time required for completion of the test battery is approximately 2 hours. To date, only four subjects have completed the in-hospital phase of the study. Although we do not know at this time whether these subjects received drug or placebo, evidence of toxicity was not observed in any case (Figs. 19-4 and 19-5). Nevertheless, we will continue to emphasize a prompt and accurate analysis of individual test results, with the goal of early detection of any toxic effects that might appear in any subject. Presumably, slight degrees of toxicity will be detectable only when the study is completed and scores are averaged within the placebo and drug groups. Analysis at that time should also indicate which tests or combinations of tests are most effective in detecting vestibular toxicity.

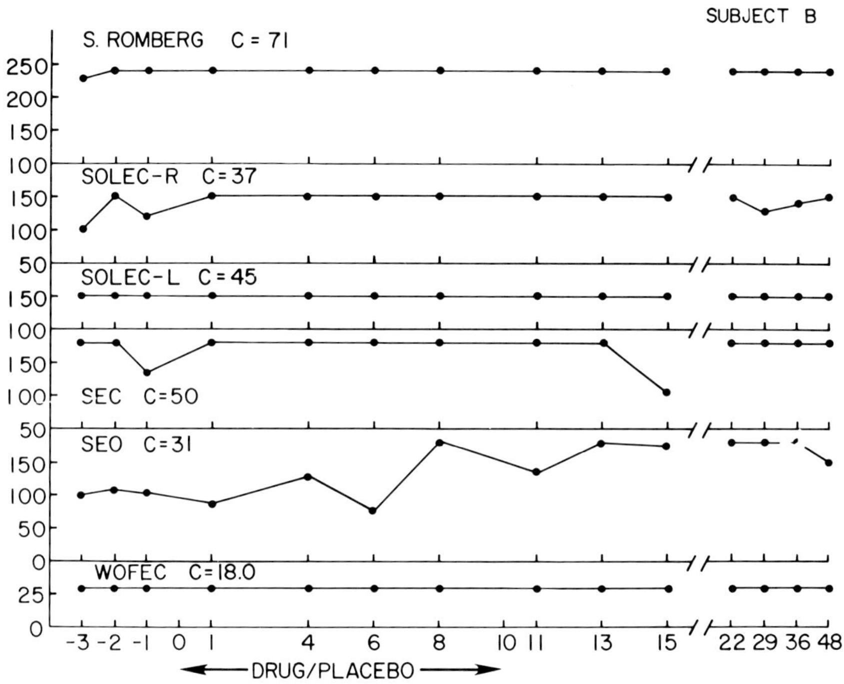

Figure 19-5. Posture and ataxia test results (cf. Table 19-1) for second subject in study. There was a slight improvement in performance of the STAND, EYES OPEN (SEO) test during the hospital stay. Drug or placebo was administered from day 0 to day 10. (C = criterion level for toxicity, based on percentage of baseline performance. Abscissa: Time [days]. Ordinate values are in seconds except for WOFEC, which is scored in number of steps.)

References

1. Baloh, R. W., and Honrubia, V. *Clinical Neurophysiology of the Vestibular System.* Philadelphia: Davis, 1979.
2. Coats, A. C., Hebert, F., and Atwood, G. R. The air caloric test: A parametric study. *Arch. Otolaryngol.* 102:343, 1976.
3. Collins, W. E., Crampton, G. H., and Posner, J. B. Effects of mental activity on vestibular nystagmus and the electroencephalogram. *Nature* 190:194, 1961.
4. Dayal, V. S., Chait, G. E., and Fenton, S. S. A. Gentamicin vestibulotoxicity: Long term disability. *Ann. Otol. Rhinol. Laryngol.* 88:36, 1979.
5. Dayal, V. S., Smith, E. L., and McCain, W. G. Cochlear and vestibular gentamicin toxicity: A clinical study of systemic and topical usage. *Arch. Otolaryngol.* 100:338, 1974.
6. Fleming, P. M., Proctor, L. R., Dix, R. C., and Metz, W. A. Results of new air caloric testing method among normal subjects. I. Biphasic testing. *Ann. Otol. Rhinol. Laryngol.* 87:248, 1978.
7. Fregly, A. R., and Graybiel, A. An ataxia test battery not requiring rails. *Aerospace Med.* 39:277, 1968.

8. Fregly, A. R., Graybiel, A., and Smith, M. J. Walk on floor eyes closed (WOFEC): A new addition to an ataxia test battery. *Aerospace Med.* 43:395, 1972.
9. Honrubia, V. Katz, R. D., Strelioff, D., and Ward, P. H. Computer analysis of induced vestibular nystagmus: Rotatory stimulation of normal cats. *Ann. Otol. Rhinol. Laryngol* [*Suppl. 3*], 1971.
10. Jongkees, L. B. W. The caloric test and its value in evaluation of the patient with vertigo. *Otolaryngol. Clin. North Am.* 6:73, 1973.
11. Lidvall, H. F. Vertigo and nystagmus responses to caloric stimuli repeated at short intervals. *Acta Otolaryngol.* 53:33, 1961.
12. Meyers, R. M. Ototoxic effects of gentamicin. *Arch. Otolaryngol.* 92:160, 1970.
13. Nashner, L. M. Vestibular and Reflex Control of Normal Standing. In R. B. Stein et al. (Eds.), *Control of Posture and Locomotion.* New York: Plenum, 1973. P. 291.
14. Proctor, L. R. Testing the Vestibular System: Value of the Caloric Test. In R. F. Naunton (Ed.), *The Vestibular System.* New York: Academic, 1975. P. 249.
15. Proctor, L. R., Fleming, P. M., and Little, R. J. Results of new air caloric method among normal subjects. II. Monophasic testing. *Acta Otolaryngol.* 84:178, 1977.
16. Proctor, L. R., Walters, G. J., and Glackin, R. N. The stimulus-controlled caloric test: A reliability study. *Am. J. Otolaryngol.* 1:39, 1979.
17. Robinson, D. A. Adaptive gain control of vestibulo-ocular reflex by the cerebellum. *J. Neurophysiol.* 39:954, 1976.
18. Tjernström, O., Banck, G., Belfrage, S., et al. The ototoxicity of gentamicin. *Acta Pathol. Microbiol. Scand.* [*B*] 241:73, 1973.
19. Torok, N. The effects of arousal upon vestibular nystagmus. *Adv. Otorhinolaryngol.* 17:76, 1970.
20. Wall, C., and Black, F. O. Algorithms for the clinical analysis of nystagmic eye movement. *I.E.E.E. Trans. Biomed. Eng.* In press.
21. Winkel, O., Hansen, M. M., Kaaber, K., and Rozarth, K. A prospective study of gentamicin ototoxicity. *Acta Otolaryngol.* 86:212, 1978.

20. Methods of Vestibular Testing in Infants and Children Exposed to Ototoxic Drugs

Lydia Eviatar and Abraham Eviatar

The major problem in the evaluation of vestibular toxicity of aminoglycosides in children is to find a simple, reliable, and noninvasive method of assessing vestibular function. Such a method should be safe, as well as nonthreatening to the children tested and to the parents who witness the testing procedures. A short test is preferable to a prolonged one, since it will be accepted and tolerated better by the children. Test results depend upon the state of consciousness of the child at the time of testing. Drowsiness and sleep may inhibit vestibular responses, whereas irritability and crying may produce significant muscular artifacts that compromise the interpretation of results. It is, therefore, the examiner's task to keep the patient alert and comfortable throughout most of the test by providing the baby with a pacifier or a bottle of sweetened water, if possible, and by reciting nursery rhymes or singing for the toddler. Infants should be tested midway between meals.

Taking into account all of the difficulties encountered in vestibular testing of infants and children, we designed a method of examination that evaluates the various levels of maturation of the nervous system at different stages of development. It provides a complete evaluation of the child's postural responses as well as the mechanisms of adaptation to changes of position in space and to shifts in the center of gravity during body movements. Tonic neck reflexes, which depend in part on adequate labyrinthine input, reflect the most prominent movement pattern in the neonate up to 4 months of age. These patterns of behavior are controlled primarily by the subcortical nuclei. The developing cerebral and cerebellar cortex exerts a gradual inhibitory influence on primitive movement patterns, and by 6 to 8 months highly integrated patterns such as righting responses will emerge, which are largely dependent upon labyrinthine and visual input. The righting reflexes, which remain present throughout life, are the cornerstone for the development of more sophisticated and highly integrated equilibrium responses.

The normal individual relies heavily on both labyrinthine and proprioceptive stimuli for the development of righting and equilibrium responses. When labyrinthine function is impaired, the patient's vision gradually compensates for the deficit. If the patient is tested blindfolded, however, he becomes totally disoriented and unable to sustain abrupt changes in the center of gravity without losing balance. One can thus obtain an indirect evaluation of labyrinthine function by evaluating the primitive tonic neck reflexes in the infant until the age of 4 months, and by looking for righting reflexes in the infant from 6 months on. In children more than 4 years old, equilibrium responses on a tilting board or in response to abrupt changes in the body's center of gravity can be evaluated. In addition, head control should be assessed with the patient prone, supine, when pulled up from supine, and in the sitting position. The infants are divided into four groups according to age and level of maturation of the central nervous system.

Group One: Birth to 4 Months

In this group, tonic neck reflexes predominate. They are obtained by passive or active motions of the head, relative to fixed positions of the body which elicit movement of the endolymphatic fluid in the semicircular canals and stimulate the sensory nerve endings in the cristae ampullares. At the same time, proprioceptive stimuli arise from the cervical vertebrae and muscles. Appropriate tonic neck responses will depend on the integrity of the vestibular and proprioceptive afferents and on the efferent motor pathways. Although one cannot separate proprioceptive from labyrinthine stimuli, a well-coordinated reflex indicates a normal overall integrated response.

The primitive tonic neck reflexes are neck righting, asymmetric tonic neck reflex, symmetric tonic neck reflex, and the Moro reflex. A detailed description of these reflexes appears elsewhere [2]. Specific vestibular reflexes in this age group are vertical acceleration (introduced by the authors) and the "doll's-eye" phenomenon.

Vertical Acceleration

The baby is held in the supine position on the examiner's extended forearms. The head and trunk are aligned and parallel to the floor. The examiner bends rapidly on his knees to a crouched position, producing a rapid downward acceleration of the baby's horizontal head and body. A normal response consists of slight dorsiflexion of the head with abduction and extension of the arms.

Doll's-Eye Phenomenon

The baby is held vertically under the axillae with his head bent forward 30 degrees over his chest. He is rotated for 360 degrees around a vertical axis passing through the examiner's head for 10 consecutive rotations in one direction during 1 minute. After a pause of 5 minutes, 10 rotations in the opposite direction are performed for 1 minute. The normal response is deviation of the eyes and head in the direction opposite the direction of rotation. The reflex persists for the first weeks of life in full-term neonates and up to 6 weeks in full-term babies small for their gestational age. Premature babies may have persistent doll's-eye responses until 3 months of age. Gradually, as vestibular responses mature, nystagmus is superimposed, with a fast component in the direction of rotation. This latter response can be recorded by electronystagmography. In most cases, it is sufficient to observe the response visually during and following rotation.

Group Two: 4 to 6 Months

Babies in this age group vary in terms of their developmental achievements. Many normal infants still have residual primitive tonic neck reflexes, whereas others begin to show righting responses. Both conditions are normal.

Group Three: 6 to 18 Months

This is a period of rapid motor and sensory development. Myelination of the pyramidal tract proceeds, as well as dendritic arborization of the cerebral cortex and cerebellar cortical differentiation. Integration of visual, labyrinthine, and proprioceptive stimuli occurs, resulting in more elaborate motor responses to changes in head position. These are called righting reflexes. They are elicited by an abrupt tilt of the patient and change in his center of gravity. The acceleration imposed on the labyrinth elicits stimuli that bring about righting of the head and protective reactions of the extremities in the direction of tilt. Since optical and vestibular righting responses are identical, the individual must be tested blindfolded so that visual cues are eliminated. The most important reflexes are the head-righting responses. They can be obtained in the infant who is picked up from the prone or supine position and brought to the upright position, or by tilting of the seated infant sideways, forward, or backward. Every abrupt change of the head position in space elicits vestibular head-righting responses in which the mouth and eyes of the infant become parallel to the ground. At the same time, propping reactions of the extremities may be noticed, especially in the sitting position. The presence of this reflex enables the child to maintain his equilibrium during sitting [2].

Group Four: 4 Years to Adult

Equilibrium Responses

Although equilibrium reactions may be present before the age of 4 years, it is difficult to test them in the very young child who may be too frightened to cooperate and relax when major changes in the center of equilibrium are imposed. The equilibrium responses are essentially more sophisticated and highly integrated righting reactions, involving the whole body. They can be tested in the sitting or kneeling position with the examiner pulling the child by his arm sideways. The normal response consists of righting of the head and extension with abduction of the extremities on the side opposite the direction of tilt. Postural reactions can also be elicited by tilting of the patient on a tilting board in the prone or supine position. The angle of tilt of the board is about 45 degrees sideways. The examiner looks for righting responses of the head and extension with abduction reactions of the extremities. Righting and equilibrium responses in the blindfolded child appear to be excellent gauges of the integrity of the vestibular channels and of their influence on myostatic and static reflexes, provided the child does not suffer from a neuromuscular deficit.

Additional information on the vestibular apparatus may be obtained from recording of oculomotor responses to rotation, positional changes, and irrigation with ice-cold water. Electronystagmography provides a permanent recording of the nystagmus elicited, which is available for further analysis of the nystagmic beats. The quality of the nystagmus can be evaluated by measurement of (1) the amplitude of the beats; (2) the speed of the slow component of nystagmus (true vestibular component), measured in degrees of eye movement per second; (3) the number of beats per 10 seconds; (4) the duration of the response; and (5) the latency of the response.

Details of the method of testing and recording vestibular responses in neonates have been reported by the authors [2, 4]. We have described the developmental aspects of vestibular function as reflected in electronystagmography and have published normative data for vestibular responses in different gestational groups [3, 5]. These norms may serve as a basis for the evaluation of vestibular responses in infants treated with aminoglycosides.

Two hundred seventy-six normal infants were tested for per-rotatory nystagmus and ice-cold caloric responses at 3-month intervals from birth until 12 months of age, and at 6-month intervals from 12 months to 24 months. Positional nystagmus was never found in normal infants; therefore, if positional nystagmus appears after treatment with an ototoxic drug, it may be the first indicator of possible ototoxicity. About 50 percent of the infants will develop nystagmus during per-rotatory stimulation within 10 to 20 days after birth, whereas 95 percent of infants will have nystagmus in response to per-rotatory stimulation within 20 to 30 days after birth. There is a delay of up to 90 days of age, however, before the appearance of nystagmus in premature infants subjected to torsion swing stimulation [4]. These maturational factors, which are correlated with gestational age and weight at birth, should be considered in the evaluation of the per-rotatory response in infants treated with aminoglycosides. Indeed, one of the effects produced by aminoglycoside treatment may be a delay in acquisition of per-rotatory responses, as shown by the authors in Chapter 21.

In normal infants and children, values for the speed of the slow component, amplitude, and number of beats per torsion swing excursion are identical for right- and left-beating nystagmus. The total number of beats of nystagmus to the right and to the left is also identical. Directional preponderance is considered when the total number of beats in one direction exceeds the number of beats in the other direction by 25 percent. Directional preponderance on torsion swing stimulation was never found in normal infants. A directional preponderance may be present, however, in association with a strong positional nystagmus and may be secondary to it. When present during or following aminoglycoside treatment, directional preponderance may be a sign of vestibular dysfunction.

The mean amplitude and number of beats per torsion swing excursion for per-rotatory nystagmus do not increase significantly with age. In our observations, the speed of the slow component of per-rotatory nystagmus increased significantly from the time of its appearance until age 4 years, from 29.5 ± 7.0 degrees per second to 40.0 ± 7.3 degrees per second. Sleep and drowsiness were shown to inhibit the responses significantly [5].

Per-rotatory nystagmus represents the combined response of both labyrinths. When information is required from each labyrinth separately, a 10-second ice-cold caloric irrigation of each ear canal can be performed. During this test, the blindfolded baby is placed in the supine position and restrained in a papoose board, and the head is ventroflexed at 30 degrees. A 10-second irrigation of one ear with ice water is the stimulus used (the temperature at the spout is around 5°C). Recording of the oculomotor response starts at the onset of irrigation. The direction of nystagmus will be opposite the ear stimulated. As soon as a good response appears, the baby is turned to the prone position, and the direction of nystagmus is reversed if the labyrinth is intact. When this new response begins to fade, the baby is turned back to the supine position. The direction of nystagmus reverts to the initial direction, away from the ear stimulated. If the child is sleepy or very irritable during the test, the response may be inhibited or incomplete (response only in supine or prone position, for example). The test is performed in three positions with each irrigation so that false responses, such as intensification of a latent nystagmus or a response from the other labyrinth, are eliminated. Ten minutes should elapse before the ear canal is stimulated with ice-cold water.

Twenty-five percent of the full-term infants tested had a positive response to caloric stimulation within 10 to 20 days after birth, and the majority of infants responded within the first month. Only about 40 percent of small-for-date babies responded by 1 month of age, however, and although the majority responded by 6 to 8 weeks, many premature infants did not respond until they were 3 months old. It is thus important not to confuse the absence of a positive nystagmic response caused by delayed maturation with the lack of response brought on by ototoxic damage from aminoglycosides. When a positive response is present, its quality becomes an indicator of the maturity of vestibular responses, or of possible damage incurred as the result of treatment.

A maturational pattern manifested by increases in the frequency (number of beats per 10 seconds), amplitude, and speed of the slow component is striking in the first 3 months of life for all gestational groups (premature infants, small-for-date babies, term babies appropriate for gestational age, and term babies large for gestational age) [3]. Full-term babies, both appropriate and large for gestational age, acquire a mature pattern of nystagmus within 3 to 6 months of age. Premature and small-for-date babies, however, show progressive maturation of caloric responses throughout the first year of life.

The frequency and speed of the slow component are the most reliable variables in the qualitative evaluation of induced caloric nystagmus. In the first 6 months of life, these variables are directly proportional to gestational age and birth weight. Whereas the intensity of the evoked nystagmus increases with age, the latency of response decreases with the duration of gestation and the weight at birth. Latency provides an additional estimate of the maturity of vestibular responses. Because of the method used, which involves changing the baby's position from supine to prone and back to supine, the total duration of the evoked nystagmus might give a less reliable estimate of the degree of maturation. Since normative values are available, however, one can estimate the dysfunction by evaluating the total duration of response as well as the other parameters.

Optokinetic stimulation with a rotating film strip at speeds of 3 degrees per second and 16 degrees per second can be used in infants 5 months old and older for eliciting of optokinetic nystagmus. This provides additional information on oculomotor responses, visual pathways, and supranuclear control of visual function [1].

Children 4 years old and older can be tested in the same way as adults. In addition to positional, per-rotatory, and optokinetic stimulation, a bithermal caloric irrigation of the ear canals may be performed after appropriate calibration of eye movements. It is likely that no significant differences exist between evoked nystagmus in the young child and in the adolescent, but we are still collecting data for comparison and statistical analysis.

Until more sensitive methods of testing become available, it appears that the combined evaluation of postural control, developmental reflexes, and electronystagmography provides a fairly comprehensive method for testing of vestibular function in children.

References

1. Benitez, J. T. Eye tracking and optokinetic tests: Diagnostic significance in peripheral and central vestibular disorders. *Laryngoscope* 80:834, 1970.
2. Eviatar, L., and Eviatar, A. Neurovestibular examination of infants and children. *Adv. Otorhinolaryngol.* 23:169, 1978.
3. Eviatar, L., and Eviatar, A. The normal nystagmic response of infants to caloric and perrotatory stimulation. *Laryngoscope* 89:1036, 1979.
4. Eviatar, L., Eviatar, A., and Naray, I. Maturation of neurovestibular responses in infants. *Dev. Med. Child Neurol.* 16:435, 1974.
5. Eviatar, L., Miranda, S., et al. Development of nystagmus in response to vestibular stimulation in infants. *Ann. Neurol.* 5:508, 1979.

21. Vestibular Effects of Aminoglycosides in Infants

Lydia Eviatar and Abraham Eviatar

The evaluation of aminoglycoside ototoxicity in infants is a complex problem. Unlike experiments on healthy animals, which can be planned and the results of which can be compared with those in controls, clinical observations on aminoglycoside toxicity generally involve patients who are seriously ill, with multiple systems affected. It may be difficult, therefore, to conclude which symptoms should be attributed to drug therapy rather than to the underlying disease. More often than not, testing for ototoxicity is performed during drug administration or after therapy, and not as part of a planned prior examination. Moreover, whereas cochlear toxicity can be evaluated by a battery of hearing tests that can detect early damage, vestibular disturbances are usually discovered late, mainly because the vestibular tests in use are cumbersome. Since these tests may inflict additional suffering on the patient, the physician may decide to avoid them and to spare the patient the discomfort.

The evaluation of vestibular toxicity is not standardized. There is no formula or universal method of testing agreed upon by all investigators. Although there is general agreement when severe vestibular damage is diagnosed, smaller changes in test results are open to a variety of interpretations as to their pathologic significance. It may be difficult, therefore, to compare results of clinical studies performed by different authors on the vestibular toxicity of aminoglycosides.

A method of testing the vestibular system in infants and children and normative data on infants' responses to vestibular stimulation have been reported [5, 6]. The method described in the previous chapter was employed in the examination of 43 neonates treated with aminoglycosides mainly because of suspected neonatal sepsis. The infants were tested repeatedly over a period of 2 to 4 years. Of these 43 infants, 26 were treated by intramuscular injection with kanamycin and 17 with gentamicin.

Of the kanamycin-treated babies, 16 were premature, with birth weights between 1,350 and 2,000 g; 10 were full-term babies. Of the latter, 8 had neonatal jaundice, with a maximum bilirubin level which did not exceed 12 mg/dl. There was no significant bilirubin elevation among the prematures. None had evidence of renal disease. The average dose of kanamycin administered was 15 mg/kg per day. The average duration of treatment with kanamycin was between 5 and 7 days. Trough blood levels were usually determined once in every patient and ranged between 15 and 24 μg/ml. Follow-up of vestibular function in most cases was for 2 to 3 years, with a maximum of 6 years for 3 children.

Of the gentamicin-treated infants, 7 were full-term, with weights appropriate for their gestational age, according to the classifications devised by Battaglia and Lubchenco [1]; 8 were premature, with birth weights between 1,000 and 2,500 g; and 2 were full-term and small for their gestational age. None of the babies had evidence of renal failure. Sixteen of the 17 infants were treated with gentamicin, 7.5 mg/kg per day for a minimum of 5 days and a maximum of 28 days. One infant was treated with 10 mg/kg per day for 9 days. Trough values never exceeded 2 μg/ml. The gentamicin-treated babies had at least 2 vestibular tests after the end of treatment and were followed for an average of 2 years.

The examinations of all children included a general physical examination and a neurologic evaluation with special emphasis on head and postural control and developmental reflexes, based on the method previously described by the authors [5]. Vestibular responses to per-rotatory (torsion swing) and caloric stimulation were tested in all children. The tests were performed in a semidarkened room with the infant blindfolded so that optokinetic nystagmus or fixation of gaze was eliminated. The test started with recording of positional nystagmus in the supine, prone, and right and left lateral positions. Positional nystagmus recorded by electronystagmography is considered pathologic in children. The infants were subsequently tested for per-rotatory responses in a torsion swing. They were seated in the mother's lap with the head ventroflexed at 30 degrees, so that the horizontal semicircular canals were parallel to the floor. Alternating 90-degree excursions to the right and left were performed at an average speed of 7 excursions per minute. Nystagmus was analyzed for the number of beats per excursion to the right and left. When the number of beats in one direction exceeded by 25 percent the number of beats in the other direction, directional preponderance was established. Directional preponderance is considered pathologic in infants and children.

Caloric testing was performed with the child restrained in a papoose board in the supine position, with the head ventroflexed at 30 degrees. A 10-second caloric irrigation was performed, with the temperature at the irrigating spout at or below 5°C. Responses were recorded on the electronystagmograph from the start of irrigation. The nystagmus recorded was analyzed for amplitude of beats (an average of 4 beats at the peak of response), the number of beats per 10 seconds (an average of 40 seconds), the speed of the slow component (average of 4 maximal beats), and total duration of nystagmus. As in our previous studies, when the nystagmus in the supine position was fading, the child was turned to the prone position and the nystagmus in the opposite direction was observed and recorded. At the end of the response in the prone position, the infant was returned to the supine position, and the electronystagmograph tracing was analyzed until the response had ended. We used this technique in order to eliminate the possibility of recording latent nystagmus or a nystagmus originating from the opposite labyrinth.

In addition to responses to caloric irrigation, infants were tested for optokinetic nystagmus. The child was placed in the mother's lap and allowed to follow a film strip at speeds of 3 degrees per second and 16 degrees per second. The distance between the infant's eyes and the film strip was kept constant at 6 feet. Optokinetic stimulation was first attempted at the age of 4 months, and results were satisfactory in all infants by 6 to 8 months.

Of the 26 infants treated with kanamycin, 6 showed evidence of transient vestibular dysfunction, manifested by positional nystagmus. Subsequent neuromuscular development as well as head and postural control were normal. Only one child had a more significant vestibular abnormality at 2 months of age, manifested by left positional nystagmus and left directional preponderance on per-rotatory stimulation. These abnormalities were no longer present by 4 months. At 5 and 8 months, optokinetic stimulation showed a normal response to the right and reversed nystagmus on left optokinetic stimulation. By 39 months, the response to right optokinetic stimulation remained normal, and no response to left optokinetic stimulation was recorded. At 43 months, spontaneous left-beating nystagmus on straight gaze was first noted during examination of the cranial nerves. This reaction was more pronounced in the right eye. By 5 years, a normal response to left optokinetic stimulation was recorded for the first time. Ice-cold caloric stimulation produced responses bilaterally at 2 months; at 4 months, the response to the left ice-cold caloric irrigation was stronger than that to the right. In addition to the vestibular dysfunction mentioned, this child developed a high-frequency sensorineural hearing loss bilaterally. His neuromuscular development and his head and postural control were slightly delayed, as was the appearance of righting and equilibrium responses.

Of the 17 infants treated with gentamicin, 10 developed positional nystagmus at the end of treatment. In three of the children, this was a transient phenomenon. In the other seven, additional signs of vestibular dysfunction appeared; these are listed in Table 21-1. The total dose of gentamicin used, the amounts of any aminoglycoside subsequently administered, and the results of vestibular testing are also listed in this table.

Four of the seven children had directional preponderance on per-rotatory stimulation, in addition to positional nystagmus (Fig. 21-1). One infant showed delayed maturation of per-rotatory responses, manifested by a doll's-eye pattern at 7 months of age (conjugate eye deviation in the direction opposite to the swing rotation). At 14 months, he developed a good response to torsion swing stimulation, with increased amplitude of the nystagmic beats. The delayed maturity of vestibular responses was also manifested by an absent response to right ice-cold caloric stimulation at 7 months of age and a fair response to left ice-cold irrigation at the same age, as determined from the

Table 21-1. Abnormal Vestibular Responses in Gentamicin-Treated Infants

Drug	Duration of Treatment (Days)	Daily Dose (mg/kg)	Total Dose (mg)	Gestational Group	Positional Nystagmus	Torsion Swing	R.I.C.C.	L.I.C.C.
Gentamicin	8	7.5	132	Premature	←N	R. Dir. Prep.	FR	←N
Amikacin	15	10.5	517					
Gentamicin (Heroin withdrawal)	10	7.5	140	FT	N→	R. Dir. Prep.	N→	GR
Gentamicin	46	7.5	616	Premature	←N	GR	NR	PR
Tobramycin	3	12.5	375					
Gentamicin	26	7.5	495	Premature	N→	R. Dir. Prep.	NR	PR
Tobramycin*	21	4.0	126					
Gentamicin	30	7.5	495	Premature	⟷N	GR	PR	FR
Gentamicin	9	10.0	270	FT	←N	R. Dir. Prep.	PR	FR
Gentamicin	26	7.5	500	Premature				
				7 mo	—	DEP	NR	FR
				14 mo	N→	FR	GR	GR

*Infant died.
R.I.C.C. = right ice-cold caloric; L.I.C.C. = left ice-cold caloric; FT = full-term; FR = fair response; NR = no response; PR = poor response; GR = good response; DEP = doll's-eye pattern; N→ = nystagmus to the right; ←N = nystagmus to the left; ⟷ N = nystagmus in both directions; R. Dir. Prep. = right directional preponderance.

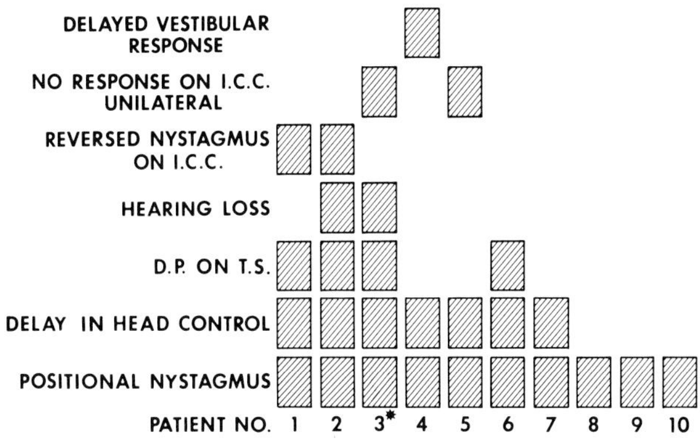

Figure 21-1. Gentamicin vestibular toxicity in 10 of 17 infants tested. (I.C.C. = ice-cold caloric; D.P. = directional preponderance; T.S. = torsion swing. The asterisk indicates that the patient died.)

speed of the slow component of the evoked nystagmus. By 14 months, he had developed good responses bilaterally.

In two children, ice-cold caloric stimulation produced nystagmus in a direction opposite to that expected (reversed nystagmus). Two children had no response unilaterally and poor response on the opposite side (> 2 SD from normal).

Aminoglycosides are known to cause sensorineural hearing loss in newborn children [2, 3, 7, 8]. Little is known, however, about the effects of aminoglycosides on the vestibular apparatus of the newborn. Elfving and co-workers [4] studied 30 children 2 to 4 years old who had been treated with gentamicin, 1 to 14 mg/kg per day, during the first 13 days of life. Two infants showed evidence of mild vestibular dysfunction upon rotary stimulation, which could have been related to the gentamicin treatment. In 1979, a long-term follow-up study of 347 neonates treated with gentamicin and kanamycin was reported by Finitzo-Hieber et al. [7]. The infants were tested for per-rotatory vestibular responses 3 or 4 years after the end of aminoglycoside treatment, and no evidence of vestibular dysfunction was found.

The results of our study differ from those reported by the other authors. None of the children studied had renal failure or was treated with diuretics. Of the 26 infants treated with kanamycin, however, 7 developed transient positional nystagmus. None of the children had a total dose larger than the 500-mg/kg dose that has been implicated in ototoxicity [9]. The infants treated with gentamicin who developed vestibular toxicity were very ill and received not only gentamicin, but other aminoglycosides as well. It is difficult to determine whether the damage incurred was the result of the total dose of gentamicin, the combined effect of two aminoglycosides, or the effect of the underlying disease. In one case, it is possible that the relatively high dose of gentamicin (10 mg/kg/day) contributed to the damage, although the only trough value available does not substantiate this hypothesis. In the only child for whom both the dose per kilogram and the total dose of gentamicin were small, the etiology of the vestibular damage may have been related to CNS damage secondary to maternal heroin addiction. Among the gentamicin-treated babies without ototoxicity, one had *Escherichia coli* meningitis and received gentamicin for 37 days in daily doses of 5 mg/kg intramuscularly and 3 mg gentamicin intrathecally. He was followed for 5 years and had no signs of cochlear or vestibular disturbances. Thus, the high total dose and the addition of intrathecal treatment did not produce ototoxicity in this child.

It is clear that further observations are needed before final conclusions on vestibular toxicity caused by aminoglycosides in infants can be drawn. The vestibular examinations in use at present are not sufficiently refined to reveal early vestibular dysfunction, and the damage may already be serious at the time when all tests become positive. Early clinical warnings of vestibular dysfunction in adults or older children may be dizziness or inability to stand on one foot, to walk on a line, or to make sharp turns, long before nystagmus appears. In infants and children, abnormal postural reflexes, delayed head control, and the presence of positional nystagmus on electronystagmography may be the first signs of dysfunction. Until better vestibular tests are developed, these signs may be helpful and should be looked for.

References

1. Battaglia, F. C., and Lubchenco, L. O. A practical classification of newborn infants by weight and gestational age. *J. Pediatr.* 71:159, 1967.
2. DeBeukelaer, M. M., Travis, L. B., Dodge, W. F., et al. Deafness and acute tubular necrosis following parenteral administration of neomycin. *Am. J. Dis. Child.* 121:250, 1971.
3. Eichenwald, H. F. Some observations on dosage and toxicity of kanamycin in premature and full-term infants. *Ann. N.Y. Acad. Sci.* 132:984, 1966.
4. Elfving, J., Pettay, O., and Raivio, M. A follow-up study on the cochlear, vestibular and renal function in children treated with gentamicin in the newborn period. *Chemotherapy* 18:141, 1973.
5. Eviatar, L., and Eviatar, A. Neurovestibular examination of infants and children. *Adv. Otorhinolaryngol.* 23:169, 1978.
6. Eviatar, L., and Eviatar, A. The normal nystagmic response of infants to caloric and perrotatory stimulation. *Laryngoscope* 89:1036, 1979.
7. Finitzo-Hieber, T., McCracken, G. H., Jr., Roeser, R. J., et al. Ototoxicity in neonates treated with gentamicin and kanamycin: Results of a four year controlled follow-up study. *Pediatrics* 63:443, 1979.
8. McCracken, G. H., Jr., and Nelson, J. D. *Antimicrobial Therapy for Newborns: Practical Application of Pharmacology to Clinical Usage.* New York: Grune & Stratton, 1977. P. 44.
9. Yow, M. O., Tengg, N. E., Bangs, J., et al. The ototoxic effects of kanamycin sulfate in infants and children. *J. Pediatr.* 60:230, 1962.

Discussion of Chapter 21

Dr. I. Tabachnick (Schering Corporation, Bloomfield, New Jersey): Have you administered gentamicin intrathecally to any neonates, and did you see anything unusual?

Dr. L. Eviatar: Yes. We did administer gentamicin intraventricularly, in a case of *E. coli* meningitis, and, fortunately for that baby, there were no vestibular abnormalities or any hearing deficit when the child was tested 5 years later.

22. Serial Vestibular Testing of Normal Subjects

James W. Roeder, Harris J. Mowry, Gregory J. Matz, and Stephen A. Lerner

The question as to which nystagmus parameter best describes the function of the vestibular system in caloric testing is a subject of controversy. Three parameters, frequency [5, 6], duration [4], and slow-phase velocity [2], have been advocated as providing the greatest validity. These have been evaluated in many studies, but great intersubject variability in caloric responses has been observed. We lack studies in which the intertest variation of nystagmus parameters is evaluated by serial caloric testing of a given individual.

In a prospective study of aminoglycoside ototoxicity (see Chap. 23), patients were evaluated with serial caloric vestibular testing. Because of the large intersubject variability and because of the lack of information on serial caloric testing, it was difficult to determine how much change in the nystagmus parameters indicates vestibular toxicity and not merely normal day-to-day variability. In our study, we performed serial caloric tests on normal subjects to determine which, if any, of the commonly used measures of nystagmus are sufficiently reliable to indicate vestibular toxicity when applied to a patient population.

Method

Standard vestibular caloric tests were performed on 20 normal volunteer subjects who had no history of disease of the auditory or vestibular system. The subjects ranged in age from 21 to 58 years. They had ingested no medications or alcohol for 24 hours preceding each test. Subjects were placed in a supine position with the head of the table elevated to 30 degrees. Electrodes were arranged for recording of horizontal nystagmus only. The electronystagmograph was calibrated with the subject looking alternately at lights 10 degrees to the left and 10 degrees to the right of the midline. Two separate water baths maintained temperatures at 30°C and 44°C and delivered 250 ml of water to the ear canal during 30 seconds. All of the data were obtained from AC recordings with a time constant of 3 seconds. During recording, the subjects had their eyes closed in a quiet, dimly lit room. The sequence of irrigations in all cases was 30°C left, 30°C right, 44°C left, and 44°C right, with 8-minute intervals between irrigations. The subjects performed mental arithmetic tasks aloud to maintain mental alertness.

Three tests were given to each of the subjects approximately at 1-week intervals. In all of the recordings, the following five parameters were evaluated:

Frequency The number of beats of nystagmus during the 10-second interval in which the nystagmus was most intense

Slow-phase velocity The average slow-phase velocity, in degrees per second, of all of the beats in the 10-second interval in which the response was most intense

Amplitude The average rapid-phase amplitude of all beats in the 10-second interval used for determination of frequency and slow-phase velocity

Duration The interval from the start of the irrigation until nystagmus was no longer detectable

Latency The interval from the start of irrigation to the start of definite nystagmus.

The correlation coefficients were calculated as described by Blommers and Lindquist [3] for comparison of the first with the second test and of the first with the third test for all five parameters.* All of the parameters were calculated manually with the technique used in the routine interpretation of electronystagmograms in our vestibular laboratory.

Results

Calculation of the correlation coefficients showed that frequency and slow-phase velocity had the smallest intertest variation in a given subject (Table 22-1). The overall correlation coefficient for both frequency and slow-phase velocity was 0.86 (a coefficient of 1.0 would indicate a perfect correlation). The latency parameter had the greatest variability, whereas amplitude and duration had intermediate values. The scatter diagrams in Figs. 22-1 through 22-10 provide a graphic representation of the results.

The mean, standard deviation, and range for each parameter for all recordings in this study are shown in Table 22-2. The mean frequency was 19 beats

*The correlation coefficient is given by

$$r = \frac{\Sigma x_i y_i - \frac{(\Sigma x_i)(\Sigma y_i)}{N}}{\sqrt{\left[\Sigma x_i^2 - \frac{(\Sigma x_i)^2}{N}\right]\left[\Sigma y_i^2 - \frac{(\Sigma y_i)^2}{N}\right]}}$$

where x = baseline value, y = subsequent test value, and N = number of irrigations.

Table 22-1. Correlation Coefficients (r) for Nystagmus Parameters in Repeated Caloric Tests

Parameter	r (1 vs. 2)	r (1 vs. 3)	r (total)
Frequency	0.87	0.86	0.86
Slow-phase velocity	0.88	0.83	0.86
Amplitude	0.74	0.67	0.70
Duration	0.58	0.59	0.58
Latency	0.40	0.05	0.23

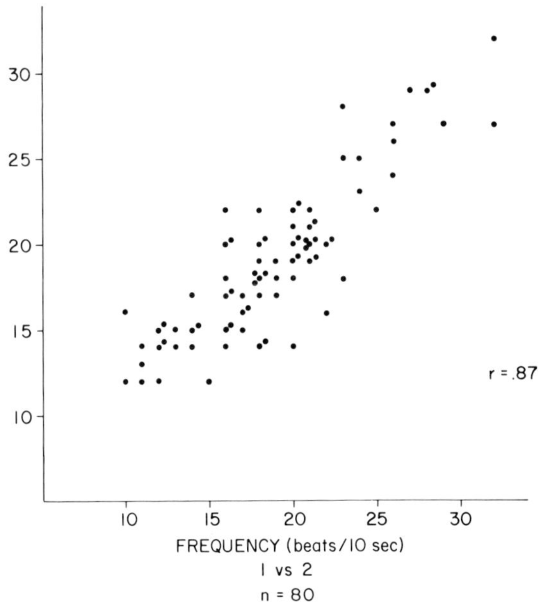

22-1

Figures 22-1 through 22-10. In all of these scatter diagrams, the subjects' first test is plotted on the horizontal axis and the subsequent test is plotted on the vertical axis. The following units were used: frequency, beats/10 sec; slow-phase velocity, degrees/sec; amplitude, degrees; duration, seconds; latency, seconds.

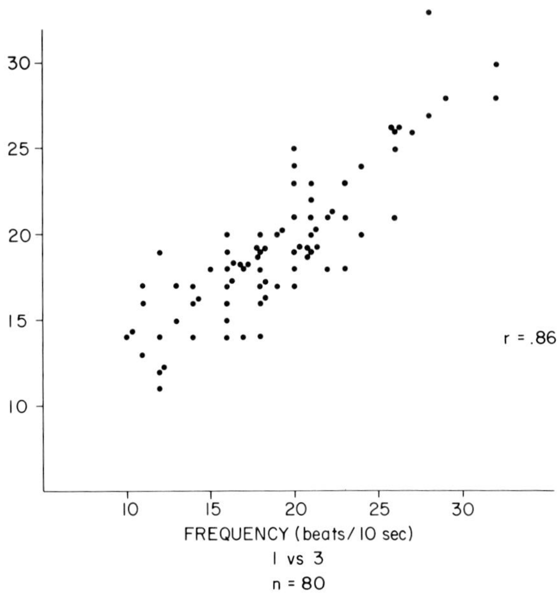
30
25
20
15
10
r = .86
10
15
20
25
30
FREQUENCY (beats/ 10 sec)
1 vs 3
n = 80

22-2

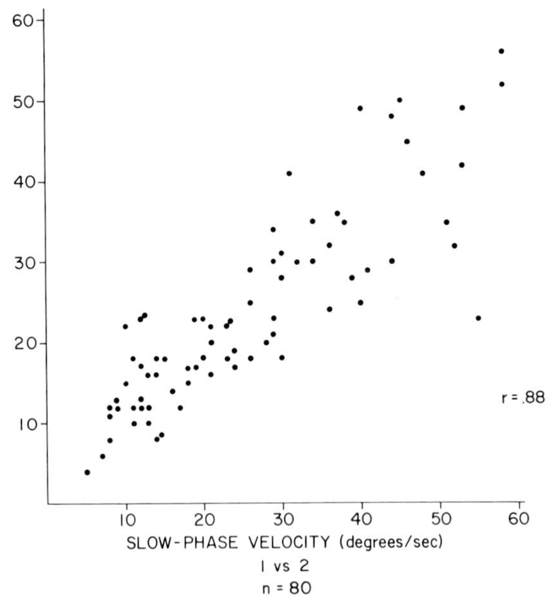
60
50
40
30
20
10
r = .88
10
20
30
40
50
60
SLOW-PHASE VELOCITY (degrees/sec)
1 vs 2
n = 80

22-3

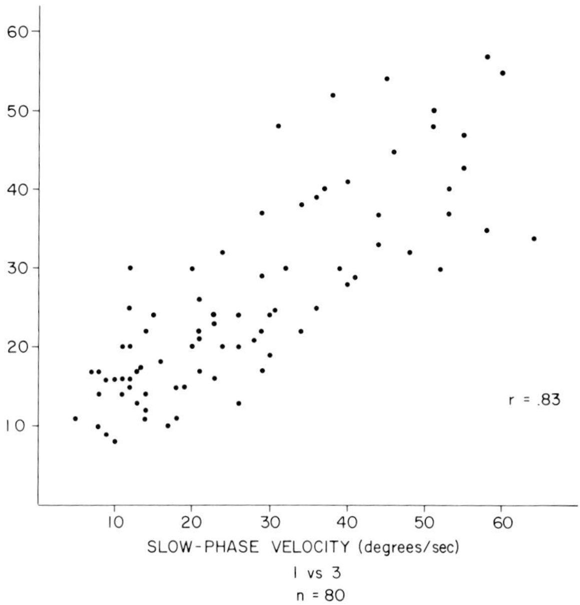
60
50
40
30
20
10
r = .83
10 20 30 40 50 60
SLOW-PHASE VELOCITY (degrees/sec)
1 vs 3
n = 80

22-4

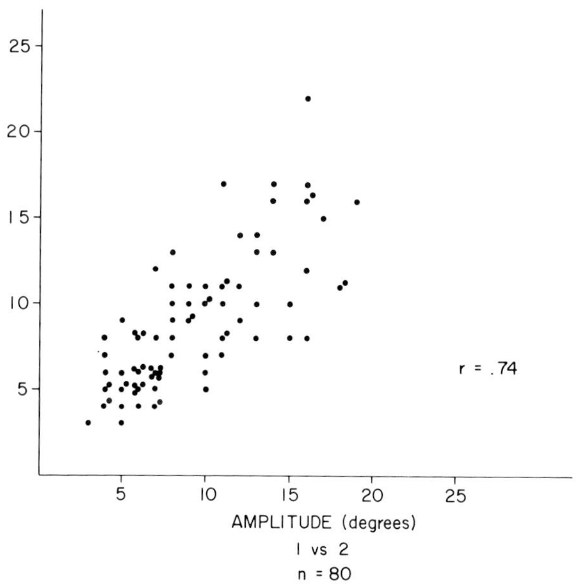
25
20
15
10
5
r = .74
5 10 15 20 25
AMPLITUDE (degrees)
1 vs 2
n = 80

22-5

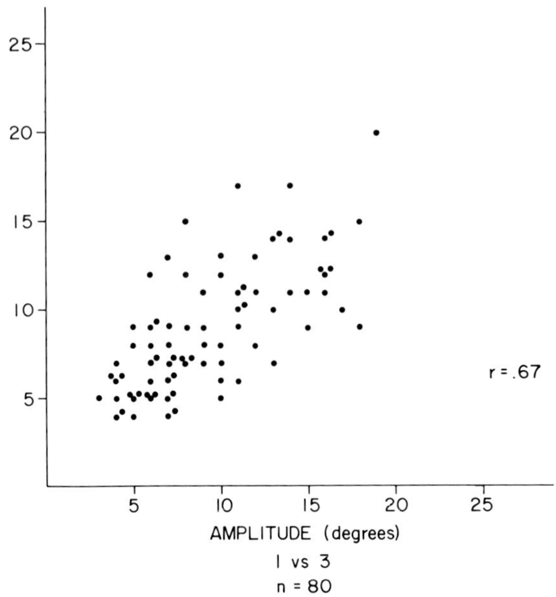
25
20
15
10
5
5
10
15
20
25
r = .67
AMPLITUDE (degrees)
1 vs 3
n = 80

22-6

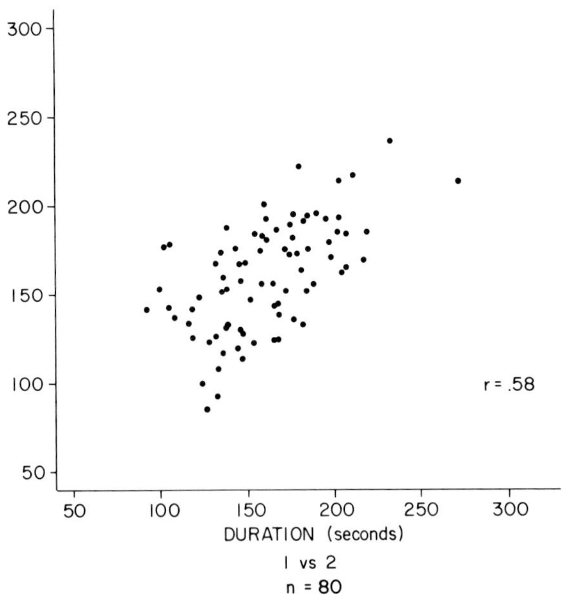
300
250
200
150
100
50
50
100
150
200
250
300
r = .58
DURATION (seconds)
1 vs 2
n = 80

22-7

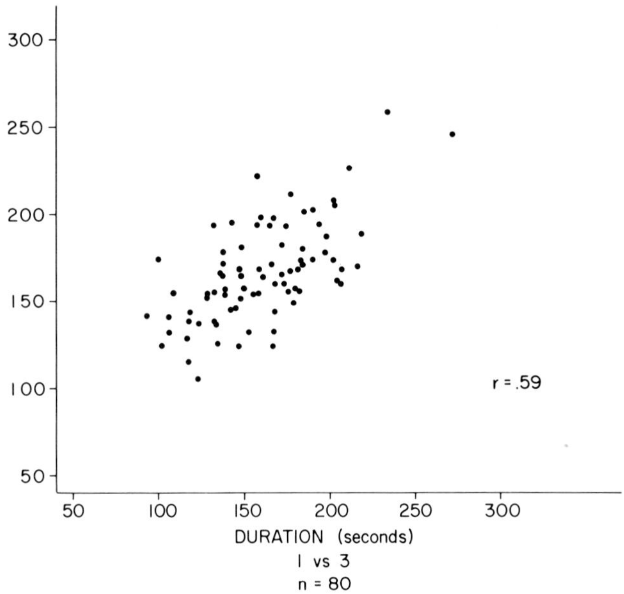
300
250
200
150
100
50
r = .59
50
100
150
200
250
300
DURATION (seconds)
1 vs 3
n = 80

22-8

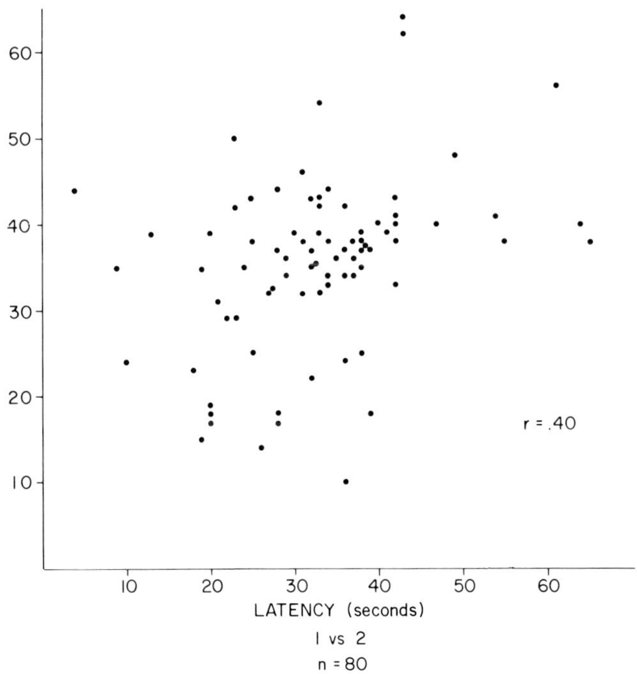
60
50
40
30
20
10
r = .40
10
20
30
40
50
60
LATENCY (seconds)
1 vs 2
n = 80

22-9

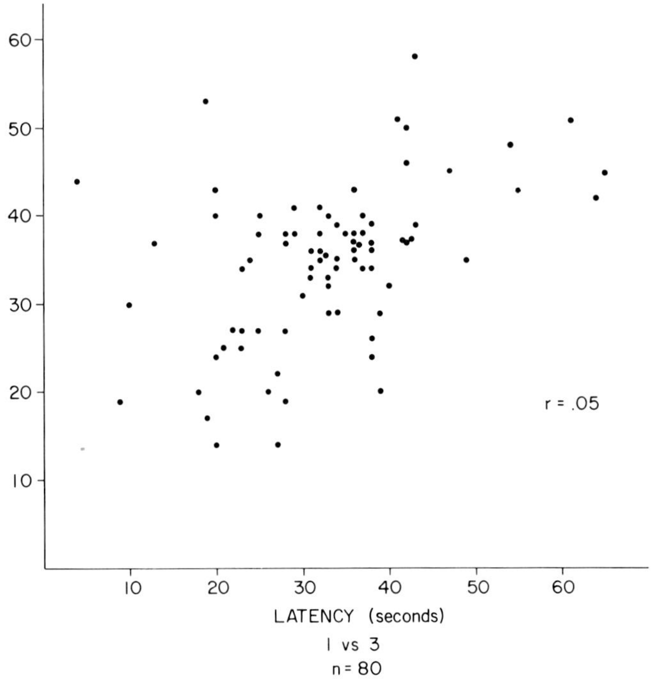

22-10

per second, the slow-phase velocity, 26.4 degrees per second, and the mean amplitude, 9.0 degrees. The mean values for latency and duration were 34.2 seconds and 163.8 seconds, respectively. There was no evidence of habituation of responses in this study (Table 22-3).

The serial recordings during the 10-second interval of most intense nystagmus for 2 of the subjects are shown in Figs. 22-11 and 22-12. They illustrate the similarity of the tracings from test to test in a given individual.

Comments

The problem that prompted this study was well summarized by Baloh and Honrubia [1], who stated that, because of the wide range of normal values for nystagmus parameters, the values for an individual could decrease several-fold and still be within the normal range. They advocated the use of serial measurements on the same individual for identification of early vestibular impairment, such as might result from the ototoxic effect of drugs. Therefore, we examined the consistency of the various nystagmus parameters in serial tests. In our normal subjects, the parameters of frequency and slow-phase velocity were found to be consistent when the subjects were tested at weekly intervals. This indicates that a significant decrease in either of these parameters in the

Table 22-2. Mean Values and Variability Measures for the Parameters in the Electronystagmogram

	Mean	Standard Deviation	Range
Frequency (beats/10 sec)			
Left 30°	18.4	3.9	10–29
Left 44°	19.1	5.4	11–32
Right 30°	19.6	4.3	11–32
Right 44°	18.8	4.7	10–33
Slow-phase velocity (degrees/sec)			
Left 30°	28.0	14.3	6–62
Left 44°	24.8	14.5	9–64
Right 30°	25.2	10.4	8–49
Right 44°	26.8	16.9	4–59
Amplitude (degrees)			
Left 30°	9.7	4.2	4–20
Left 44°	8.7	4.0	4–22
Right 30°	8.7	3.4	4–17
Right 44°	9.1	3.9	3–17
Duration (sec)			
Left 30°	171.1	38.2	93–271
Left 44°	154.7	26.2	93–207
Right 30°	63.1	30.5	86–222
Right 44°	63.2	26.6	100–211
Latency (sec)			
Left 30°	33.6	11.0	9–58
Left 44°	37.6	9.9	4–64
Right 30°	33.3	10.7	15–65
Right 44°	33.1	8.4	10–52

Table 22-3. Mean Values for Each Parameter in the Electronystagmogram

Parameter	Mean Values		
	Test 1	Test 2	Test 3
Frequency (beats/10 sec)	18.9	19.0	19.2
Slow-phase velocity (degrees/sec)	27.4	25.6	26.0
Amplitude (degrees)	9.3	8.8	9.1
Duration (sec)	161.2	161.2	164.3
Latency (sec)	32.9	35.2	34.6

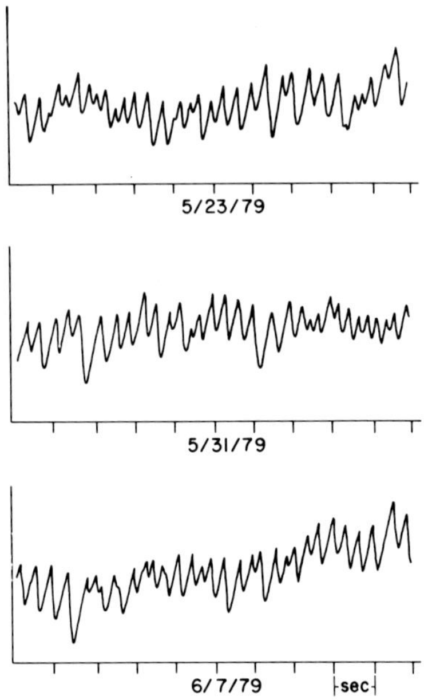

Figure 22-11. Recordings of the 10-second intervals of most intense nystagmus in response to 44°C irrigations of the left ear canal in subject 6. The dates of the tests are indicated below each tracing.

course of serial caloric tests may reflect decreased vestibular function. It is assumed, however, that the individual remains cooperative and that disease, medications, or both did not alter his or her mental alertness.

The question then arises as to what constitutes a significant decrease in frequency or slow-phase velocity. In the prospective study of aminoglycoside ototoxicity discussed in Chapter 23, a 50 percent decrease in the slow-phase velocity from a patient's baseline value was taken to indicate vestibular toxicity. None of the normal subjects in our present study showed a 50 percent decrease in either frequency or slow-phase velocity during his or her serial tests.

Therefore, we also evaluated the data to determine how many subjects showed a decrease of 33 percent during serial testing. If a 33 percent decrease in the parameters could be used as an indication of vestibular toxicity, caloric testing might become a more sensitive tool for detection of early toxic effects. Three of the 20 normal subjects (15%), who were not on vestibulotoxic medication, showed a decrease in slow-phase velocity of more than 33 percent, however, and 1 of the 20 subjects (5%) had a decrease in frequency of more than 33 percent in serial tests. This seems to indicate that using a 33 percent decrease in frequency or slow-phase velocity as an indicator of vestibular toxicity would result in a small number of false-positive findings in our vestibular laboratory.

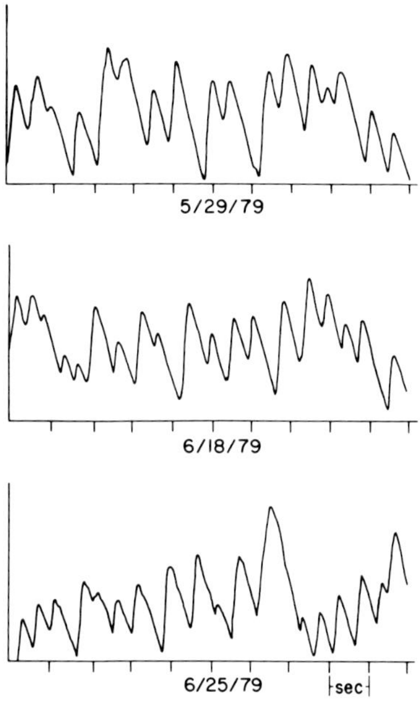

Figure 22-12. Recordings of the 10-second intervals of most intense nystagmus in response to 44°C irrigation of the right ear canal in subject 12. The dates of the tests are indicated below each tracing.

Conclusion

Twenty normal subjects underwent serial vestibular caloric testing. Frequency and slow-phase velocity were found to have a high intertest reliability in a given subject. We conclude that a 50 percent decrease in the frequency or the slow-phase velocity of nystagmus during serial caloric testing is an appropriate criterion for vestibular toxicity.

References

1. Baloh, R., and Honrubia, V. *Clinical Neurophysiology of the Vestibular System.* Philadelphia: Davis, 1979.
2. Barber, H., and Stockwell, C. *Manual of Electronystagmography.* St. Louis: Mosby, 1976.
3. Blommers, P., and Lindquist, E. F. *Elementary Statistical Methods.* Boston: Houghton Mifflin, 1960. P. 391.
4. Brash, T., and Falbe-Hansen, J. Electronystagmography on normal persons. *Acta Otolaryngol.* 77:412, 1974.
5. Torok, N. Nystagmus frequency versus slow-phase velocity—rotatory and caloric nystagmus. *Ann. Otol. Rhinol. Laryngol.* 78:625, 1969.
6. Torok, N. Quantitative parameters in nystagmography. *ORL* 36:37, 1973.

Discussion of Chapters 19, 20, 21, and 22

Dr. L. Nordström (Malmö General Hospital, Malmö, Sweden): Dr. Eviatar, how many of the children whom you tested were known to have preexisting vestibular dysfunction? I want to emphasize the importance of making such an observation, especially since so many people say that children tolerate the aminoglycosides better than do adults.

Did the 4-year-old child have two courses of ototoxic drugs? Was this the child who received amikacin for 15 days?

Dr. L. Eviatar: Those were all neonates who were treated with aminoglycosides because of sepsis or suspected sepsis. Clinically, one could not detect or predict vestibular dysfunction, since head control is not a good measure of vestibular function and can be altered for a variety of reasons. Therefore, the only way we could detect vestibular abnormalities was by doing specific vestibular tests. In older children receiving gentamicin, initial examination includes posture, gait, and walking on a balance beam or the stepping test.

As to your question about the 4-year-old child, this was a full-term 4-kg baby who was treated for 6 days with 15.5 mg kanamycin per kg per day. It was thought that this patient had aseptic meningitis. No other aminoglycosides were given. That child initially passed all audiologic behavioral tests, and, by age 2, we thought was getting well and developing speech reasonably well. By age 4, we detected the hearing loss by doing audiometric tests.

Dr. Wersäll: Is there a standardized method for vestibular testing that can be used at the bedside for patients treated with ototoxic antibiotics?

Dr. Proctor: If I had to perform an examination at the bedside of someone who was ambulatory, I might consider asking the patient to walk each day across a mattress with his eyes closed. Most bedside tests are of limited value as quantitative measures of vestibular function. Designing a test battery that could be applied within the time frame specified was quite a challenge, even though our subjects were healthy. Testing patients is a more difficult task. Responsiveness of ill subjects may be modified by fatigue or drowsiness.

Dr. Cohen: The basic problem, it seems, is that the gain of the vestibular part of the vestibulo-ocular reflex varies widely in normal subjects, from 20 percent to as much as 90 percent. As a result of the variation in gain, one would anticipate that retrospective studies to determine whether patients had vestibular dysfunction from results of caloric tests would have a relatively low yield. It has been demonstrated many times that the absolute values for the caloric response are not good indexes of the integrity of the vestibular system. On the other hand, in a prospective study, you might have a very sensitive index by doing a frequency analysis of the response to rotation, with the eyes open and with the eyes closed. In contrast to the relatively low gain of the vestibulo-ocular reflex in darkness, the gain is close to unity in light for head and body turning. These kinds of tests may yield valuable data on changes in the vestibular system.

The question how to assess the vestibular system at the bedside after the damage has occurred is very difficult. Nobody has mentioned positional nystagmus, which becomes obvious in testing with Frenzel glasses. I am not aware of any other bedside vestibular tests that are worthwhile. If one is doing serial testing, one can establish a gain for the vestibular part of the vestibulo-ocular reflex that can be followed carefully. Of course, after labyrinthine compensation, even the gain of the vestibulo-ocular reflex goes back to 1, as people learn to compensate with neck reflexes and central nervous system reflexes.

If we intend to establish a sensitive measure that will indicate a sudden drop in vestibular function, one would think this would be the way to go. I was thinking specifically of Dr. Proctor's study of patients before and after administration of aminoglycosides.

Dr. Honrubia: The visual reflexes dominate the vestibular reflexes, so that, if you want to evaluate vestibular function, it is necessary to take the visual reflexes into consideration.

Dr. A. Eviatar: We are now recording nystagmus with computers. However, a much more sensitive test is to have a patient stand on one foot or walk a line.

I want to ask Dr. Proctor about his new test because I think it is very interesting the way he applies hot followed immediately by cold caloric stimulation. One would expect that they would somehow cancel each other out. Maybe you can explain the technique.

Dr. Proctor: The conventional test with a 30-second irrigation results in an objectionably prolonged stimulation. The studies of Cawthorne and Cobb* and Hood† support the idea that the temperature difference takes about 10

*T. Cawthorne and W. A. Cobb, Temperature changes in the perilymph space in response to caloric stimulation in man. *Acta Otolaryngol.* 44:580, 1954.

†J. D. Hood, Persistence of response in the caloric test. *Aerospace Med.* 44:444, 1973.

minutes to equilibrate to insignificant levels. This prolonged action can be avoided if the first irrigation pulse is followed by a short pulse of opposing temperature, as described in our report. The second pulse serves the purpose of terminating the stimulus after it has reached a desired level of intensity. Thus, a monophasic stimulation is produced. The duration of each pulse is based on a mathematical model of heat flow in the temporal bone.‡

Dr. Honrubia: You don't use the sinusoidal hot-cold test anymore? I thought that was a sensible approach. With your present test, you would have the same problem, namely, the difficulty in evaluating the transmission of heat through the temporal bone. The concept of this test is not much different from earlier ones. In the test you used 1 or 2 years ago, you were driving the ampulla back and forth so that one would expect to see a sinusoidal output. I thought that test was a good one. What happened?

Dr. Proctor: The "sinusoidal biphasic" caloric test produces an initial hot stimulus, then a cold stimulus that is balanced with the hot stimulus.§ However, the monophasic stimulus described above appears to provide a superior technique; this method has been used routinely for the past 9 months on about 600 patients, as well as in the aminoglycoside study.

We tried both the sinusoidal and monophasic tests in our laboratory. The monophasic test is much more acceptable to patients because it is so brief. Furthermore, it is very helpful to stop after each stimulus in order to assess the reaction, talk to the patient, and make logical decisions about the next stimulus. For example, if the initial stimulus produces severe vertigo, we can conveniently reduce the intensity of subsequent stimulations by adjusting the duration of the irrigation pulse.

Dr. Honrubia: I conclude that your experience with the biphasic test is unsatisfactory—that you have decided the benefits that would result are not worth the inconvenience to the patient and the technician.

Dr. Proctor: In my judgment, the monophasic test is superior to the biphasic test for clinical purposes.

Dr. Igarashi: Dr. Eviatar, I understand the necessity of using a battery of tests for younger patients. You said that the positional nystagmus test is the most sensitive indicator of vestibular function. Is that true? Also, is there any reason for your use of the 3-degrees-per-second optokinetic stimulus?

Dr. L. Eviatar: Positional nystagmus is not the most sensitive test. I would say it is the first abnormality to appear when you prospectively study patients who are receiving aminoglycosides, especially infants, who are unable to verbalize vestibular symptoms until the age of 3 or 4. Positional tests can be done easily and practically at the bedside. Electrodes are applied to the head, and recording is done with a portable electronystagmograph. Positional

‡J. H. Young, Analysis of vestibular system responses to thermal gradients induced in the temporal bone. University of Michigan, Ann Arbor, Thesis, 1972.

§L. R. Proctor, G. H. Walters, and R. N. Glackin, The stimulus-controlled caloric test: A reliability study. *Am. J. Otolaryngol.* 1:39, 1979.

nystagmus will be the first abnormality detected. Later abnormalities following torsion swing stimulation will be noted in patients with aminoglycoside ototoxicity. These data were obtained in a pilot study. It seems to me that, once directional preponderance is detected, a significant irreversible deficit may be present in the vestibular system.

For optokinetic stimulation in children, we use a 3-degrees-per-second and a 16-degrees-per-second speed. A film strip showing animals is rotated at these frequencies. We get good optokinetic nystagmus at both speeds.

Clinical Studies of Ototoxicity

Much of the available information on ototoxicity of aminoglycosides in man has been obtained from anecdotal accounts of patients who have experienced toxicity, from drug trials in normal subjects, and from multicenter treatment trials in which the focus was primarily on drug efficacy. It is difficult to derive either the incidence or the characteristics and risk factors of ototoxicity from such sources. Gregory Matz and Stephen Lerner provide a critical review of ototoxicity studies in hospitalized patients treated with various aminoglycosides. As an example of a prospective comparative study of aminoglycoside ototoxicity, they describe their evaluation of ototoxicity in gentamicin- and amikacin-treated patients.

It has been the experience of pediatricians that ototoxicity is no more frequent in neonates than in adults. Jane Siegel and George McCracken provide a well-documented review of ototoxicity studies in children of different ages and with various risk factors. They point out the potential of the methods described by Terese Finitzo-Hieber and the Eviatars for evaluation of aminoglycoside effects on the inner ear in children.

Current knowledge of aminoglycoside pharmacokinetics in animals has been summarized by Tran Ba Huy et al. (Chap. 5) and by Federspil (Chap. 6). In order to determine whether the pharmacokinetics of aminoglycosides is comparable in man, Stephen Lerner and his co-workers measured the concentration of gentamicin in the perilymph and serum of patients who died during a course of therapy. As in animals, gentamicin in perilymph was found to equilibrate slowly with that in the serum.

Ototoxicity in animals treated with an aminoglycoside and a loop diuretic has been examined by Brummett et al. (Chap. 4). In the following section, Cedric Quick provides clinical observations on the ototoxic effect of these two types of drugs, which are often administered concurrently to patients.

23. Prospective Studies of Aminoglycoside Ototoxicity in Adults

Gregory J. Matz and Stephen A. Lerner

Prior to the evaluation of gentamicin, most reports on aminoglycoside ototoxicity in man were retrospective, i.e., patients were identified only after the appearance of ototoxicity. Generally, the numbers of patients in these studies were small, and most of the patients had poor renal function or had received large, sometimes excessive doses of aminoglycoside antibiotics. Little information was available on the total population of patients treated with aminoglycosides, on the risk factors which were associated with ototoxicity, and on the incidence or characteristics of more subtle, subclinical ototoxicity.

Prospective studies of patients who receive aminoglycoside antibiotics provide opportunities for more comprehensive evaluation of the ototoxicity of these drugs in man. Studies of toxicity during the early experimental phase of the development of individual aminoglycosides have involved short-term experiments in human volunteers. Later studies, however, have been performed on patients who were seriously ill with infections and required aminoglycoside therapy. These are the patients who, in actual practice, are subjected to the risk of ototoxicity. Large numbers of patients in many centers have been studied by numerous investigators; however, drug efficacy has been the major focus of such studies, although possible toxic effects have also been examined whenever possible. Such multicenter studies have the advantage of including large numbers of patients. Later studies in single centers have sometimes focused more consistently on testing for ototoxicity and on monitoring of renal function and serum aminoglycoside levels for appropriate adjustment of dosage. Conditions for testing of inner ear function vary among institutions, as do criteria for ototoxicity. Thus, given the lack of standardization of protocols for clinical research on ototoxicity, results obtained by different investigators may not be strictly comparable.

A well-designed prospective study brings together a multidisciplinary team that can coordinate careful otologic evaluation with the administration of aminoglycoside antibiotics. This may provide opportunities to refine and extend methods of testing inner ear function for evidence of toxicity. Furthermore, in prospective studies, histopathologic findings in the cochlear and vestibular systems of patients who die during or after aminoglycoside therapy can be correlated with the treatment course and with premortem examinations of inner ear function.

Gentamicin Studies

Jackson and Arcieri [2] found a probable incidence of ototoxicity of about 2 percent in reports from many medical centers, furnished by investigators who considered inner ear toxicity as part of an overall evaluation of gentamicin. Methods of auditory and vestibular testing were not described. The predominant risk factor was renal impairment. The authors also pointed out that high serum levels of gentamicin would enhance the risk of ototoxicity.

Nordström et al. [9] and Tjernström et al. [12] were among the first to perform a prospective clinical study on the inner ear function of patients treated with gentamicin. In careful tests of cochlear function by audiometry and of vestibular function by caloric testing with electronystagmographic recording, they showed that, of 45 patients, 7 exhibited a pathologic decline in vestibular function (3 were asymptomatic), whereas none suffered cochlear impairment. The authors underscored the importance of assessing vestibular toxicity by formal testing of vestibular function rather than by relying on subjective assessment of vertigo or dizziness. As in the findings of Jackson and Arcieri [2], preexisting renal impairment appeared to be a risk factor for development of ototoxicity. A history of previous treatment with an ototoxic drug was also more common among patients who developed ototoxicity. Despite concern about enhancement of ototoxicity by elevated serum levels of gentamicin, there were no levels above 10 μg/ml in ototoxic patients. These authors [9, 12] demonstrated that ototoxicity could appear several weeks after completion of gentamicin therapy, and therefore they recommended that late follow-up inner ear testing should be carried out. Also, they documented that vestibular function can occasionally recover following damage caused by gentamicin.

Subsequently, we [6] studied 33 gentamicin-treated patients, 5 of whom (15%) developed ototoxicity. Two patients had auditory toxicity (one, asymptomatic and irreversible; the other, symptomatic and reversible); two patients had vestibular toxicity (one, symptomatic and of indeterminate duration; the other, symptomatic and reversible); and one patient had both auditory and vestibular toxicity (asymptomatic and reversible).

Noone et al. [8] observed no cases of auditory toxicity in 23 audiometrically monitored patients; however, 4 of 22 patients (18%) tested for vestibular function had a unilateral deficit.

A higher incidence of ototoxicity was reported by Winkel et al. [13] in 10 of 20 patients who received gentamicin. Audiometric and vestibular tests were performed at the time of treatment, and again up to 19 weeks after the cessation of treatment. The mean duration of therapy for these patients was 8 days.

Seven patients developed only auditory toxicity and one patient, only vestibular toxicity; two patients had toxic effects on both auditory and vestibular function. Cochlear toxicity was noted in 3 patients within a few days after the end of gentamicin therapy, and delayed auditory toxicity occurred in 6 patients 3 to 19 weeks after cessation of therapy. Two of the cases of vestibular toxicity were evident at the first follow-up test; the third was apparent at the second follow-up test. This study again points out the need for follow-up inner ear tests from which the actual incidence of ototoxicity can be determined. In four instances, the ototoxicity was transient. In most of the cases of ototoxicity, the effects were unilateral. Elevated trough levels were noted in four of the ototoxic patients, but similarly elevated trough levels were also present in four of the patients without ototoxicity. In one ototoxic patient, an elevated peak level was detected. Total dose given, concomitant furosemide therapy, and age were not significant risk factors.

Tobramycin Study

In a study by Lehmann et al. [4], the auditory and vestibular function of 18 patients treated with tobramycin was evaluated by audiometry and caloric testing with electronystagmographic recording at the beginning of, during, and at the end of therapy, and again 4 and 9 months later. The dose of tobramycin in the 13 patients with normal renal function was relatively low (2–3 mg/kg/day), but the range of duration of treatment courses was 10 to 49 days, with a mean of 18 days. There were no complaints of tinnitus, and the repeated audiograms of all patients showed no loss greater than 10 dB. The three patients with symptoms of vertigo developed bilateral impairment of nystagmic responses during therapy. These symptoms disappeared during or shortly after therapy, and in all three cases progressive recovery of vestibular function was shown by vestibular testing. The three patients with vestibular toxicity were among five with renal failure. Furthermore, the mean maximal peak serum level and the mean minimal trough level of tobramycin were significantly higher in toxic patients than in those without ototoxicity. Vestibular toxicity was also correlated with longer duration of therapy, although not with total dose, probably because the dose was reduced in the patients with impaired renal function.

Amikacin Studies

Amikacin, a semisynthetic derivative of kanamycin, is effective against most gram-negative aerobes that are resistant to gentamicin and tobramycin. Coordinating clinical studies on amikacin, Lane et al. [3] analyzed data from many centers on 1,548 patients who had been given this drug. Of 328 of these patients who had audiograms, 3.4 percent were found to have cochlear toxicity. Apparently no vestibular tests were carried out. Statistically significant risk factors were a higher total dose of amikacin and a history of previous aminoglycoside therapy.

Black et al. [1] reported that 13 of 44 patients treated with amikacin in 55 treatment courses showed evidence of toxicity by comparison of pre- and post-treatment audiograms. They identified the following statistically significant risk factors for auditory toxicity: duration of therapy, total dose of amikacin, history of aminoglycoside therapy, and elevated peak and trough levels of amikacin in serum. Whereas among patients with peak levels less than or equal to 32 μg/ml the incidence of auditory toxicity (toxic patients per number of treatment courses) was 13 percent, the incidence among patients with at least one peak level greater than 32 μg/ml was an astonishing 57 percent. Similarly, whereas only 19 percent of patients with amikacin trough levels all less than or equal to 10 μg/ml had auditory toxicity, 55 percent of patients with at least one trough level greater than 10 μg/ml had significant audiometric changes.

Yu et al. [14] reported a 20 percent incidence of auditory toxicity in the 15 amikacin-treated patients who underwent serial audiometry in a study of amikacin efficacy in 21 patients. None of the three patients evaluated by electronystagmography had evidence of vestibular toxicity. The mean peak serum level of amikacin was 20.8 μg/ml in the 24 treatment courses given. No comparison was made between the serum levels or other possible risk factors in the three patients who developed auditory toxicity and the characteristics of the other patients and their treatment courses.

In a study of efficacy in 20 amikacin-treated patients, Leonard et al. [5] reported 1 case of auditory toxicity in a patient with renal failure who developed moderate bilateral high-frequency hearing loss and eventually became deaf in the right ear. This patient also had markedly elevated serum levels of amikacin; on the eleventh day of therapy, the predialysis concentration of amikacin in serum was 49 μg/ml. There was no report of vestibular function testing in this study.

Comparative Studies

Some recent randomized, prospective studies [7, 10, 11] have focused on the toxicity as well as the efficacy of aminoglycoside antibiotics in comparative trials. Patients had serial audiograms, and the authors reported careful monitoring of serum aminoglycoside peak and trough levels, as well as renal function tests. Newer aminoglycosides were compared with a previously well-studied aminoglycoside antibiotic such as gentamicin. The incidence of ototoxicity obtained could then be evaluated with careful attention to risk factors such as age, duration of therapy, total dose, peak and trough serum levels, renal function, previous aminoglycoside therapy, concomitant administration of furosemide, and baseline sensorineural hearing deficit.

In a study of granulocytopenic patients with cancer, Love et al. [7] found audiologic evidence of toxicity in 2 of 32 patients treated with gentamicin, 1 of 29 treated with amikacin, and 1 of 29 treated with netilmicin. All of the patients with hearing loss were asymptomatic.

In a prospective, randomized, double-blind trial of gentamicin and amikacin by Smith et al. [10], audiograms showed toxicity (decrease in thresholds of > 10 dB) in 3 of 30 gentamicin-treated patients and in 2 of 34 patients treated with amikacin. The magnitude of these asymptomatic deficits in both groups of patients was comparable (20–30 dB).

In a similarly constructed study of auditory toxicity in patients treated with gentamicin or tobramycin, Smith et al. [11] reported that 5 of the 47 gentamicin-treated patients exhibited audiologic evidence of toxicity, and this was seen in 5 of the 44 tobramycin-treated patients. The average decrease in hearing threshold in these patients was comparable in the 2 groups (mean, 22 dB; range, 15–35 dB), and the effects were seen at 4.0 or 8.0 kHz or both in all but 1 of the patients.

Our Comparative Study on Gentamicin and Amikacin

In an effort to define further the characteristics of aminoglycoside ototoxicity in a patient population well monitored for renal and inner ear function and to compare the toxicity of amikacin to the standard, gentamicin, we conducted a prospective, randomized, double-blind comparative study of patients treated with one or the other of these two drugs. The emphasis of this study was on ototoxicity rather than efficacy, and, unlike other comparative studies previously described, it included an attempt to test patients for vestibular as well as auditory function.

Patients were considered for entry into the study if they were likely to require aminoglycoside therapy for at least 1 week and had received no aminoglycoside for at least 14 days previously. Additional requirements for patient entry were the ability to cooperate in audiometric testing and give consent for randomization to gentamicin or amikacin therapy.

The initial gentamicin dose was 1.7 to 2.0 mg/kg every 8 hours, and the initial amikacin dose was 5 to 6 mg/kg every 8 hours. Peak serum levels were determined by radioenzymatic assays carried out 15 minutes after the end of a 30- to 60-minute intravenous infusion (most of the patients were treated intravenously) or 60 minutes after intramuscular injection. Trough levels were measured in serum samples obtained 30 minutes before a dose was administered. The doses were adjusted to maintain peak gentamicin levels in the range of 4 to 8 μg/ml and peak amikacin levels of 15 to 30 μg/ml. Peak levels for both drugs were determined at least 2 to 3 times per week and trough levels, 1 to 2 times per week.

The patients' auditory pure-tone function was tested at 0.25, 0.50, 1.0, 2.0, 4.0, 6.0, and 8.0 kHz. Vestibular function was tested with water irrigation at 30°C and 44°C for 30 seconds in each ear. Responses were recorded on an electronystagmogram (ENG) with the patient's eyes closed. Baseline tests were carried out within 72 hours after initiation of treatment. Audiometry (and vestibular testing if the patient could cooperate) was performed every 1 to 2 weeks during therapy and 1 to 2 weeks after discontinuation of the aminoglycoside antibiotic. Patients were examined by a physician and ques-

Table 23-1. Patient Populations Under Study for Ototoxicity of Gentamicin and Amikacin

	No. of Patients Treated	
Major Underlying Disorder	Gentamicin	Amikacin
None	12	8
Hematologic malignancy	14	9
Lymphoproliferative malignancy	12	14
Solid tumor	4	4
Marrow aplasia	1	—
Hemoglobinopathy	1	4
Genitourinary	3	3
Collagen vascular disease	—	2
Sarcoidosis	—	1
Inflammatory bowel disease	—	1
Diabetes	3	2
Alcoholism	2	3
Drug Abuse	2	3
Total	54	54
Age (years) (mean ± standard deviation)	46.0 ± 22.6 (Range 4–85)	40.9 ± 17.6 (Range 6–83)
Elevated baseline serum creatinine (> 1.4 mg/100 ml)	5	2

tioned at least 4 times per week for symptoms of decreased hearing, tinnitus, or vertigo. If patients had such symptoms, more frequent inner ear testing was done.

Only patients with serial audiograms that could be evaluated for auditory toxicity are included in this report. Some patients were unable to cooperate with vestibular testing, and others had inadequate vestibular responses. Thus, not all of these patients could be evaluated for vestibular toxicity. Auditory toxicity was defined as a decrease of at least 15 dB in the threshold at 2 or more frequencies in either ear. Vestibular toxicity was defined as a decrease of at least 50 percent from the baseline average maximum slow-phase velocity of the caloric response in the ENG for either ear.

Table 23-1 lists the major underlying disorders of the 54 patients treated with gentamicin and the 54 patients treated with amikacin who were evaluable for ototoxicity. About half of the patients had malignant disease. Only five gentamicin patients and two amikacin patients had impaired renal function during the baseline period.

Thirty-one (57%) of the 54 gentamicin-treated patients could be evaluated for vestibular as well as auditory toxicity. Six patients (11%) developed ototoxicity (four auditory and two vestibular). Other characteristics of the toxicity in each of these six patients are also listed here:

1. Auditory: Bilateral, asymptomatic
2. Auditory: Unilateral, asymptomatic, delayed onset
3. Auditory: Bilateral, symptomatic, preceded by nephrotoxicity
4. Auditory: Bilateral, symptomatic, delayed onset
5. Vestibular: (Unilateral testing), asymptomatic, delayed onset
6. Vestibular: Bilateral, symptomatic, delayed onset, persistent, preceded by nephrotoxicity

Three of the patients were asymptomatic, and there were examples of unilateral inner ear deficits and of delayed onset (usually within 7 to 20 days after the end of therapy).

Thirty-five (65%) of the 54 amikacin-treated patients could be evaluated for vestibular as well as auditory toxicity. Seven patients (13%) developed ototoxicity (four auditory, two vestibular, and one both auditory and vestibular). Only one of the patients was symptomatic. Unilateral toxicity and delayed onset were again seen:

1. Auditory: Unilateral, asymptomatic, delayed onset, reversible
2. Auditory: Unilateral, asymptomatic, delayed onset, reversible
3. Auditory: Unilateral, symptomatic, persistent
4. Auditory: Unilateral → bilateral, asymptomatic → symptomatic, persistent
5. Auditory: Unilateral, asymptomatic, delayed onset, persistent
   Vestibular: (Unilateral testing), asymptomatic, delayed onset
6. Vestibular: Bilateral, asymptomatic, delayed onset, reversible
7. Vestibular: Bilateral, asymptomatic, delayed onset

Reversibility of the toxicity was documented in the audiograms of two patients with auditory toxicity and in the ENGs of one with vestibular toxicity.

Possible risk factors for ototoxicity in gentamicin-treated patients are given in Table 23-2. The only statistically significant differences between ototoxic and non-ototoxic patients were the higher mean trough serum levels of gentamicin and the higher incidence of a history of previous treatment with an aminoglycoside in the patients who developed toxicity. The same risk factors were considered for ototoxicity in amikacin-treated patients (Table 23-3). In this group, the mean age was significantly higher among patients who developed ototoxicity, but there was no correlation with ototoxicity of higher mean trough serum levels of amikacin or a history of previous aminoglycoside therapy. The mean course of therapy and mean total dose among non-ototoxic patients were skewed upward by 1 patient who received amikacin for 43 days.

In both the gentamicin and amikacin groups, furosemide treatment was not correlated with ototoxicity. We did not evaluate the concomitant use of ethacrynic acid, since this loop diuretic is seldom used in our hospital.

As others have also noted, audiometric testing reveals many cases of auditory toxicity in patients who are asymptomatic. In some of our patients, toxicity was first detected 7 to 20 days after cessation of therapy. The actual date of onset of detectable toxicity is not known. We were unable to test many of our

Table 23-2. Possible Risk Factors for Ototoxicity in 54 Gentamicin-Treated Patients

Risk Factor	Ototoxic (6)*	Non-ototoxic (48)*	*p*
Mean age (years)	46.7	50.0	ns
Mean course of therapy (days)	19.0†	10.3	ns
Mean total dose (mg/kg)	77.6†	43.9‡	ns
Mean of mean peak levels (μg/ml)	6.2†	6.3	ns
Mean of highest peak levels (μg/ml)	7.7†	7.6	ns
Mean of mean trough levels (μg/ml)	2.1†	1.3	< 0.05
Elevated baseline serum creatinine (> 1.4 mg/100 ml)	0%	10%	ns
Development of nephrotoxicity	33%	8%	ns
Previous aminoglycoside therapy	83%	23%	0.01
Peak level ≥ 10.0 μg/ml	0%	10%	ns
Trough level ≥ 2.5 μg/ml	50%	23%	ns
Concomitant furosemide	33%	12.5%	ns
Baseline sensorineural auditory deficit	33%	44%	ns

ns = not significant.
*Number of patients.
†Until onset of ototoxicity.
‡Patients with elevated baseline serum creatinine were excluded.

Table 23-3. Possible Risk Factors for Ototoxicity in 54 Amikacin-Treated Patients

Risk Factor	Ototoxic (7)*	Non-ototoxic (47)*	*p*
Mean age (years)	49.6	39.6	< 0.025
Mean course of therapy (days)	8.9†	11.3	< 0.05
Mean total dose (mg/kg)	135.7†	189.3‡	< 0.05
Mean of mean peak levels (μg/ml)	22.3†	20.9	ns
Mean of highest peak levels (μg/ml)	26.6†	27.0	ns
Mean of mean trough levels (μg/ml)	4.5†	3.7	ns
Elevated baseline serum creatinine (> 1.4 mg/100 ml)	0%	4%	ns
Development of nephrotoxicity	0%	0%	—
Previous aminoglycoside therapy	29%	21%	ns
Peak level ≥ 30 μg/ml	29%	28%	ns
Trough level ≥ 7.5 μg/ml	29%	15%	ns
Concomitant furosemide	0%	17%	ns
Baseline sensorineural auditory deficit	71%	38%	ns

ns = not significant.
*Number of patients.
†Until onset of ototoxicity.
‡Patients with elevated baseline serum creatinine were excluded.

patients later than a few days into the posttreatment period. Thus, we may have missed the development of auditory toxicity in some of these patients, and our figures for incidence may be underestimates. For purposes of comparison, we would expect the randomization used in the study protocol to make the effects of underestimation equivalent in the two treatment groups.

Comments

Efforts to refine and extend the techniques for assessment of auditory function in man are likely to aid research on ototoxicity. Testing of auditory thresholds at frequencies above 8.0 kHz (see Chaps. 15 and 16) should detect ototoxic auditory deficits at an earlier stage. Many seriously ill patients treated with aminoglycosides cannot be tested audiometrically because their level of consciousness does not permit them to cooperate adequately. In some of these patients, auditory function could perhaps be tested by means of evoked brainstem response (see Chap. 18).

Vestibular testing can be arduous, and many of the patients in our study could not participate because they could not be moved to the ENG laboratory or because they were too ill. Furthermore, some patients had such poor nystagmic responses to caloric irrigation in baseline studies that subsequent decreases could not be evaluated. In some cases, narcotic and hypnotic medications contributed to these depressed responses. For these reasons, only about 60 percent of our patients could be evaluated for the development of vestibular toxicity. Studies with sophisticated vestibular testing of normal subjects, such as those described in Chapter 19, should lead to improvements in the evaluation of vestibular toxicity. Whether such studies in normal volunteers can be extrapolated to seriously ill patients treated with aminoglycosides is not yet clear.

References

1. Black, R. E., Lau, W. K., Weinstein, R. J., Young, L. S., and Hewitt, W. L. Ototoxicity of amikacin. *Antimicrob. Agents Chemother.* 9:956, 1976.
2. Jackson, G. G., and Arcieri, G. Ototoxicity of gentamicin in man: A survey and controlled analysis of clinical experience in the United States. *J. Infect. Dis.* 124 [*Suppl.*]:S130, 1971.
3. Lane, A. Z., Wright, G. E., and Blair, D. C. Ototoxicity and nephrotoxicity of amikacin. *Am. J. Med.* 62:911, 1977.
4. Lehmann, W., Häusler, R., and Waldvogel, F. A. A clinical study on the ototoxic effects of tobramycin. *Arch. Otorhinolaryngol.* 212:203, 1976.
5. Leonard, J. M., McGee, Z. A., and Alford, R. H. Gentamicin-resistant bacillary infection. *Arch. Intern. Med.* 138:201, 1978.
6. Lerner, S. A., Verma, S. K., and Matz, G. J. Prospective clinical studies of ototoxicity of gentamicin. 9th International Congress of Chemotherapy (London), Abstract M-271, 1975.
7. Love, L. J., Schimpff, S. C., Hahn, D. M., Young, V. M., et al. Randomized trial of empiric antibiotic therapy with ticarcillin in combination with gentamicin, amikacin or netilmicin in febrile patients with granulocytopenia and cancer. *Am. J. Med.* 66:603, 1979.
8. Noone, P., Parsons, T. M. C., Pattison, J. R., Slack, R. C. B., et al. Experience in

monitoring gentamicin therapy during treatment of serious gram-negative sepsis. *Br. Med. J.* 1:477, 1974.

9. Nordström, L., Banck, G., Belfrage, S., Juhlin, I., et al. Prospective study of the ototoxicity of gentamicin. *Acta Pathol. Microbiol. Scand.* [*B*] 81 [Suppl. 241]:58, 1973.
10. Smith, C. R., Baughman, K. L., Edwards, C. Q., Rogers, J. F., and Lietman, P. S. Controlled comparison of amikacin and gentamicin. *N. Engl. J. Med.* 296:349, 1977.
11. Smith, C. R., Lipsky, J. J., Laskin, O. L., Hellmann, D. B., et al. Double-blind comparison of the nephrotoxicity and auditory toxicity of gentamicin and tobramycin. *N. Engl. J. Med.* 302:1106, 1980.
12. Tjernström, Ö., Banck, G., Belfrage, S., Juhlin, I., et al. The ototoxicity of gentamicin. *Acta Pathol. Microbiol. Scand.* [*B*] 81 [Suppl. 241]:73, 1973.
13. Winkel, O., Hansen, M. M., Kaaber, K., and Rozarth, K. A prospective study of gentamicin ototoxicity. *Acta Otolaryngol.* 86:212, 1978.
14. Yu, V. L., Rhame, F. S., Pesanti, E. L., and Axline, S. G. Amikacin therapy; use against infections caused by gentamicin- and tobramycin-resistant organisms. *J.A.M.A.* 238:943, 1977.

Discussion of Chapter 23

Dr. L. Nordström (Malmö General Hospital, Malmö, Sweden): The efficacy and toxicity of netilmicin were clinically evaluated in Malmö, Sweden. We studied 81 patients with a median age of 64 years. These were patients from the Infectious Diseases Clinic, and some of them had renal abnormalities. The average course of netilmicin therapy was 13 days. Seventy-four of the 81 patients were examined with audiograms before, during, and after the course of netilmicin. We discovered a low-frequency hearing loss due to netilmicin therapy in one patient.

The vestibular function of 76 of the 81 patients was also studied by electronystagmography and caloric testing before, during, and after the course of netilmicin therapy, and for up to 3 months after the drug was discontinued. One patient had a slightly abnormal electronystagmogram after treatment. This patient did not experience any dizziness or episodes of vertigo.

This netilmicin study was done in the same way as our gentamicin study in 1973 (Chap. 23, refs. 9, 12); therefore, the results obtained for netilmicin toxicity can be compared with those for gentamicin toxicity. However, we did find less ototoxicity with netilmicin than in our 1973 gentamicin study.

Dr. N. G. Toremalm (Malmö General Hospital, Malmö, Sweden): I would like to comment on 29 cases from the Renal Clinic in Malmö. All of the patients had severe kidney disease. Twenty-five of the 29 had electronystagmograms performed during gentamicin treatment. We found that, of the 29 patients, 5 had vestibular toxicity. However, 4 of the 5 had pretreatment vestibular function abnormalities; this emphasized the importance of baseline studies within the first 24 to 48 hours.

Dr. M. Barza (Tufts University, Boston): We have just completed a comparative study of netilmicin and amikacin. These drugs were not significantly different in their ototoxicity, but interestingly, all of the 10 patients with ototoxicity were males, in a study in which two-thirds of the subjects were male. I wonder whether anyone else has noticed a sex difference in ototoxicity.

Dr. Matz: We haven't found that in our study. I agree with Dr. Toremalm; we would not accept a patient for our study unless we had a baseline audiogram and vestibular test. We define baseline values as having been obtained within 72 hours of the start of therapy. It is desirable to perform the tests before the aminoglycoside is started, but that is not generally possible.

Dr. Smith: In our studies, the two patients with the most severe auditory toxicity were women. In most of the studies that have been reported by Dr. Matz, only relatively large differences in ototoxicity could have been determined—that is, differences of 20 or 25 percent. So, there may be smaller differences that went undetected in the small number of patients tested.

Dr. P. A. Bernard (Laval University, Quebec): What do you think about the possible age bias in the interpretation of high-frequency hearing loss following ototoxic drugs? Recently, I had the opportunity to review the charts of patients with urologic diseases who were treated with the newer aminoglycoside antibiotics, and I noticed that most of the patients were more than 60 years old. The pretreatment audiograms of a number of these patients showed high-frequency hearing loss (above 4 kHz). Since aminoglycosides cause high-frequency hearing loss, how is it possible to detect ototoxicity in these older patients who have presbycusis?

Dr. Lerner: It is true that, if you have a major preexisting hearing deficit, the possibility of detecting an additional deficit is compromised. There were some patients in our study, particularly very elderly patients, who were so deaf to begin with, or who had so little electronystagmographic response, that we did not include them in our study. If there is not much function to begin with, you simply cannot evaluate these patients. You may recall, however, that Dr. Matz mentioned that there did not seem to be an increased risk of ototoxicity in patients who had some preexisting hearing deficit, but who could be evaluated for toxicity.

Dr. Brummett: Dr. Matz, how long was the delay in the onset of ototoxicity?

Dr. Matz: It was usually detected about 7 to 20 days after the end of therapy. Most of these patients were asymptomatic. Some did not have audiograms performed immediately at the end of therapy, so we were not sure of the exact time of onset of hearing loss in these "delayed" cases. In our study, we did not find the classical delayed ototoxicity that had been observed with dihydrostreptomycin. The delayed toxicity that we found is probably something that we had missed in a previous examination.

Dr. Brummett: How long after the initiation of therapy did you first notice ototoxicity?

Dr. Matz: The earliest onset of toxicity that I have come across occurred on the sixth or seventh day in a patient given an accidental neomycin overdose.* In our prospective study, probably the earliest symptoms of toxicity

*L. Lowry, M. May, and P. Pastore, Acute histopathological inner ear changes in deafness due to neomycin: A case report. *Ann. Otol. Rhinol. Laryngol.* 82:876, 1973.

were seen at 10 days. Moffat and Ramsden† reported a case of ototoxicity at 3 days.

Dr. Brummett: I would exercise caution in regard to the continuous infusion of aminoglycosides. It has been shown by several people at our university and by others that if you give aminoglycosides to rats at the same total dose in two or three injections per day, you get more nephrotoxicity than you would if you gave the drug as a single bolus dose. This also occurs with ototoxicity in the guinea pig, but we may not be able to extrapolate that to man. However, I don't think we want to start giving patients aminoglycosides by continuous infusion.

Dr. Matz: We are not planning continuous-infusion therapy.

Dr. Lerner: Bodey's group at M. D. Anderson Hospital is the only one that has used continuous-infusion therapy in large numbers of patients (Chap. 25, ref. 8). In their neutropenic patients, the effectiveness of aminoglycosides given alone by continuous infusion is comparable to that of the combination of aminoglycoside and carbenicillin. If it is true that you have a patient who is penicillin-allergic and neutropenic and has an organism for which one can use only an aminoglycoside, one might consider continuous drug therapy. But I think there is probably an increased risk of ototoxicity.

†D. A. Moffat and R. T. Ramsden, Profound bilateral sensorineural hearing loss during gentamicin therapy. *J. Laryngol. Otol.* 91:511, 1977.

24. Aminoglycoside Ototoxicity in Children

Jane D. Siegel and George H. McCracken, Jr.

Pediatric Pharmacology

The aminoglycosides have been used for the past 2 decades as first-line drugs for treatment of serious infections in 5 groups of pediatric patients: the newborn, children with cystic fibrosis, oncology patients, surgery patients, and those with burn injuries. In the early years of aminoglycoside use, no information was available on differences in the metabolism and excretion of these drugs in neonates and young children, as compared with adults. Therefore, excessive doses often caused irreversible ototoxicity. As pediatric pharmacology gained recognition as a specialized field, the pharmacokinetics of these antibiotics has been defined for each age group, and safe and effective dose schedules have been established. An understanding of the unique features of aminoglycoside pharmacology in pediatric patients is necessary for the detection and prevention of drug-induced ototoxicity.

The earliest exposure to aminoglycosides may occur in utero when these drugs are administered to pregnant women. Transplacental transport of amikacin [2], gentamicin [34], kanamycin [14], streptomycin [15], and tobramycin [3] has been documented (Table 24-1). Passage of drugs across the placenta is greatest during the first and third trimesters and when the drug is administered very rapidly to the mother. Cord serum levels may vary from 15 to 70 percent of the concentrations in maternal serum. Although the fetal kidney does not function as an organ of elimination of waste products, therapeutic levels of aminoglycosides are present in the fetal kidney and urine for as long as 12 to 30 hours after a dose of the drugs. Drug concentrations in the fetal inner ear have not been reported. Renal failure, concomitant use of diuretics, and a prolonged course of therapy are the most important factors in the development of fetal ototoxicity.

The young infant may be exposed to aminoglycosides that are excreted into the breast milk. Kanamycin and dihydrostreptomycin levels have been measured in human milk [20, 24]. Following the intramuscular administration of

Table 24-1. Transplacental Transport of Aminoglycosides

Drug	Dose and Route	Peak Serum Concentration: μg/ml (hrs after dose)		Concentration: μg/ml (hrs after dose)		
		Maternal	Cord	Amniotic Fluid	Fetal Kidney	Fetal Urine
Amikacin [2]	7.5 mg/kg IM	18.0 (1)	3.4 (2)	1.04 (≥ 3.5)	22 (12)	24 (3)
Gentamicin [34]	40 mg IM prior to delivery	3.65 (0.5)	1.25 (1–2)	—	—	—
Kanamycin [14]	500 mg IM prior to delivery	18.6 (1)	9.0 (1.75)	5.5 (6)	—	—
Streptomycin [15]	100,000 units SC prior to delivery	7.6 units/cc (1.5)*	5.9 units/cc (1.5)*	—	—	—
Tobramycin [3]	2 mg/kg IM	4.0 (1)	0.6 (2.5)	0.25 (≥ 4)	7.2 (34)	3.4 (25)

*Not peak value; this was the only time that samples were obtained.

1 g kanamycin, the average concentration of kanamycin in milk was 18.4 μg/ml at 1 hour after injection, compared to 0.3 to 1.3 μg/ml after a similar dose of dihydrostreptomycin. There are, however, no documented cases of aminoglycoside toxicity in a suckling infant of a mother receiving aminoglycoside therapy. This is probably the result of the low total amount of drug ingested and the poor absorption of aminoglycosides from the uninflamed gastrointestinal tract.

Because the volume of distribution of aminoglycosides approximates that of the extracellular fluid space, and because these drugs do not penetrate well into cells, it has been assumed that they are distributed primarily in this space [1]. The variation of the extracellular fluid volume best explains the age-related dose response to aminoglycosides. The extracellular fluid space is approximately 40 to 44 percent of body weight during the newborn period, 26 percent from 6 months to 5 years, and 18 percent in older children and adults [12]. Therefore, when doses are based on body weight, they must be higher in the infant and young child than in the adult to provide the same therapeutic serum concentrations.

The aminoglycosides are excreted in unaltered form by glomerular filtration. Therefore, an understanding of neonatal kidney function is essential for the prediction of drug levels in the serum and the risk of renal toxicity and ototoxicity. Induction of new nephrons is completed by 34 weeks' gestation, but the glomerulus in a full-term neonate has only one-third of its adult diameter. The renal plasma flow and consequently the glomerular filtration rates are low at birth, but increase substantially by 3 days of age. As the kidney continues to mature, creatinine clearance increases to a level of 113 mg/min per 1.73 m^2, achieved by 3 years of age. Any factor that decreases renal plasma flow will delay drug elimination. For example, a prolonged serum half-life of amikacin has been observed in hypoxemic infants [22].

Serum creatinine is the most convenient index of renal function in the newborn infant. At birth, creatinine levels reflect maternal renal function; these levels decrease rapidly over the first 24 to 48 hours of life. The serum creatinine remains at or below 1 mg/dl after 2 days of age in term babies, but may be as high as 1.8 mg/dl during the first 10 days of life in preterm infants. This may explain why prolonged serum half-life values and elevated peak serum concentrations of aminoglycosides after an average of 10 doses have been observed in infants with very low birthweight [7].

Studies of Ototoxicity in Children

Interpretation of studies of aminoglycoside ototoxicity in children is limited by the following factors:

1. Most studies were performed prior to the development of dose schedules appropriate for infants and children; therefore, the reported incidence of ototoxicity cannot be applied to presently recommended dose schedules.

2. With the traditional methods used for detection of hearing loss, only major impairment could be measured in children 2 years of age or older. The recent introduction of auditory evoked brainstem potentials for assessment of auditory function [30] has enabled the pediatrician to identify abnormalities within the first month of life and does not require the patient to be in an alert state of consciousness. Insufficient data have been gathered to date, however, to allow a confident prediction of permanent hearing impairment.
3. In most studies, vestibular function has not been evaluated carefully.
4. Few studies have been prospective, randomized, and controlled, with adequate follow-up. A review of the studies of aminoglycoside ototoxicity in children will provide the basis for future investigations and for the development of guidelines for the prevention and detection of ototoxicity.

Intrauterine Exposure

The introduction of streptomycin and dihydrostreptomycin was a major advancement in the therapy of tuberculosis. Although it was not long before impairment of auditory function was recognized as an adverse effect of dihydrostreptomycin, and to a lesser extent of streptomycin, the effect on children born of tuberculous mothers who had been treated with one of these drugs during pregnancy was not immediately apparent. Robinson and Cambon [28] suggested that the greatest risk for ototoxicity should be during the first half of pregnancy, because the inner ear reaches complete maturation by midterm. Yet there are reports of ototoxicity that occurred with exposure during the last trimester only [28, 32].

It is difficult to determine the incidence of ototoxicity in children exposed in utero because most authors have reported only isolated cases. Robinson and Cambon studied 300 preschool children with hearing loss and found 2 whose mothers had received prolonged therapy with streptomycin (total dose 16 and 32 g) during pregnancy [28]. Conway [6] studied 17 children whose mothers had received streptomycin or dihydrostreptomycin during pregnancy and found no hearing loss at the speech frequencies. Four children did, however, have a threshold below 20 dB at 8,000 Hz unilaterally, and 6 had abnormal responses to caloric testing. The authors suggest that children who have been exposed in utero receive audiologic evaluation before successive exposures to ototoxic agents so that a preexisting hearing loss can be ruled out.

A remarkable case of ototoxicity associated with exposure in utero was reported by Jones in 1973 [18]. At 28 weeks' gestation, the mother received 4.5 g of kanamycin over 5 days for a *Klebsiella* urinary tract infection; 3 days after initiation of antimicrobial therapy, ethacrynic acid was prescribed for induction of diuresis because the serum creatinine had increased to 5.4 mg/dl. Within 2 weeks, the mother was deaf, and her child had severe sensorineural hearing loss when first tested at age 3 years. The toxicity of kanamycin for this infant was apparently enhanced by maternal renal insufficiency and the addition of a second drug known to contribute to ototoxicity.

Familial Predisposition

In their studies of ototoxicity caused by streptomycin and dihydrostreptomycin, Pražić et al. [25] and Johnsonbaugh et al. [17] observed a familial predisposition toward developing toxicity upon exposure to these two drugs. Pražić et al. cite seven family members whose hearing was tested. In the four members who had not received either drug, the audiometric findings were normal. Three sisters, however, became deaf after receiving 5 daily doses of 1 g of streptomycin. Similarly, Johnsonbaugh et al. reported a mother and infant who developed bilateral sensorineural loss in the speech range after receiving 138 g and 350 mg of streptomycin, respectively. Tinnitus was noted by the mother 11 months after streptomycin therapy for tuberculosis was begun. Bilateral sensorineural hearing loss was documented 2 months later. Her son received a total dose of 350 mg of streptomycin as a neonate, but hearing loss was not documented until his first audiogram was performed at age 5 years. Although this phenomenon has not been reported for other aminoglycosides, these drugs should be avoided, if possible, in patients who have a positive family history of ototoxicity.

Immaturity

The major studies of ototoxicity caused by aminoglycosides have been performed on neonates. The newborn infant, especially if premature, is at the greatest risk for ototoxicity because of his renal immaturity and the presence of underlying conditions that may act alone or synergistically with drugs to damage the inner ear. In 1958, Campanelli et al. [5] reported sensorineural hearing loss in 15.9 percent of 44 premature infants tested at 72 to 84 months of age. Low birthweight and prolonged exposure to incubator noise were significantly associated with abnormal hearing; drug therapy was not evaluated. Apnea, hypoxia, hyperbilirubinemia, hypotension, electrolyte imbalance, and gram-negative meningitis have also been implicated as etiologic factors in hearing impairment.

The studies of aminoglycoside ototoxicity in neonates are listed in Table 24-2. Early studies in which an increased incidence of ototoxicity in treated infants was reported generally included fewer patients than did a later group of studies that showed no differences in the occurrence of ototoxicity between groups of treated infants and comparable controls.

Yow et al. [35] reported a retrospective study of 30 children who were at least 22 months of age, 8 of whom had received kanamycin during the first 2 months of life. Three of the eight infants were premature, and two of these three had bilateral sensorineural hearing loss. These children received large total doses, 865 mg/kg and 975 mg/kg, and showed evidence of drug accumulation that was attributed to reduced renal function. The third premature infant who had received a comparable dose of kanamycin did, however, have normal hearing. All of the controls for this age group had normal auditory function.

Elfving et al. [10] studied 28 children 2 years old or older who had received

Table 24-2. Ototoxicity Studies in Neonates Who Received Parenteral Aminoglycosides

Study	Drug	Total Number	Number Impaired (%)	
Ototoxicity present				
Yow et al., 1962 [35]	K	8	2	(25)
Elfving et al., 1973 [10]	G	28	2	(7.5)
Bernard et al., 1979 [4]	G, T	15	15	(100)
Ototoxicity absent				
Johnsonbaugh et al., 1966 [17a]	S	98	16*	(16.3)
Eichenwald, 1966 [9]	K, S	236	12*	(5.1)
Sanders et al., 1967 [29]	K	20	0	(0)
Winkel et al., 1978 [33]	K + incubator	54	10*	(18.5)
Finitzo-Hieber et al., 1979 [11]	G, K	118	11*	(9.3)

G = gentamicin; K = kanamycin; T = tobramycin; S = streptomycin.
*No difference from control groups.

gentamicin as neonates; they found only 1 infant with a severe bilateral sensorineural hearing loss and mild impairment of vestibular function that could be attributed to gentamicin. Admittedly, the role of prematurity, hypoglycemia, and septicemia cannot be overlooked as contributing factors. This child, however, had received the largest dose of gentamicin in the series. An additional patient with slight vestibular dysfunction had a course complicated by asphyxia, aseptic meningitis, and cerebral concussion at age 10 months. The doses of gentamicin given to all of these infants were substantially lower than those used today: 0.9 to 4.3 mg/kg per day versus 5.0 to 7.5 mg/kg per day.

Recently, Bernard et al. [4] reported the use of brainstem response audiometry for assessment of auditory function in 15 neonates treated with either gentamicin or tobramycin at a daily dose of 7.5 mg/kg for 6 to 10 days. The latency of the prominent wave V was significantly delayed in all 15 after 5 and 10 days of therapy, compared with those measured in a control group of 14 neonates. Further follow-up is required, however, to establish how accurately these changes will predict functional impairment.

Marcus et al. [19] examined 35 deaf children who had been born prematurely and looked specifically for an etiologic noxious agent. Auditory function was absent in 30 and markedly reduced (> 60 dB to 100 dB at most frequencies) in 5 cases. Similarly, vestibular function was absent in 26, markedly reduced (< 5 seconds of post-rotatory nystagmus) in 8, and normal in 1. Twenty-nine of the 35 children had received dihydrostreptomycin in the premature nursery in doses of 125 to 250 mg per day for an average of 5 to 7 days. Because these doses greatly exceeded the recommended daily dose of 40 mg/kg in 21 of these infants, the authors infer a cause-and-effect relationship between auditory and vestibular dysfunction and dihydrostreptomycin therapy. This does not, however, explain the impairment observed in the 6 children who did not receive aminoglycoside therapy.

Four of the five studies performed that did not implicate the aminoglycosides as causative agents of ototoxicity in premature infants included a reasonably well-matched control population. The incidence of hearing impairment varied from 5 to 20 percent, but showed no difference from that in the untreated controls within each study. The studies performed by Eichenwald [9] and by Finitzo-Hieber et al. [11] are noteworthy for their prospective controlled design.

Eichenwald enrolled 212 untreated infants as controls, 165 infants treated with 15 mg/kg per day of kanamycin for an average of 8 days, and 111 infants treated with 40 mg/kg per day of streptomycin for an average of 10 days; 30 percent of the infants in each group were born prematurely. The dropout rate varied from 13 to 20 percent; there were 170, 143, and 93 infants, respectively, in each group, who underwent audiometric testing at age 4 to 5 years. The percentage of infants with hearing deficit defined as a loss $\geq$ 30 dB in at least 2 frequencies was essentially the same in each group: 4.4, 5.1, and 5.6 percent, respectively. Vestibular function was not evaluated.

In the study of kanamycin and gentamicin conducted by Finitzo-Hieber et al. [11], infants treated with either of these two drugs and appropriately matched untreated controls were enrolled at the time of their hospitalization in the newborn nursery. There were 347 infants enrolled in the study: 116 in the gentamicin group received 5 to 6 mg/kg per day for a mean of 8.2 days, 118 in the kanamycin group received 15 mg/kg per day for a mean of 7.4 days, and 113 were untreated controls. Conventional tests of auditory and vestibular function were performed at yearly intervals for 4 years. This yearly follow-up was intended to provide an accurate assessment of function and identify any interim events beyond the period of treatment that could affect auditory function. The methods of assessment used for each age group in this study are listed in Table 24-3. Because of minimal stimulus control during the first-year auditory examination, only infants with severe bilateral impairment could be identified. This evaluation, however, provided a general comparison of the auditory capabilities between the two drug-treated groups and the control infants. At the second-year examination, tympanometry and acoustic reflex measures for pure tones at 500, 1,000, 2,000, and 4,000 Hz were obtained for each ear. Vestibular function was estimated by the Bárány rotational test. At the third-year examination, pure-tone thresholds were obtained for each ear under earphones, and impedance and vestibular function were tested. Audiometric evaluation was repeated at the fourth-year examination only in children who had failed at the third-year examination. Psycholinguistic ability, visual-motor integration, and picture vocabulary ability were evaluated at the age of 4 years.

The average total dose per patient was 38 mg/kg of gentamicin and 100 mg/kg of kanamycin. Peak serum concentrations were greater than the hypothesized toxic level of 10 μg/ml of gentamicin in 2 patients. All kanamy-

Table 24-3. Methods Used for Evaluation of Hearing and Vestibular Function in Children in 4-Year Follow-Up Study after Treatment with Kanamycin or Gentamicin

1. First-year examinations
   - Taped filtered environmental sounds at 70–90 dB sound pressure level in quiet room
   - Parental report of response to sound, vocalization
2. Second-year examinations
   - Behavioral observation audiometry
   - Visual reinforcement audiometry
   - Impedance testing
   - Tympanometry
   - Bárány rotational test
3. Third-year examinations
   - Pure-tone thresholds for each ear, determined by conditioned play audiometry
   - Speech and music awareness responses
   - Bárány rotational test
4. Fourth-year examinations
   - Illinois Test of Psycholinguistic Abilities (ITPA)
   - Beery Test of Visual Motor Integration (VMI)
   - Peabody Picture Vocabulary Test (PPVT)

Source: T. Finitzo-Hieber et al., Ototoxicity in neonates treated with gentamicin and kanamycin: Results of a four-year controlled follow-up study. *Pediatrics* 63:443, 1979.

cin peaks were below 30 μg/ml. The proportion of the original population that returned for follow-up decreased substantially each year: 62, 49, 37, and finally 25 percent at the fourth-year examination. Although there was an insignificantly increased incidence of acute renal toxicity in the gentamicin group, no significant differences in auditory (see Fig. 24-1) and vestibular function were demonstrated among the gentamicin-treated, kanamycin-treated, and control groups at the third-year follow-up. There were, however, four major limitations of this study: (1) a high yearly dropout rate characteristic of a transient population; (2) the length of time required for definitive evaluation of auditory and vestibular function; (3) the imprecision of the methods available at the time; and (4) the doses used in this study, which were lower than those currently recommended. Therefore, the failure to demonstrate ototoxicity at the doses employed does not completely assure the safety of the larger doses.

Drs. Finitzo-Hieber and McCracken are now engaged in a prospective, randomized, controlled study in which they are using brainstem response audiometry to determine the relative ototoxic effect of amikacin and netilmicin in neonates. To date, 103 infants have been enrolled. Because this is a blind study, the code has not been broken and no results are available at present.

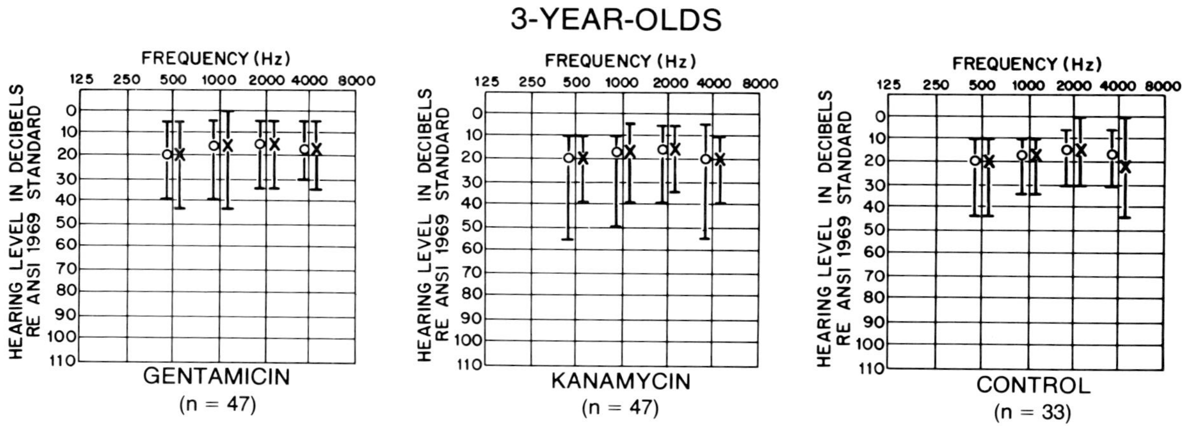

Figure 24-1. Pure-tone audiometric test results for the right (○) and left (×) ears for each subject group (mean and range) at 3-year examination. (From T. Finitzo-Hieber et al., Ototoxicity in neonates treated with gentamicin and kanamycin: Results of a four-year controlled follow-up study. *Pediatrics* 63:443, 1979. Reprinted by permission.)

Clinical Conditions Associated with Increased Risk of Aminoglycoside Ototoxicity in Children

Most of the following underlying clinical conditions have not been assessed for their individual contributions to the development of aminoglycoside ototoxicity in children because it is difficult to study them independently:

Apnea
Hypoxia
Hyperbilirubinemia
Electrolyte imbalance
Hypotension
Sepsis/meningitis
Maintenance in incubator
Diuretic therapy
Renal failure

Noise related to prolonged maintenance of premature infants in an incubator has, however, been studied by Winkel et al. [33]. In this study, audiometric and vestibular functions of ninety-one 4- to 6-year-old children with birth weights below 2,000 g were evaluated. The same incidence of sensorineural hearing loss (19%) was found in 54 children treated as neonates with 10 mg/kg per day of kanamycin as in a group of 37 infants who did not receive kanamycin. There were no signs of synergism between incubator noise and kanamycin when 54 children who were both treated with kanamycin and placed in an incubator were compared with a group of 16 children placed in an incubator only. Although all five of the cases of moderate or severe hearing loss occurred in the group subjected to both incubator and kanamycin, these children also had more severe neonatal complications. These findings are in contrast to the animal studies of Dayal et al. [8] and Jauhiainen et al. [16], which demonstrated conclusively that the hair cells of the guinea pig cochlea were sensitized by neomycin and kanamycin, resulting in increased susceptibility to the damaging effects of low-intensity noise (68 to 72 dB at 125 Hz), which is comparable to that of a standard nursery incubator. These studies suggest that incubator noise warrants further evaluation of its role in ototoxicity.

Route of Administration

Patients who receive aminoglycosides by the oral, intrathecal, or intraventricular routes may be at increased risk of developing ototoxicity because of the unexpectedly high serum and CSF levels that are sometimes attained. Nunnery and Riley [23] administered gentamicin orally to a group of infants below 1 year of age who had *Shigella* dysentery. More than 10 percent of the drug was excreted in the urine during the acute phase of illness, compared to only 2 percent after acute inflammation had subsided. Similarly, Ritter et al. [27] have demonstrated a significant increase in peak serum levels of gentamicin in infants with necrotizing enterocolitis who received 15 mg/kg per day of gentamicin by nasogastric tube in addition to 7.5 mg/kg per day intramuscularly. Four of 9 patients in the study achieved peak serum gentamicin levels above 10 μg/ml; none of the 9 control infants reached this level. Auditory function was not evaluated in these infants. Ranta [26] has implicated the intrathecal administration of streptomycin to children with tuberculous meningitis in the development of ototoxicity. Eighteen percent of 124 children with nonmeningitic tuberculosis developed mild hearing loss; they had received a total dose of 40 to 50 g dihydrostreptomycin. In contrast, 62 percent of 101 children with tuberculous meningitis developed hearing loss. These children received 1 to 3 mg/kg per day of streptomycin sulfate intrathecally in addition to 10 to 50 mg/kg per day of dihydrostreptomycin parenterally. Because the incidence of both hearing and vestibular loss decreased in the later years of the study, concomitant with both abandonment of intrathecal streptomycin and reduction in dose of dihydrostreptomycin, the ototoxicity has been attributed to drug therapy rather than to the disease process. It is difficult to determine to what extent other factors such as earlier diagnosis contributed to this reduction in toxicity.

In infants with coliform meningitis, gentamicin concentrations above 30 μg/ml have been measured in the lumbar and ventricular fluid 2 to 4 hours following intrathecal and intraventricular therapy. One might anticipate that this would produce a substantial elevation of drug levels in the inner ear fluid, resulting in toxicity; however, such levels have not been measured. Data from the first Neonatal Meningitis Cooperative Study [21] indicated that only one (1.3%) of 79 infants who received gentamicin for a minimum of 3 weeks (5–7.5 mg/kg/day) and were followed for 2 to 6 years had hearing impairment that may have been related to gentamicin. Analysis of patients in the second study who received intraventricular gentamicin has not been completed. The development of distinctive toxic lesions in the brainstem following intrathecal therapy with gentamicin in an adult patient with *Pseudomonas aeruginosa* meningitis has been reported [31]. This effect was reproduced in rabbits after intracisternal injection of 2.5 mg/kg of gentamicin. A greatly increased risk of ototoxicity might be expected in such a patient. Presently, this is more a theoretical than a practical consideration, because intrathecal and intraventricular administration of aminoglycosides are no longer recommended for the treatment of coliform meningitis in neonates [21]; intrathecal therapy offers no advantage, and intraventricular therapy is associated with increased mortality.

Total Dose

Ranta [26] concluded from his study of the therapy of tuberculous meningitis in children that a daily dose of 10 to 20 mg/kg and a total dose of 50 g of dihydrostreptomycin were not associated with the development of hearing loss. In their study of 30 children 14 years of age or younger who received 10 to 100 mg/kg per day of kanamycin, Yow et al. [35] indicated that the total dose that can be administered safely to children is comparable to that for adults

[13]: 500 mg/kg. Three of 12 children who received total doses above 500 mg/kg developed hearing loss, compared with only 2 of 18 in the group that received less than 500 mg/kg. There are no other aminoglycoside studies in children that define a range of relatively safe total doses.

Conclusion

The major pediatric reviews of aminoglycoside ototoxicity indicate that, in spite of the many high-risk factors present, it is difficult to implicate these drugs during the neonatal period as a single cause of substantial sensorineural hearing impairment. This is consistent with the recent clinical experience of pediatricians who have used these agents with apparent impunity. The major limitation of these studies, however, has been the inability to detect mild to moderate auditory dysfunction in very young infants and to determine a definitive relationship to drug therapy. Studies such as those described in this volume by Finitzo-Hieber on brainstem evoked response and by the Eviatars on vestibular testing will assist the clinician in developing guidelines needed for evaluation of the safety of routinely used drugs as well as of investigational drugs newly introduced into the nursery. More importantly, the use of brainstem response audiometry should permit detection of hearing loss early enough to prevent speech impairment.

References

1. Arant, B. S., Jr. Developmental patterns of renal functional maturation compared in the human neonate. *J. Pediatr.* 92:705, 1978.
2. Bernard, B., Abate, M., Threlen, P. F., Attar, H., Ballard, C. A., and Wehrle, P. F. Maternal-fetal pharmacological activity of amikacin. *J. Infect. Dis.* 135:925, 1977.
3. Bernard, B., Garcia-Cázares, S. J., Ballard, C. A., Thrupp, L. D., Mathies, A. W., and Wehrle, P. F. Tobramycin: Maternal-fetal pharmacology. *Antimicrob. Agents Chemother.* 11:688, 1977.
4. Bernard, B., Pechere, J. C., Hebert, R., Dery, P., and Carrier, C. Detection of aminoglycoside antibiotics induced ototoxicity in newborns using brainstem response audiometry. 19th Interscience Conference on Antimicrobial Agents and Chemotherapy (Boston), Abstract 939, 1979.
5. Campanelli, P. A., Pollock, F. J., and Henner, R. An otoaudiological evaluation of forty-four premature children. *Arch. Otolaryngol.* 67:609, 1958.
6. Conway, N. Streptomycin in pregnancy: Effect on the foetal ear. *Br. Med. J.* 2:260, 1965.
7. Coyer, W. F., Wesbey, G. E., Cech, K. L., and Robinson, J. A. Intravenous gentamicin pharmacokinetics in the small preterm infant. *Pediatr. Res.* 12:Abstract 240, 1978.
8. Dayal, V. S., Kokshanian, A., and Mitchell, D. P. Combined effects of noise and kanamycin. *Ann. Otol. Rhinol. Laryngol.* 80:897, 1971.
9. Eichenwald, H. F. Some observations on dosage and toxicity of kanamycin in premature and fullterm infants. *Ann. N.Y. Acad. Sci.* 132:984, 1966.
10. Elfving, J., Pettay, O., and Raivio, M. A follow-up study on the cochlear, vestibular and renal function in children treated with gentamicin in the newborn period. *Chemotherapy* 18:141, 1973.
11. Finitzo-Hieber, T., McCracken, G. H., Jr., Roeser, R. J., Allen, D. A., Chrane, D. F., and Morrow, J. Ototoxicity in neonates treated with gentamicin and kanamycin: Results of a four-year controlled follow-up study. *Pediatrics* 63:443, 1979.

12. Friis-Hansen, B. Body water compartments in children: Changes during growth and related changes in body composition. *Pediatrics* 28:169, 1961.
13. Frost, J. O., Hawkins, J. E., and Daly, J. F. Kanamycin. II. Ototoxicity. *Am. Rev. Respir. Dis.* 82:23, 1960.
14. Good, R. G., and Johnson, G. H. The placental transfer of kanamycin during late pregnancy. *Obstet. Gynecol.* 38:60, 1971.
15. Heilman, D. H., Heilman, F. R., Hinshaw, H. C., Nichols, D. R., and Henell, W. E. Streptomycin: Absorption, diffusion, excretion and toxicity. *Am. J. Med. Sci.* 210:576, 1945.
16. Jauhiainen, T., Kohonen, A., and Jauhiainen, M. Combined effect of noise and neomycin on the cochlea. *Acta Otolaryngol.* 73:387, 1972.
17. Johnsonbaugh, R. E., Drexler, H. G., Light, I. J., and Sutherland, J. M. Familial occurrence of drug-induced hearing loss. *Am. J. Dis. Child.* 127:245, 1974.
17a. Johnsonbaugh, R. E., Drexler, H. G., Sutherland, J. M., and Light, I. J. Audiometric study of streptomycin-treated infants. *Am. J. Dis. Child.* 112:43, 1966.
18. Jones, H. C. Intrauterine ototoxicity. *J. Natl. Med. Assoc.* 65:201, 1973.
19. Marcus, R. E., Small, H., and Emanuel, B. Ototoxic medication in premature children. *Arch. Otolaryngol.* 77:198, 1963.
20. McCracken, G. H. Clinical Pharmacology of Antibacterial Agents. In J. S. Remington and J. O. Klein (Eds.), *Infectious Diseases of the Fetus and Newborn Infant.* Philadelphia: Saunders, 1976. P. 1029.
21. McCracken, G. H., Jr., Mize, S. G., and Threlkeld, N. Intraventricular gentamicin therapy in gram-negative bacillary meningitis of infancy. *Lancet,* April 12, 1980, p. 787.
22. Myers, M. G., Roberts, R. F., and Mirhij, N. J. Effects of gestational age, birthweight and hypoxemia on pharmacokinetics of amikacin in serum of infants. *Antimicrob. Agents Chemother.* 11:1027, 1977.
23. Nunnery, A. W., and Riley, H. D., Jr. Gentamicin: Pharmacologic observations in newborns and infants. *J. Infect. Dis.* 119:402, 1969.
24. O'Brien, J. E. Excretion of drugs in human milk. *Am. J. Hosp. Pharm.* 31:844, 1974.
25. Pražić, M., Salaj, B., and Subotić, R. Familial sensitivity to streptomycin. *J. Laryngol. Otol.* 78:1037, 1964.
26. Ranta, L. J. Acoustic and vestibular disturbances following streptomycin-treated tuberculous meningitis in children. *Acta Otolaryngol. (Stockh.)* [Suppl. 136], 1958.
27. Ritter, D. A., Hansen, T. N., Speer, M. E., and Kenny, J. D. Absorption of oral gentamicin in infants with necrotizing enterocolitis. 19th Interscience Conference on Antimicrobial Agents and Chemotherapy (Boston), Abstract 109, 1979.
28. Robinson, G. C., and Cambon, K. G. Hearing loss in infants of tuberculous mothers treated with streptomycin during pregnancy. *N. Engl. J. Med.* 271:949, 1964.
29. Sanders, D. Y., Eliot, D. S., and Cramblett, H. B. Retrospective study for possible kanamycin ototoxicity among neonatal infants. *J. Pediatr.* 70:960, 1967.
30. Starr, A., Amlie, R. N., Martin, W. H., and Sanders, S. Development of auditory function in newborn infants revealed by auditory brainstem potentials. *Pediatrics* 60:831, 1977.
31. Watanabe, I., Hodges, G. R., Dworzack, D. L., Kepes, J. J., and Duensing, G. F. Neurotoxicity of intrathecal gentamicin: A case report and experimental study. *Ann. Neurol.* 4:564, 1978.
32. Watson, E. H., and Stow, R. H. Streptomycin therapy. *J.A.M.A.* 137:1599, 1948.
33. Winkel, S., Bonding, P., Larsen, P. K., and Roosen, J. Possible effects of kanamycin and incubation in newborn children with low birth weight. *Acta Paediatr. Scand.* 67:709, 1978.
34. Yoshioka, H., Monma, T., and Matsuda, S. Placental transfer of gentamicin. *J. Pediatr.* 80:121, 1972.
35. Yow, M. D., Tengg, N. E., Bangs, J., Bangs, T., and Stephenson, W. The ototoxic effects of kanamycin sulfate in infants and children. *J. Pediatr.* 60:230, 1962.

Discussion of Chapter 24

Dr. Anniko: Dr. Siegel, you have presented a very thorough review of the literature. Is there any difference in ototoxicity if you administer an aminoglycoside early or late during pregnancy? Can you separate ototoxic and teratogenic effects on the developing inner ear?

Dr. Siegel: We have not looked at that, and I don't know of any reports in the literature.

Dr. Smith: Can anyone else comment on that?

Dr. Brummett: I can't make any comments about the teratogenicity, but we have been looking at the guinea pig as a model, and if you give a drug during the last 2 weeks of gestation, you do find some ototoxic effects on the fetus. I don't know how that relates to the developing ear. Other people have shown that, if you give an aminoglycoside to guinea pigs early in pregnancy, during organogenesis of the ear, you do observe ototoxic effects.

Dr. Lerner: In your review of those studies that looked at children treated with intraventricular or intrathecal aminoglycosides, were any of the children followed prospectively?

Dr. Siegel: Dr. McCracken's neonatal cooperative meningitis study followed the patients prospectively. These patients were followed developmentally, with neurologic evaluations, and if any abnormalities were noted, audiometry was carried out. Approximately one percent of the patients had audiograms.

Dr. L. Eviatar: I would like to concur with some of your findings and mention that we have tested several hundred babies who were treated with gentamicin. I did not include these data in my paper because these patients were not adequately followed. However, when we later examined these children, we did not find a higher incidence of hearing loss.

In my experience, it is not the total dose that is important. For example, we have followed children who had received a total of 500 mg of gentamicin, and we observed no ototoxicity. Simultaneous use of two aminoglycosides in large amounts produces more deficit than gentamicin alone. We studied several 1,000-g premature babies with meningitis who were treated with gentamicin, and vestibular and auditory studies gave normal results after 5 years. The same results were noted when gentamicin was given intrathecally. Noise does not seem to increase the ototoxic effect.

Dr. R. Amlie (University of California at Irvine, Irvine, California): We have examined several babies with meningitis and found transient auditory changes. This may be due to meningitis or to aminoglycosides. We have measured evoked brainstem potentials within 1 or 2 days after the diagnosis of meningitis and noticed a return to normal of these potentials over 4 to 6 weeks. These findings were the same in preterm, 1,000-g babies, and also in term infants.

25. Pharmacokinetics of Gentamicin in the Inner Ear Perilymph of Man

Stephen A. Lerner, Robert Seligsohn, Ishan Bhattacharya, Raúl Hinojosa, and Gregory J. Matz

The exact route by which aminoglycosides reach the hair cells of the inner ear from the bloodstream is not known. From the bloodstream, they may enter the perilymph and pass into the endolymph; alternatively, they may first enter the endolymph and then pass into the perilymph. Other fluid compartments may be involved as well. Despite our ignorance of the exact details, we do know from studies in animals that there is a direct relationship between the intensity of aminoglycoside ototoxicity and the level of drug reached in the perilymph after systemic administration [2, 3, 5], and that aminoglycosides perfused directly into the perilymphatic space can induce toxic effects (see Chap. 3). We also know that there is a pharmacokinetic relationship among aminoglycoside levels in perilymph (see Chaps. 5, 6), endolymph [5] (see also Chap. 5), and serum.

The correlation of aminoglycoside pharmacokinetics in serum with that in perilymph may be investigated under various conditions, such as altered renal function. Such correlation may further our ability to predict concentrations of aminoglycosides in the inner ear, which is relatively inaccessible, from concentrations of these drugs in serum, which is easily sampled. This information may permit the administration of aminoglycosides in dose regimens that may reduce their ototoxic potential without compromising their antibacterial efficacy.

Animal studies designed to examine the question of aminoglycoside ototoxicity have some obvious advantages. In studies of aminoglycoside pharmacokinetics in the inner ear, large numbers of animals can be killed for sampling of perilymph and endolymph at any time relative to the administration of a drug, whereas human perilymph can be sampled only during autopsy

We wish to express our deep appreciation to Theodore Karrison for his advice and assistance with the methodology of statistical analysis and to Elisabeth F. Lanzl for her collaboration in the writing of this chapter.

following death for other reasons. A wide variety of aminoglycosides and an unlimited range of dosages may be used in animal studies, whereas in man we are limited to the use of aminoglycosides that either are approved for general use or are under clinical investigation, and in dosages that are medically indicated and not excessive.

Study of inner ear pharmacokinetics of aminoglycosides directly in man seemed desirable, however, for a number of reasons. First, toxic effects of these agents may differ among various animal species. Furthermore, animal studies of the pharmacokinetics and toxic effects of aminoglycosides usually employ much larger doses (corrected for body weight) than those administered clinically, producing much higher levels in serum than are usually achieved in man [3, 5] (see also Chaps. 2, 4, 6, 8, 12, 13; Table 5-1). Moreover, chronic experiments in animals often suffer from the fact that dosage usually is not adjusted according to measurements of renal function and serum aminoglycoside levels [2, 3, 5] (see also Chaps. 1, 8, 12, 13; Table 5-1). In other studies in animals, the pharmacokinetics is examined after only a single dose of the drug has been given (see Chap. 6 and Table 5-1). None of these types of animal experiments simulates the usual treatment course in patients.

In an effort to evaluate the pharmacokinetics of aminoglycoside antibiotics in the perilymph of man, we have assayed the concentration of such drugs in serum and perilymph obtained at autopsy from patients who have died during or shortly after a course of treatment with one of these agents. Since the aminoglycoside used most extensively in our hospital is gentamicin, most of the patients studied had received that drug. Therefore, this initial report presents the results for gentamicin-treated patients only.

Materials and Methods

Patients who died during or shortly after a treatment course of gentamicin were considered suitable for study. Within several hours of death, either the autopsy was carried out or the cadaver was refrigerated for later examination. At autopsy, blood was obtained from the heart, and serum aspirated from a centrifuged specimen was frozen at −20°C. The cranium was opened, and after removal of the brain, both cochleas encased in their temporal bones were removed. Fluid was aspirated through the oval window into fine-tipped micropipettes by means of gentle mouth suction. Any specimen with visible contamination by red blood cells or with a volume less than 4.5 μl was discarded. The perilymph specimens were frozen at −20°C until they were assayed for gentamicin. In most cases, both temporal bones were sampled for perilymph; however, in some instances, only one of the temporal bones was sampled, and the other was instead preserved for unrelated studies. If sampling was not done immediately, the bone was refrigerated at 4°C until later removal of the perilymph.

The concentration of gentamicin in serum or perilymph was assayed radioenzymatically, as modified from the method of Smith et al. [6]. Adenylylation of the aminoglycoside was carried out with ^{14}C-ATP (0.2 mM) at a specific activity of 8 or 16 μCi/μmole. Under conditions of the assay, the minimum detectable amount of gentamicin was about 2.0 ng. When perilymph from both ears of a patient was available, the samples were assayed separately. Unless otherwise indicated, the concentration of gentamicin in perilymph is reported as the mean of bilateral measurements or as the single determination of a unilateral sample.

The following information was recorded from each patient's chart: duration of gentamicin treatment, time from last dose to death, and whether the patient received furosemide during gentamicin treatment. No information on ototoxicity was available. Renal function was estimated from the calculated creatinine clearance according to the method of Cockcroft and Gault [4], which uses age, sex, body weight, and serum creatinine level. Renal function was considered abnormal if the calculated creatinine clearance was less than 70 ml/minute.

The data on gentamicin concentrations in perilymph and in serum were normalized by construction of three-parameter lognormal distributions* [1]. The expression ln(level in μg/ml + 2.8) was used to transform the perilymph levels; the expression ln(level in μg/ml + 2.3) was used to transform the serum levels. Except as indicated, all statistical analyses were performed on transformed data.

Welch's modification of Student's t-test was used for comparison of the levels of gentamicin in perilymph and serum in patients who had normal renal function with the levels in patients who had abnormal renal function. The ratios of the concentration of gentamicin to that in serum were compared in a similar manner in these two patient groups.

Multiple regression and stepwise multiple regression were carried out with programs provided by SAS Institute, Inc., Raleigh, North Carolina.

Results

Of the 36 gentamicin-treated patients who were studied, most had deteriorating renal function prior to death (Table 25-1). The 30 patients with abnormal

*Positive skewing of the data was apparent in histograms constructed from the original serum and perilymph concentrations. Rank-it plots suggested that a more nearly normal distribution could be achieved by a logarithmic transformation of the data. A three-parameter lognormal distribution was used because of the presence in the original data of a few slightly negative calculated values for serum and perilymph concentrations. The appropriate constant, y_0', was obtained from

$$y_0' = \frac{s}{c} - \bar{y}',$$

where

s = standard deviation of original data

$\bar{y}'$ = mean of original data

$$c = 0.7937 \left(\sqrt[3]{g_1 + \sqrt{g_1^2 + 4}} + \sqrt[3]{g_1 - \sqrt{g_1^2 + 4}} \right),$$

where g_1 = Fischer's statistic of skewness. The actual y_0' used in the transformation of both serum and perilymph concentrations was a weighted average of y_0' obtained separately for patients with abnormal and those with normal renal functions.

Table 25-1. Age and Various Independent Variables Affecting Gentamicin Perilymph Levels in 36 Gentamicin-Treated Patients

	Renal Function		
	Normal	Abnormal	p
Number	6	30	na
Mean age (years)	28.0 ± 28.2* (Range ⅔–67)	58.8 ± 16.6 (Range 21–94)	< 0.025
Renal function at death			
Normal	6		na
Abnormal, stable		9	
Abnormal, deteriorating		20	
Hemodialysis		1	
Mean duration of therapy (days)	8.8 ± 8.5	6.9 ± 5.5	ns
Mean time from last dose to death (hours)	43.0 ± 66.7	31.9 ± 47.6	ns

na = not applicable; ns = not significant.
*Mean ± standard deviation.

renal function (ARF) were significantly older ($p < 0.025$) than the 6 patients with normal renal function (NRF). Serum levels of gentamicin were determined for only 29 of the 30 ARF patients, since the serum from 1 patient was inadvertently discarded.

Volumes of perilymph assayed for gentamicin ranged from 4.7 to 25.0 μl, with a mean and standard deviation of 15.6 ± 6.1 μl. Perilymph was obtained from both ears of 25 patients and from one ear of 11 patients. Figure 25-1 compares the gentamicin levels in the perilymph of one ear with that in the other for the patients from whom bilateral samples were obtained. The differences between levels in the two ears exceeded 1.0 μg/ml in only four patients; the lower level in each of these patients was at least 2.0 μg/ml.

Figure 25-2 indicates the gentamicin concentration in the perilymph of the 6 NRF patients and the 30 ARF patients. Only 2 of the NRF patients had perilymph concentrations > 0.35 μg/ml, whereas 22 of the ARF patients had concentrations of gentamicin exceeding that level. As shown in Table 25-2, the mean perilymph concentrations in the NRF and ARF patients, 0.84 μg/ml and 2.45 μg/ml, respectively, differed significantly ($p < 0.05$). The mean serum levels and the ratios of gentamicin concentrations in perilymph and serum at death were also significantly higher ($p < 0.05$) in the ARF patients than in those with NRF. The concentration of gentamicin in perilymph exceeded that in serum in 10 of the 29 ARF patients tested, but was less than that in serum in all 6 NRF patients.

A plot of perilymph levels versus serum levels (data not shown) gave no indication of an association between the two. We then examined the possible effects of other variables, separately and together, on the concentration of

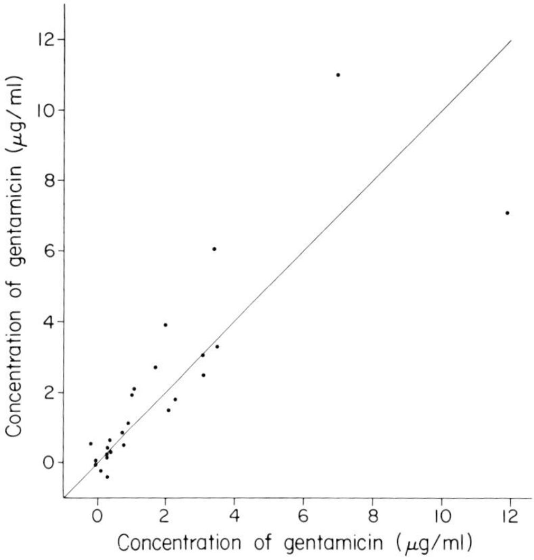

Figure 25-1. Concentration of gentamicin in the perilymph of the left ear (abscissa) and right ear (ordinate) in the 25 patients from whom both ears were sampled. A theoretical line of equality between the concentrations in both ears is shown.

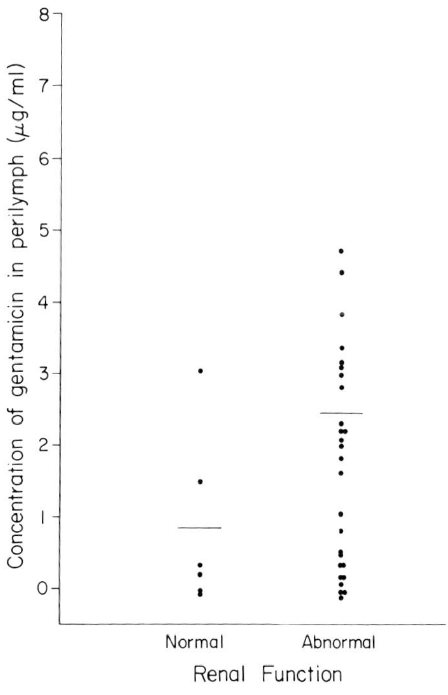

Figure 25-2. Concentration of gentamicin in the perilymph of the 6 patients with normal renal function and the 30 patients with abnormal renal function. The mean level for each subpopulation is indicated as a horizontal line.

Table 25-2. Gentamicin Levels in Perilymph and Serum

	NRF	ARF	p*
Perilymph†	0.84 ± 1.24	2.45 ± 2.61	< 0.05
Serum†	1.45 ± 2.00	3.30 ± 2.07	< 0.05
Perilymph/serum‡	0.45 ± 0.23	1.14 ± 1.67	< 0.05

NRF = normal renal function; ARF = abnormal renal function.
*Statistical analysis on transformed data, as described in section on materials and methods.
†Mean ± standard deviation, in μg/ml.
‡Mean ± standard deviation of the ratios of gentamicin concentrations in perilymph and serum from each patient.

gentamicin in perilymph and serum at death. We analyzed the data for all patients as well as for NRF and ARF patients separately (Table 25-3). In addition to the independent variables listed, we considered age and concomitant furosemide therapy.

In Fig. 25-3A, the concentrations of gentamicin in perilymph are plotted as a function of the duration of treatment. Analysis of the transformed data by linear regression showed no significant correlation of gentamicin perilymph levels with duration of treatment when all patients or only the NRF patients were considered. For the ARF patients, however, there was a significant positive correlation ($p = 0.004$) of gentamicin concentration with duration of treatment. A plot of gentamicin concentrations in serum as a function of the duration of treatment is shown in Fig. 25-3B. Similar statistical analysis again demonstrated a significant positive correlation ($p = 0.05$) only in the ARF patients.

The concentration of gentamicin in perilymph as a function of the time from the last dose until death is shown in Fig. 25-4A. Linear regression analysis of the transformed data revealed no significant correlation of the gentamicin perilymph level with the time from last dose to death for all patients or for ARF or NRF patients. A plot of concentration of gentamicin in serum as a function of the time from last dose to death is shown in Fig. 25-4B. Similar statistical analysis demonstrated a significant negative correlation for all patients taken together ($p = 0.007$) and for the ARF patients alone ($p = 0.02$), but not for the NRF patients.

In order to examine the relative influence of various factors on gentamicin concentrations in serum and perilymph, we carried out both multiple regression and stepwise multiple regression analysis. Among the factors considered were renal function (NRF versus ARF), duration of treatment, time from last dose to death, age, and whether furosemide had been administered concurrently with gentamicin.

By multiple regression analysis, the concentration of gentamicin in perilymph was positively correlated with the duration of therapy ($p = 0.007$), and the presence of abnormal renal function ($p = 0.02$). An inverse relationship, however, was found between the gentamicin concentration in perilymph

Table 25-3. Results of Statistical Analysis[a] Correlating Serum and Perilymph Gentamicin Levels with Various Independent Parameters

	Linear Regression		Multiple Regression		Stepwise Multiple Regression	
Independent Variable	Serum	Perilymph	Serum	Perilymph	Serum	Perilymph
Presence of ARF	—	—	0.002	0.02	0.007	0.06
Duration of therapy						
ARF patients	0.05	0.004	—	—	—	—
NRF patients	ns	ns	—	—	—	—
All patients	ns	0.06	0.03	0.007	0.09	0.01
Time from last dose to death						
ARF patients	0.02*	ns	—	—	—	—
NRF patients	ns	ns	—	—	—	—
All patients	0.007*	ns	0.002*	0.06*	0.003*	0.08*

ARF = abnormal renal function; NRF = normal renal function; ns = not significant.
[a]p values < 0.10 are shown. An asterisk indicates an inverse correlation.

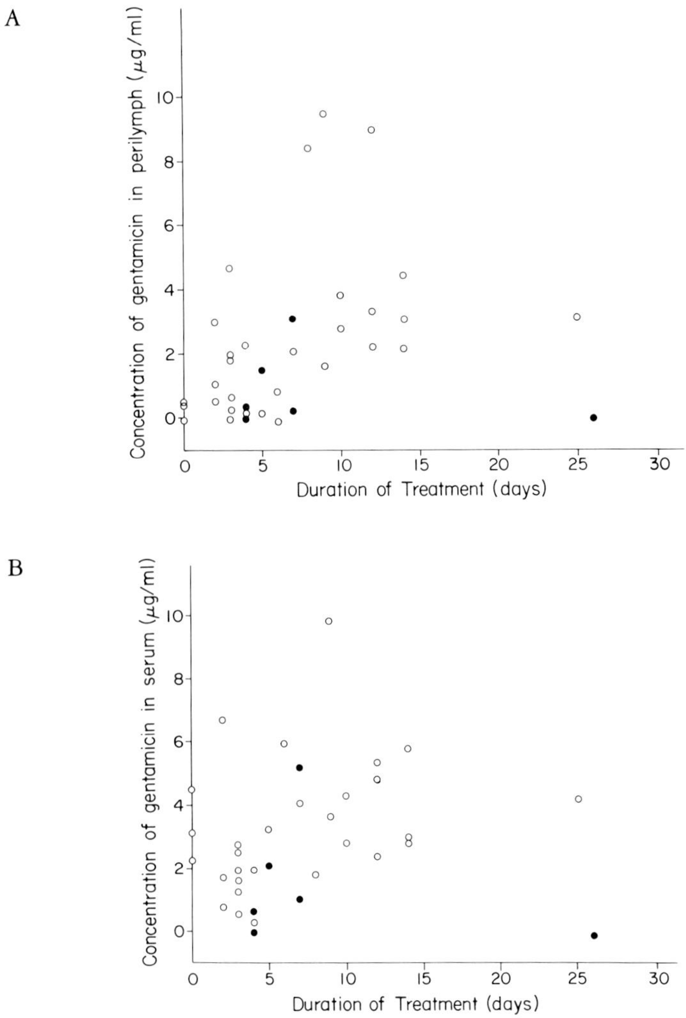

Figure 25-3. Concentration of gentamicin in (A) perilymph and (B) serum as a function of duration of the gentamicin treatment course. (○ = Patients with abnormal renal function; ● = patients with normal renal function.)

A

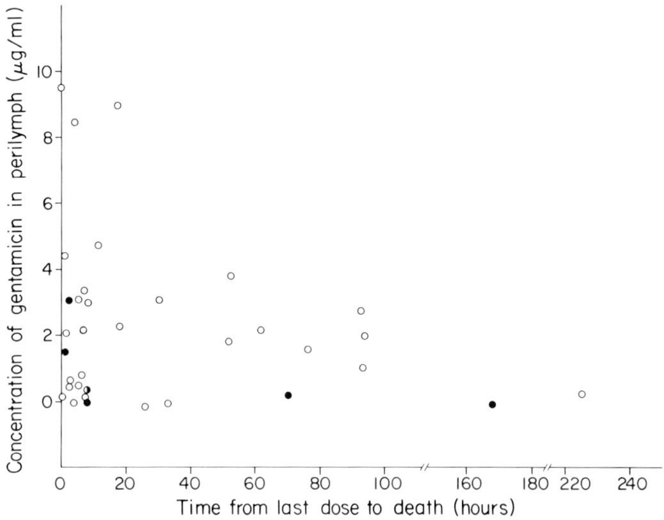

B

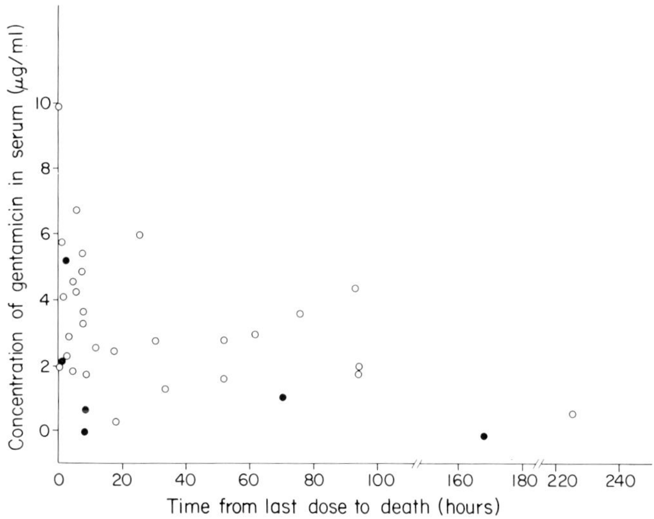

Figure 25-4. Concentration of gentamicin in (A) perilymph and (B) serum as a function of time from the last dose to death. (○ = Patients with abnormal renal function; ● = patients with normal renal function.)

and the time from last dose to death ($p = 0.06$). By stepwise multiple regression analysis, the concentration of gentamicin in perilymph showed a positive correlation with duration of treatment ($p = 0.01$) and the presence of abnormal renal function ($p = 0.06$), and a negative correlation with the time from last dose to death ($p = 0.08$).

By multiple regression analysis, the concentration of gentamicin in serum showed a positive correlation with the presence of abnormal renal function ($p = 0.002$) and duration of treatment ($p = 0.03$) and an inverse relationship with time from last dose to death ($p = 0.002$). Stepwise multiple regression analysis showed a positive correlation of serum gentamicin level with the presence of abnormal renal function ($p = 0.007$) and with the duration of treatment ($p = 0.09$), and a negative correlation with time from last dose to death ($p = 0.003$).

When considered independently of other variables in multiple or stepwise multiple regression procedures, neither age nor the presence of concurrent furosemide therapy was correlated ($p < 0.10$) with the concentration of gentamicin in perilymph or serum.

Comments

Several deficiencies in our study protocol became apparent during the course of this work; they are discussed below. We are attempting to eliminate these problems as our studies continue.

1. Although the radioenzymatic assay of aminoglycosides is specific, accurate, and precise [6, 7], radioimmunoassay [7] is preferable, since it is more sensitive and is also more precise at low drug concentrations.
2. We made no attempt to detect the possible contamination of perilymph samples with endolymph, but we know that aminoglycoside concentrations that have been measured in endolymph of animals have fallen within 25 to 100 percent of the simultaneous concentrations in perilymph (see Chap. 5). Furthermore, the volume of endolymph in each cochlea is much smaller than that of perilymph (see Chap. 5). For these reasons, we feel that possible contamination of perilymph by endolymph would have affected our results only minimally. Nonetheless, the determination of sodium and potassium concentrations in the samples obtained could be used to detect the presence of contaminating endolymph (see Chap. 5).
3. The full impact of the state of renal function on perilymph levels of gentamicin could not be assessed. In some cases, the last determination of serum creatinine was made 1 or 2 days prior to death and thus did not necessarily reflect the level of renal function immediately premortem. For this and other reasons, we assigned patients to NRF and ARF groups according to an arbitrary cutoff value of calculated creatinine clearance. It would be important to consider serum creatinine levels not only during the last 1 or 2 days of life, but also at the time of death. Measurements of creatinine in serum at death might enable us to evaluate the effect of a broad range of renal clearance rates on gentamicin levels in serum and perilymph.

4. In most of the cases, serum gentamicin levels were not determined systematically before death. More frequent premortem determinations of gentamicin concentration in the serum of each patient would aid in the correlation of the gentamicin perilymph level at death with the pharmacokinetics of gentamicin in serum.

The renal function of most of the ARF patients was deteriorating further 1 or 2 days prior to death. The preponderance of ARF in patients in our study is likely to be due in part to their advanced age and to premortem insults such as nephrotoxic drugs and diminished renal perfusion.

Since aminoglycoside ototoxicity may occur unilaterally, it was of interest to examine the difference between the levels of gentamicin in the bilateral perilymph samples. The largest differences occurred in patients with the highest perilymph levels.

In our hospital, patients with both normal and abnormal renal function are generally treated with gentamicin doses sufficient to produce peak levels in serum in the range of 4 to 8 μg/ml. Nonetheless, serum levels of gentamicin at death were higher in our ARF patients than in the NRF patients. Two factors are likely to account in large part for the difference between the two groups: (1) As renal function deteriorated further in ARF patients shortly before death, the dosage of gentamicin may not have been reduced appropriately. (2) In our hospital, aminoglycosides are administered to ARF patients at intervals such that the serum level is generally not allowed to fall to subtherapeutic concentrations for long periods before the next dose is given. Consequently, although the predose (trough) serum level of gentamicin in an NRF patient is usually less than 2.0 μg/ml, trough levels in ARF patients are usually higher. Thus, since death occurs at an unpredictable time after the last dose, the serum level at death is likely to be higher in an ARF patient than in an NRF patient.

In ARF patients, the level of gentamicin in serum at death was correlated with duration of therapy. The rise in serum gentamicin during therapy was most likely the result of premortem deterioration in renal clearance, which may have resulted in part from gentamicin toxicity. In contrast, the serum gentamicin level in NRF patients was not correlated with duration of therapy, suggesting that a steady state had been achieved rapidly.

As would be expected, the serum level of gentamicin in ARF patients fell with increasing time from last dose to death. The more rapid decline expected among NRF patients was not evident, perhaps because we lacked a sufficient number of NRF patients for whom the time from last dose to death was short.

The NRF and ARF patients were comparable in duration of therapy and time from last dose to death, but there was a dramatic difference in perilymph levels of gentamicin between these two groups. The finding that the mean perilymph gentamicin concentration in the ARF patients was higher than in the NRF patients is consistent with findings in experimental animals [5] (see also Chaps. 5, 6). In NRF patients, as in normal animals, the concentration of gentamicin in serum falls rapidly from the peak level. Since the entry of aminoglycosides into the perilymph of animals is known to be slow, there is insufficient time in animals, and presumably also in NRF patients, for equilibrium to be reached while the gentamicin concentration is at or near its peak in serum. On the other hand, in ARF patients, as in animals with compromised renal function, relatively high concentrations of gentamicin are reached in perilymph because there is sufficient time for equilibration with the more sustained elevated levels in serum.

Two factors would appear to contribute to the higher gentamicin perilymph levels observed in ARF patients with longer duration of therapy. First, as in animals with compromised renal function, longer treatment allows more complete equilibration of the perilymph levels with the sustained levels in serum. Second, since serum levels rise with duration of treatment, the level of equilibration of gentamicin in perilymph would be expected to rise with increasing duration of treatment. Since neither of these factors applies to NRF patients, it is not surprising that their perilymph gentamicin levels are not correlated with the duration of their therapy.

Data from animal experiments show that egress of gentamicin from perilymph is slower than that from serum and that a decrease in renal clearance of aminoglycosides results in a prolonged half-life of gentamicin in perilymph [5] (see also Chap. 6). Although our data suggest a decline in perilymph gentamicin concentration with increasing time from last dose to death, the relationship is only marginally significant by multiple and stepwise multiple regression analysis. This decline may have been difficult to detect because of a markedly prolonged half-life of gentamicin in the perilymph of ARF patients. In NRF patients, although the gentamicin half-life in perilymph may have been shorter, most levels were relatively low, and this may have obscured the decline.

The present study is limited by the small number of patients included and by our lack of control over their dose schedules. Our data, however, are consistent with the studies in animals that suggest that gentamicin in perilymph equilibrates slowly with that in serum.

Prolonged treatment, preexisting renal failure, and old age have been suggested as risk factors associated with an increased incidence of ototoxicity in patients receiving aminoglycosides (see Chap. 23). We found a correlation of higher perilymph levels of gentamicin with longer treatment and renal failure, but not with older age per se. Perhaps the influence of the first two risk factors on ototoxicity is due to the higher perilymph levels. Concurrent treatment with ethacrynic acid has been implicated in enhancement of aminoglycoside ototoxicity; the usual dosage of furosemide, another loop diuretic, has been found less toxic (see Chaps. 4, 23, 26). We found no association between perilymph gentamicin levels and concurrent furosemide therapy.

The data from animal studies (see Chaps. 5, 6) and this report suggest that ototoxicity might be minimized, especially in ARF patients, if a sufficiently long interval between aminoglycoside doses is set to allow for the slow clearance of the drug from the perilymph before the next dose is given. Strict compliance with such long interdose intervals may be ill-advised in some ARF patients, however, since the levels in serum may be subtherapeutic for unacceptably long periods of time.

Administration of aminoglycosides by continuous infusion appears to improve their efficacy in profoundly neutropenic patients [8]. Because of the prolonged elevation of the serum level that results, we would expect the aminoglycoside level in perilymph to be higher than with treatment by intermittent infusion. Although its increased efficacy might warrant the use of continuous infusion of an aminoglycoside in a neutropenic patient, we should be aware of the potential for higher levels in perilymph that may increase the risk of ototoxicity.

References

1. Bliss, C. I. *Statistics in Biology.* New York: McGraw-Hill, 1967. Vol. 1, sections 5.3 and 7.3.
2. Brummett, R. E., Fox, K. E., Bendrick, T. W., and Himes, D. L. Ototoxicity of tobramycin, gentamicin, amikacin and sisomicin in the guinea pig. *J. Antimicrob. Chemother.* 4[Suppl. A]:73, 1978.
3. Brummett, R. E., Fox, K. E., Brown, R. T., and Himes, D. L. Comparative ototoxic liability of netilmicin and gentamicin. *Arch. Otolaryngol.* 104:579, 1978.
4. Cockcroft, D. W., and Gault, M. W. Prediction of creatinine clearance from serum creatinine. *Nephron* 16:31, 1976.
5. Federspil, P., Schätzle, W., and Tiesler, E. Pharmacokinetics and ototoxicity of gentamicin, tobramycin, and amikacin. *J. Infect. Dis.* 134[Suppl.]:S200, 1976.
6. Smith, D. H., Van Otto, B., and Smith, A. L. A rapid chemical assay for gentamicin. *N. Engl. J. Med.* 286:583, 1972.
7. Stevens, P., Young, L. S., and Hewitt, W. L. Radioimmunoassay, radioenzymatic assay and microbioassay of gentamicin: A comparative study. *J. Lab. Clin. Med.* 86:349, 1975.
8. Valdivieso, M., Feld, R., Rodriguez, V., and Bodey, G. P. Amikacin therapy of infections in neutropenic patients. *Am. J. Med. Sci.* 270:453, 1975.

Discussion of Chapter 25

Dr. Lietman: I think you are saying that the perilymph levels were not high.

Dr. Lerner: Not in patients with normal renal function.

Dr. Lietman: Is it feasible to look at hair cells postmortem? Can you obtain enough hair cells to see whether the aminoglycosides are concentrated within the cells?

Dr. Lerner: I don't know how difficult it would be to obtain a sufficiently large number of hair cells. It would certainly be interesting. With RIA it might be possible to measure the concentration in the cells.

Dr. Brummett: We have succeeded in isolating and assaying cochlear tissue from guinea pigs for aminoglycoside content.

Dr. Schacht: Did you analyze your data for the possible influence of delay between death and sampling? Has anyone determined in animals whether the drug content in perilymph changes postmortem?

Dr. Lerner: Dr. Brummett did a pilot study which may help to answer the question.

Dr. Brummett: We didn't really do a detailed study, but our data showed only minor changes in concentration of the aminoglycoside in the perilymph.

Dr. Lerner: As I recall, the perilymph level increased.

Dr. Schacht: By what percentage?

Dr. Brummett: I don't remember; it was less than twofold.

Dr. Lerner: The increase was less than twofold; this reassured us with respect to the low levels. In our work, perilymph has been removed from different patients at various times after death, and we have not found any correlation between perilymph levels and time of sampling.

26. Ototoxic Interaction Between Aminoglycosides and Loop Diuretics in Man

Cedric A. Quick

In order to assess the impact of drug ototoxicity, one needs to determine how many high-risk patients receive ototoxic drugs, and to what extent the interaction of aminoglycosides with loop diuretics plays a role in any resulting ototoxic hearing loss. In patients with normal renal function, short courses of aminoglycoside antibiotics rarely produce symptomatic ototoxicity. The management of these patients is relatively simple. Monitoring of renal function and serum levels of the aminoglycoside reduces the risk of ototoxic damage. Of greater concern is the desperately ill patient who may have renal impairment, or who may be elderly. In seriously ill individuals, an infection may require the simultaneous use of several antibiotics, and the antibiotic regimens may need to be altered during the course of treatment. In addition, the renal function may need to be stimulated by diuretics or osmotic agents such as mannitol. The clinical picture of these patients is often complex, and frequent alteration of medications may be required to keep pace with changing hemodynamic and biochemical states. Unfortunately, such seriously ill patients, who could be at greatest risk for ototoxic damage, may not perceive the early symptoms of tinnitus or vertigo that can alert the physician to impending damage. Even if these symptoms are reported by the patient, they are often overshadowed by more acute and life-threatening problems.

No statistics are available that indicate how many of these high-risk patients are encountered. It is difficult to determine the expected incidence of hearing loss in these patients, because so many variables exist that controlled trials cannot readily be designed. In a large prospective analysis of hearing loss in 600 renal dialysis and transplant patients conducted at the University of Minnesota from 1968 through 1975 [4], upon entry into the program the patients underwent an otologic interview and examination and had a full audiologic evaluation. One-sixth of the patients surveyed had some form of hearing deficit. If renal transplantation was delayed, this evaluation was repeated prior to surgery. Patients were reevaluated after transplantation and at the onset of any symptoms referable to an otologic disorder. Hearing loss was defined as a decrease in hearing threshold of 2 readings greater than 15 dB or 1 reading of at least 25 dB in the range of frequencies from 250 Hz to 8,000 Hz.

In several patients, a reversible hearing loss was seen following the use of some ototoxic drugs, and in three patients, improvement in the hearing threshold followed a successful renal transplant. The explanation for this latter phenomenon is lacking. The following case summaries illustrate the complexity of the problems encountered in the analysis of hearing loss that occurs when several ototoxic drugs are used simultaneously.

Case 1

A 29-year-old woman weighing 31 kg, with end-stage renal failure due to juvenile-onset diabetes, underwent bilateral nephrectomy in preparation for transplantation. One month later, a cadaver kidney transplantation was performed. Audiograms prior to the transplant operation were normal. No ototoxic antibiotics or diuretics were administered perioperatively. From the ninth postoperative day, the patient had spiking fevers that eventually were shown to be caused by an infected urinary fistula. Surgical exploration of the fistula was performed 18 days after the transplantation, and on that day gentamicin therapy was started. An initial dose of 40 mg IV was given, followed by 40 mg IM every 8 hours for 8 consecutive days. Following this, the patient was given gentamicin, 30 mg every 12 hours, for another 4 days, whereupon the transplanted kidney was removed because of rejection. Gentamicin was then given at doses of 35 mg IM after hemodialysis 3 times per week for 2 weeks. Throughout the course of gentamicin therapy, peak serum levels of the drug were observed to be above 5.9 μg/ml. Furosemide therapy was commenced during the surgical exploration of the fistula, with 3 IV doses of 50 mg, 50 mg, and 30 mg. This was followed in the postoperative period by an infusion of 200 mg of furosemide in mannitol and subsequently 40 mg IM every 8 hours for 12 days until the transplanted kidney was excised. Tinnitus was reported during this 2-week period, and audiograms 6 months later showed a bilateral high-frequency hearing loss (Fig. 26-1). The combined effect of furosemide and gentamicin was thought to be responsible for this audiologic picture.

Following a second transplant, the patient's health remained good for almost 2 years; there were no further changes in hearing, and renal function was satisfactory. At 2 years, a mycotic aortic aneurysm was resected. One day prior to surgery, the patient was given gentamicin prophylactically, 60 mg IV every 12 hours, and an oral neomycin bowel preparation (1 g hourly for 4 hours, and two 1-g doses 6 hours apart). Infusion of furosemide in mannitol was commenced preoperatively at the rate of 4 mg per hour. The postoperative course

Figure 26-1. Audiograms—case 1. Hearing was normal (A and B) until after treatment with gentamicin and furosemide following the first transplantation (C). A further decrease in hearing (D) occurred 2 years later, following combined gentamicin and furosemide therapy. (○ = right ear; × = left ear.)

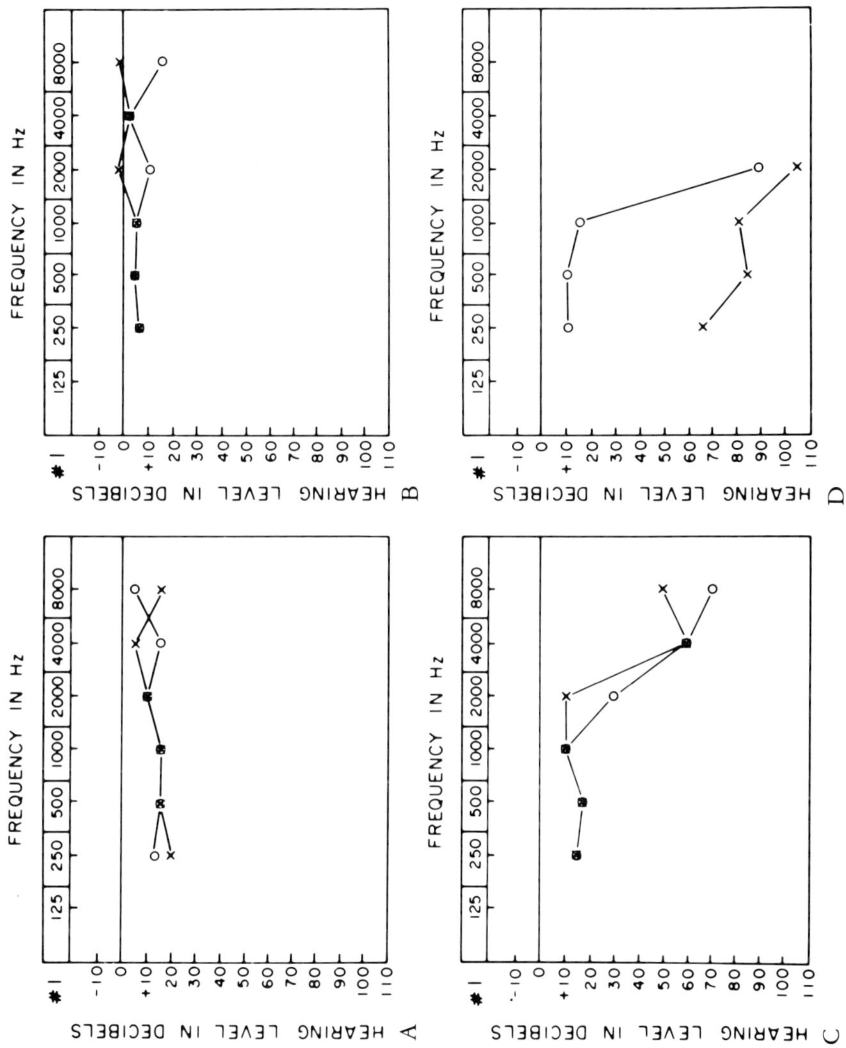
FREQUENCY IN Hz
125 250 500 1000 2000 4000 8000
HEARING LEVEL IN DECIBELS
#1
-10 0 +10 20 30 40 50 60 70 80 90 100 110
A
B
C
D

was extremely difficult, and gentamicin was administered in doses of 60 mg IM every 12 hours. Serum levels ranged between 2 and 11.5 μg per ml. Blood samples for determination of these levels were usually taken 1 hour after gentamicin administration. A total of 200 mg of furosemide was given intraoperatively, and an additional 260 mg were given in the subsequent 12 hours. Thereafter, occasional small doses of furosemide were given IV, in addition to oral administration of 40 mg twice daily. Fourteen days after the operation, the patient complained of a marked decrease in hearing, and over the subsequent few days further hearing loss occurred that ultimately stabilized as a severe sensorineural hearing loss in the right ear and virtually complete deafness in the left ear (Fig. 26-1D). Potentiation was thought to be the most likely cause of this second and more serious hearing loss, since ototoxic levels of gentamicin never reached "critical" levels. It was considered unlikely that the oral administration of neomycin contributed to the hearing loss, since hearing loss set in 12 days after neomycin administration.

Case 2

A 26-year-old woman weighing 57 kg was readmitted to the hospital with a pelvic infection following a surgical procedure performed 7 days earlier. Her condition deteriorated rapidly; septic shock, hypotension, and oliguria occurred 24 hours after her admission. She was given intensive supportive care and, on the day of admission, received gentamicin, 60 mg IM, followed by 80 mg IV 12 hours later. On the second day, in the face of decreasing renal function, she received furosemide, 40 mg IV, then 120 mg by IV push 6 hours later, followed by another 240 mg 2 hours later. After 2 hours, ethacrynic acid, 150 mg, was given by IV push. On the same day, she received 1 dose of 80 mg gentamicin IV. On the evening of the second day, the patient described a screeching tinnitus and severely decreased hearing. The next day, she was transferred to the University of Minnesota Hospital, where it was recorded that her hearing had improved clinically. No audiograms were performed because of the patient's weakened condition. She then received gentamicin, 80 mg IV daily for 2 days; this was discontinued in favor of clindamycin. Furosemide, 80 mg, was given by IV push on 2 occasions after her admission to the University Hospital. The patient subsequently complained of a further decrease in hearing and an increase in tinnitus. No further aminoglycosides or diuretics were given. Daily gentamicin levels were 5.9, 4.0, and 10.0 μg/ml 30 minutes after administration of the drug. The patient's hearing continued to deteriorate over the subsequent 5 to 7 days, and 14 days after the onset of the infection an audiogram showed a flat sensorineural hearing loss of 60 to 80 dB (Fig. 26-2). The results of electronystagmography and caloric tests were normal, indicating that there was no damage to the vestibular system. The onset of hearing loss and the type of audiometric pattern strongly suggest that the diuretics (large doses of furosemide, plus ethacrynic acid) were mainly responsible for the initial hearing loss. The later hearing loss, however, was probably the result of the combination of effects of the diuretic and aminoglycoside,

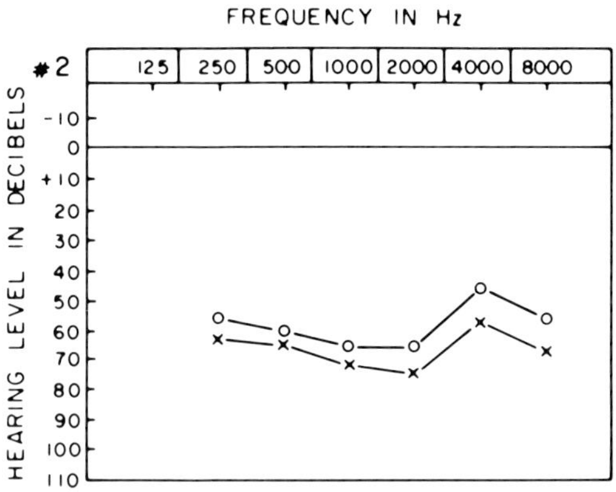

Figure 26-2. Audiogram—case 2, following severe septic shock and renal failure, which were treated with gentamicin, furosemide, and ethacrynic acid. (○ = right ear; × = left ear.)

since neither was given in what would generally be considered ototoxic amounts.

Case 3

A 34-year-old man with Goodpasture syndrome died of complications of his disease 3 years after its onset. During this time, he had received two kidney transplants, both of which were rejected and removed surgically. On his first admission, a bilateral nephrectomy was performed, and he was started on hemodialysis. At this time, a routine audiogram was normal. Eight months later, he received a cadaver kidney transplant. Furosemide was commenced prophylactically during the surgery and was administered for the following 4 weeks in an effort to stimulate the acquired kidney, until it was removed because of rejection. Doses of furosemide varied according to renal function and were between 40 and 500 mg IV daily, with occasional oral administration. At the same time, gentamicin, 60 mg IV twice daily, was given for 7 days for control of postoperative sepsis. Other drugs used at this time included lincomycin, Mycostatin, sulfisoxazole, and hydrochlorothiazide. In addition, steroids and radiation were used for control of rejection. Following this episode, tinnitus and hearing loss were reported by the patient, and an audiogram showed a moderate sensorineural loss, which was thought to be due to potentiation of gentamicin and furosemide (Fig. 26-3). Sixteen months later, transplantation of a second cadaver kidney was attempted. Gentamicin, 60 mg, was given daily for 5 days. Furosemide was commenced intraoperatively (100 mg IV) and continued for the first few postoperative days at 50 mg IM twice daily. Three weeks later, a rejection crisis and infection occurred that required intensive antibiotic therapy including gentamicin, lincomycin, sulfisoxazole, and

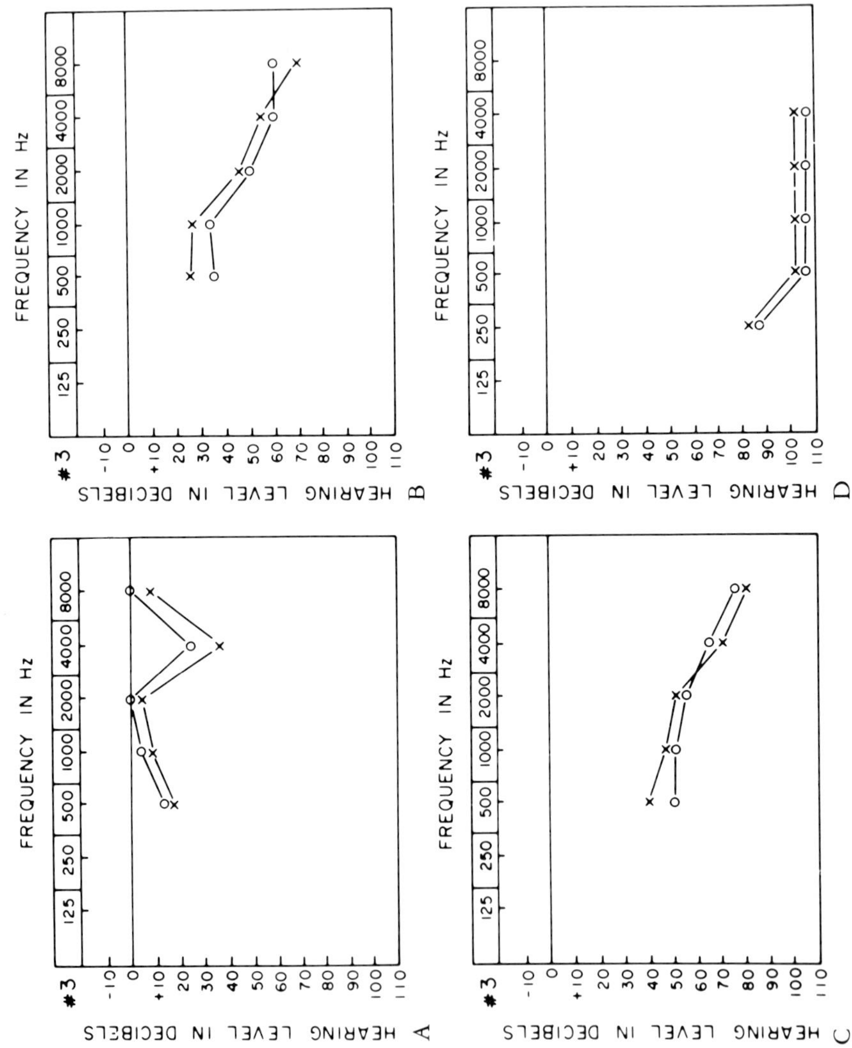
A
B
C
D
#3
FREQUENCY IN Hz
HEARING LEVEL IN DECIBELS
125 250 500 1000 2000 4000 8000
-10 0 +10 20 30 40 50 60 70 80 90 100 110

erythromycin. At the same time, furosemide and hydrochlorothiazide were given orally for 8 days. The transplanted kidney was then removed surgically. When the patient had recovered sufficiently for testing, an audiogram showed a further decline in hearing, resulting in a profound sensorineural hearing loss (Fig. 26-3D).

Case 4

Renal failure in a 49-year-old woman was caused by polycystic kidney disease. One week after bilateral nephrectomy and splenectomy, the patient received a cadaver kidney transplant. Furosemide, 60 mg IV, was given intraoperatively, and over the following 24 hours she received a total of 400 mg IV in divided doses. Thereafter, daily doses of 40 to 80 mg were given. On the second post-transplant day, the patient had spiking fevers, and gentamicin was given in doses of 50 mg IV every 8 hours. This was reduced to 30 mg every 8 hours for an additional 5 days. The transplanted kidney was rejected and removed after 8 days. One further episode of infection requiring 2 days of gentamicin treatment occurred 3 weeks later. An audiogram immediately prior to transplantation was normal, and another, performed after the transplanted kidney was removed, showed a dramatic sensorineural hearing loss at the higher frequencies (Fig. 26-4). The combination of effects of the ototoxic diuretic and ototoxic antibiotic was thought to be responsible for the resultant hearing loss, because gentamicin was given only for short periods in relatively low doses and furosemide was administered in amounts not generally considered ototoxic. The possibility of accumulation of gentamicin during the rejection period must be considered, however. Unfortunately, no serum levels of gentamicin were obtained.

Comments

It is known from animal experiments and clinical studies that ototoxic damage may develop suddenly after a few injections of an aminoglycoside, may occur for varying periods of time after cessation of therapy, and may progress even after withdrawal of the drug. The cardinal symptoms of ototoxicity are tinnitus, hearing loss, and vertigo.

Tinnitus usually accompanies acquired sensorineural hearing loss of any cause. In drug-induced cochlear damage, this symptom may precede the onset of detectable hearing loss. More commonly, the patient complains of tinnitus and is unaware of the hearing loss until it is quite significant. The quality of the

---

Figure 26-3. Audiograms—case 3. Relatively normal hearing (A) markedly deteriorated after the first transplant (B), when concomitant therapy with furosemide and gentamicin was needed. The audiogram remained stable for 16 months (C), until a second transplant was performed. Subsequent complications required gentamicin and furosemide therapy, which resulted in a further decrease in hearing (D). (○ = right ear; × = left ear.)

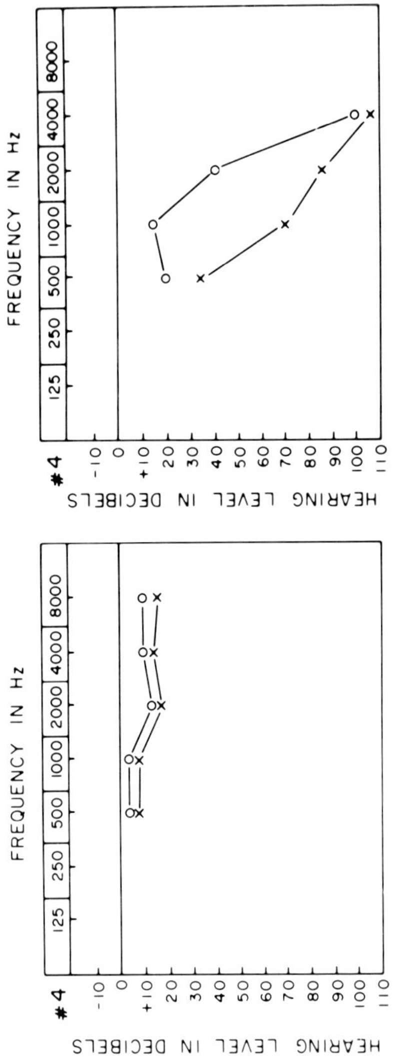

Figure 26-4. Audiograms—case 4. Hearing was normal (A) prior to renal transplantation requiring treatment with furosemide and gentamicin. The post-transplant audiogram indicated a high-frequency hearing loss (B). (○ = right ear; × = left ear.)

tinnitus with drug-induced cochlear damage is distressing in the early stages, but the patient gradually acquires tolerance. The sound is usually described as high-pitched and intense by patients who have developed ototoxicity from antibiotics, and frequently the patient states that it interferes with his ability to hear. When the sound is matched audiometrically, it corresponds to frequencies in the 4,000- to 6,000-Hz range. Tinnitus caused by the ototoxic "loop" diuretics is particularly distressing. It can occur suddenly, often within minutes following a rapid intravenous infusion. It is described as a screeching noise, like that of blaring trumpets or jet engines. The emotional response to this noise is considerable. When attempts are made to match this tinnitus audiometrically, no single frequency predominates. If the damage is less severe, the loop diuretics produce an insidious, progressive, flat or slightly sloping audiometric deficit, with only mild tinnitus. The tinnitus of patients with ototoxic damage brought on by the combined effect of diuretic and aminoglycoside has no consistent characteristics. It appears, however, that its character may reflect the more dominant ototoxic agent.

Vertigo as a result of aminoglycoside ototoxicity is insidious in onset and may occur after a few doses of a drug. The vertigo usually does not have a rotary component, is described by patients as lightheadedness or unsteadiness, and is most evident during standing or moving around, particularly in poorly lighted surroundings. It is extremely difficult to assess this aspect of ototoxicity when a combined effect of drugs is suspected. A substantial number of patients with renal failure, particularly those on dialysis or receiving antihypertensive agents, complain of some dizziness and lightheadedness. In fact, there is a definite "disequilibrium syndrome" that is associated with rapid shifts between body fluid compartments, such as occur during dialysis. In our prospective survey of 600 patients, surprisingly few had documented vestibular depression, and when this did occur, it was caused by streptomycin or gentamicin therapy [4]. We have been unable to document any changes in vestibular function in patients who had primary diuretic ototoxicity.

Hearing loss caused by aminoglycoside ototoxicity characteristically occurs at high frequencies initially [2, 3], but with continued damage it extends to all frequencies. In contrast, following diuretic ototoxicity, the audiograms show a flat or slightly sloping graph [5]. When damage is thought to have occurred because of the combined effect of diuretics and aminoglycosides, no specific audiometric pattern exists. Again, it is not known whether a flat curve or high-frequency-loss curve occurring during the combined use of diuretics and aminoglycosides indicates a predominance of damage by one agent over the other. It is my impression that the tendency for the hearing loss to progress after the drugs have been withdrawn appears to be greater when combinations of drugs are used than is the case in ototoxicity caused by single agents.

Three major classes of patients require the simultaneous administration of aminoglycosides and loop diuretics. First, there are patients who suffer an overwhelming infection that results in renal impairment. Second, infection may occur in patients with long-standing renal impairment. Third, patients may require prophylactic aminoglycosides as well as diuretics in procedures such as renal transplantation. In practice, it is unlikely that consultation on the otologic effect of combined medications will be sought prior to administration of the drugs. Occasionally, consultation is requested because of the onset of otologic symptoms such as tinnitus. Most frequently, however, an otologist is asked to evaluate the cause of a persistent hearing loss after the critical event has occurred. The cases described here illustrate the complexity of evaluation of hearing loss in such patients and the difficulty of attributing blame to any single agent when many risk factors exist.

Brummett and others have shown conclusively in animal experiments that the combined effect of an aminoglycoside and a diuretic is greater than the effect of each drug separately [1, 6]. The combined effect of these two agents may represent a simple summation of the effects or a true potentiation. The circumstances for potentiation are pharmacologically ideal. Two sites of primary action exist. Diuretics affect the stria vascularis directly, and aminoglycosides, the organ of Corti. If one assumes that the stria has a microregulatory effect on the cochlea, then the hair cells will be directly dependent upon the integrity of the stria, so that any effect on the stria would have a secondary effect on the hair cells, predisposing them to antibiotic damage. Furthermore, damage to the stria by the diuretic may allow easier passage of the antibiotic into the cochlear fluids, possibly increasing the risk of ototoxicity. In our clinical survey of patients with renal failure, eight patients were thought to have suffered hearing loss as a direct result of interaction of diuretics and aminoglycoside antibiotics, and in another five patients this interaction was thought to have contributed significantly to the hearing loss.

Although the effect of these drugs in man may represent a simple summation of factors, it is also possible that the concomitant use of these drugs results in true potentiation. The most striking result of the survey, however, was the realization that the hearing loss could rarely be clearly attributed to one cause, but stemmed from the interaction of many factors, particularly in patients who had multiple system failure (Fig. 26-4). It is not known to what extent the original systemic disease, the biochemical disorder, or the disturbance in fluid balance affects the onset or degree of ototoxic impairment.

A drug that is not ototoxic when used alone may become so when given concomitantly with another drug known to damage the cochlea. In any event, the guidelines for preventing ototoxicity may have to be restated when synergism or potentiation may be a factor. Even the newest pharmacodynamic techniques based on antibiotic peak and trough levels in the serum and on computerized calculations of available volumes of distribution of body fluids may not reflect the pharmacokinetics in the inner ear.

References

1. Brummett, R. E., Traynor, J., Brown, R., and Himes, D. Cochlear damage resulting from kanamycin and furosemide. *Acta Otolaryngol.* 80:86, 1975.
2. Jackson, G. G., and Arcieri, G. Ototoxicity of gentamicin in man: A survey and

controlled analysis of clinical experience in the United States. *J. Infect. Dis.* 124[Suppl.]:S130, 1971.
3. Lehmann, W., Häusler, R., and Waldvogel, F. A. A clinical study on the ototoxic effects of tobramycin. *Arch. Otorhinolaryngol.* 212:203, 1976.
4. Quick, C. A. Hearing loss in patients with dialysis and renal transplants. *Ann. Otol. Rhinol. Laryngol.* 85:776, 1976.
5. Quick, C. A., and Hoppe, W. Permanent deafness associated with furosemide administration. *Ann. Otol. Rhinol. Laryngol.* 84:94, 1975.
6. West, B. A., Brummett, R. E., and Himes, D. L. Interaction of kanamycin and ethacrynic acid. Severe cochlear damage in guinea pigs. *Arch. Otolaryngol.* 98:32, 1973.

Discussion of Chapter 26

Dr. Smith (Johns Hopkins University, Baltimore): In our prospective studies at Johns Hopkins, we have had a lot of trouble showing ototoxic potentiation of furosemide and the aminoglycosides. It appears that there may be a relationship, but I am not sure whether this effect occurs even with high doses of furosemide over prolonged periods of time. We have studied 2 patients who received ethacrynic acid, 1 of whom became deaf 30 to 60 minutes after the administration of ethacrynic acid. This patient had earlier received 400 mg of furosemide intravenously, and he had received an aminoglycoside for almost 10 days prior to the ethacrynic acid.

I think these observations support a difference between furosemide and ethacrynic acid in causing ototoxic potentiation. Even in large series, it is very difficult to show direct interaction between furosemide and an aminoglycoside.

Dr. Quick: I support your observations. We discontinued the use of ethacrynic acid in 1971 in favor of furosemide because the former appeared to cause hearing loss. I agree also that the high doses of furosemide may cause ototoxicity; but what is more important with respect to ototoxicity is the speed of administration of furosemide.

Dr. Brummett: One of the things you mentioned was the seeming lack of vestibular effects of the interaction of an aminoglycoside and a diuretic. That is exactly what we saw. We were not aware of vestibular toxicity for a long time because we were giving the drugs to guinea pigs, which do not ordinarily show any vestibular effects. One day, we happened to give kanamycin and ethacrynic acid to cats, and again we noted no vestibular effects. We obtained similar results with streptomycin. You can totally destroy the cochlea without any apparent damage to the vestibular system. I assume you were noting the same phenomenon in your patients?

Dr. Quick: We did not see any definite vestibular effect. However, all patients in renal failure are dizzy. These patients were difficult to test for vestibular toxicity because they had unsteadiness of gait; they were weak and very sick.

Dr. Federspil: What would be the safe maximum rate of administration of furosemide in a patient receiving aminoglycosides?

Dr. Quick: As far as the rate of administration is concerned, intravenous push has now been abandoned by most institutions. We did a study on several cases of furosemide hearing loss in which the intravenous push was the main factor in ototoxicity. Very soon afterwards, the package insert of the drug manufacturers indicated that rapid intravenous infusion was contraindicated, and that the rate should not exceed 4 mg/kg of body weight per minute.

You asked me how fast you should give the furosemide in the presence of an aminoglycoside antibiotic. I really don't know, except that one would have to give it slowly.

Dr. Igarashi: Could you explain what kind of vestibular test was performed, and how you analyzed the data?

Dr. Quick: These patients had an ENG, and a decrease of at least 30 percent in the slow-phase velocity was considered to indicate vestibular toxicity.

Histopathology of Ototoxicity

If more human temporal bones were readily available for histopathologic studies, much information could be gathered on the site of ototoxic injury in man, since efficient techniques for histopathologic evaluation of human inner ear tissues have been developed. By means of microdissection and surface preparation methods, Lars-Göran Johnsson and his group can detect degeneration in the hair cells and first-order neurons of patients with aminoglycoside ototoxicity. Joseph Nadol compares his histopathologic and clinical findings for several aminoglycosides in patients who had symptoms of ototoxicity. The work of Nadol and that of Johnsson et al. on human specimens tends to confirm the patterns of degeneration that have been noted in animals. The editors support Dr. Johnsson's plea for continued efforts to obtain human temporal bones at autopsy.

27. Aminoglycoside-Induced Inner Ear Pathology in Man, as Seen by Microdissection

Lars-Göran Johnsson, Joseph E. Hawkins, Jr., Thomas C. Kingsley, F. Owen Black, and Gregory J. Matz

Inner ear changes caused by aminoglycosides have been amply demonstrated in a variety of laboratory animals (Chaps. 12 and 13), but few cases of comparable human inner ear pathology have been reported in the literature since the advent of streptomycin, the first antibiotic of this group, some 35 years ago. This chapter concerns cochlear pathology in temporal bones obtained from five patients who had been treated with aminoglycosides by various routes of administration.

The paucity of such human material does not mean that ototoxic injury in man has been rare. Numerous reports of hearing loss or deafness and of vertigo and ataxia after aminoglycoside treatment are to be found in the clinical literature [2, 12, 23, 27, 28, 30, 49]. The otologist and the otopathologist are in an unfortunate position compared with physicians in other specialties in that temporal bones, their all-important autopsy material, are obtained only rarely. This is one of the reasons why our knowledge of inner ear pathology is still so limited. Animal models serve a useful purpose, but it should be kept in mind that the human inner ear does not necessarily respond to such insults in exactly the same fashion as does that of a laboratory animal. For example, the human ear tends to be injured more readily by drugs and less readily by noise than does the rodent ear. In man, changes associated with aging and often with noise exposure [18, 21] tend to alter or obscure damage caused by ototoxic drugs. Therefore, temporal bones obtained from young or middle-aged individuals within a reasonable time span after the insult are particularly valuable.

After the skull is opened, the temporal bone can be removed by the so-called block method with the Stryker saw. A special bone plug cutter is also available and easier to use. It is important to maintain profuse saline irrigation on the saw blade during the removal to avoid overheating of the tissues. After

This investigation was supported by USPHS Research Grants NS 05065 and NS 12706 and Program Project Grant NS 05785.

removal, the temporal bones are immersed in 10% buffered formalin (pH 7.4), in which they can be transported and stored until they are processed. Instructions for temporal bone removal are included in standard otopathology textbooks [39, 45]. Booklets and films concerning this topic are also provided by the National Temporal Bone Banks Program. No mutilation of the external ear, face, or head occurs during removal of the temporal bones.

One hopes that otologists and members of other specialties caring for patients who have problems with hearing loss or dysequilibrium will become increasingly aware of the National Temporal Bone Banks Program.* Physicians who work in neonatal care, infectious disease, nephrology, and burn units and who use aminoglycosides extensively should be aware of the fact that they can make important contributions to otopathology simply by helping to procure temporal bones at autopsy, especially from patients who have had recent audiograms and electronystagmograms.

Two methods are available for histopathologic study of the inner ear. The conventional approach [39, 45] requires decalcification of the temporal bone, followed by serial sectioning and staining of the specimen after it has been embedded in celloidin. This technique usually requires about 9 months. The technique of microdissection and surface preparations [6, 7, 14, 17], which was employed in this study, includes a "mini-autopsy" of the labyrinth after it has been stained with osmium tetroxide. It provides a three-dimensional view of the labyrinth under the dissecting microscope without the need for reconstruction from serial sections. The pattern of possible sensorineural degeneration can readily be seen and evaluated within days after autopsy. The thin, translucent cochlear tissues are examined as surface preparations (whole mounts). The entire length of Corti's organ is viewed and hair cells are counted. The number of missing hair cells and the pattern of nerve degeneration can be plotted in cytocochleograms [6, 21]. The vestibular sensory epithelia are difficult to dissect into surface preparations; we prefer to study them in man by scanning electron microscopy.

One of the first studies [12] of human inner ear pathology attributable to aminoglycoside treatment included 13 pairs of temporal bones from patients with tuberculosis meningitis who had received streptomycin intramuscularly and intrathecally. Hair cell loss and strial atrophy were observed mainly in the basal and middle turns of the cochlea. The vestibular epithelia also showed severe hair cell loss. In a second report on streptomycin ototoxicity [49], it was difficult to differentiate between pathologic changes caused by the ototoxic drugs and those caused by infection that had spread to the inner ear.

Five other reports [2, 23, 27, 28, 30] described six pairs of temporal bones in patients with poor renal function who were treated with kanamycin and neomycin and sustained labyrinthine injury. The temporal bones demonstrated various degrees of hair cell loss in the basal and middle turns of the cochlea. No significant degree of strial atrophy was reported, and few, if any, changes were seen in the first-order neurons. Vestibular changes were de-

*The Deafness Research Foundation, 336 Madison Ave., New York, NY 10017.

scribed in less detail or not mentioned at all. Vestibular sensory epithelia are particularly difficult to evaluate reliably in man by use of the conventional sectioning technique alone.

In the non-otologic literature, the term *nerve deafness* is commonly used to denote almost all forms of hearing loss caused by cochlear damage. This term, and the term *neurotoxicity* or eighth nerve toxicity, which are still sometimes used as synonyms for ototoxicity, is incorrect. In cases of ototoxicity, as in most other forms of labyrinthine injury, the initial changes involve mainly the sensory cells. As these cells and their supporting cells degenerate, secondary degeneration of cochlear nerve fibers occurs [20]. Therefore, the proper term for characterizing an aminoglycoside-induced auditory deficit is *sensorineural hearing loss.*

Material and Methods

Temporal bones were obtained at autopsy from five patients, in three of them from one side only. The specimens were processed according to the method outlined previously by Bredberg and Engström [6, 7] and Johnsson and Hawkins [17]. This method is described in detail elsewhere [14]. The middle ear is exposed, and both windows are opened. The inner ear is stained with 1% buffered osmium tetroxide solution for approximately 4 to 5 minutes by repeated perilymphatic perfusion through the oval window. The otic capsule is reduced with dental burrs to a thin shell and then removed with picks. The specimens are dissected and stored in 70% alcohol. They are transilluminated and photographed under alcohol for recording of the pattern of sensorineural degeneration (Fig. 27-1). The entire length of Corti's organ is examined systematically. The remaining hair cells and those replaced by phalangeal scars are recorded and plotted in cytocochleograms, which express the percentage of hair cells remaining per mm length of the basilar membrane.

After microdissection is completed, the temporal bones are decalcified and sectioned for evaluation of the ganglion cells in the modiolus. Only the modioli from cases 3, 4, and 5 have been processed and examined thus far.

Results

The cases studied represent different degrees and forms of aminoglycoside ototoxicity. In two of them, the respective labyrinthine injuries were caused by oral and topical administration of neomycin. The cases are presented in the order of increasing severity of sensorineural degeneration.

Case 1

HISTORY

The patient, a 45-year-old woman, died of lymphoma, regional enteritis (Crohn's disease), pulmonary infection, and endocarditis. Her renal function was normal. About 5 months before death, she was given 125 mg gentamicin 3

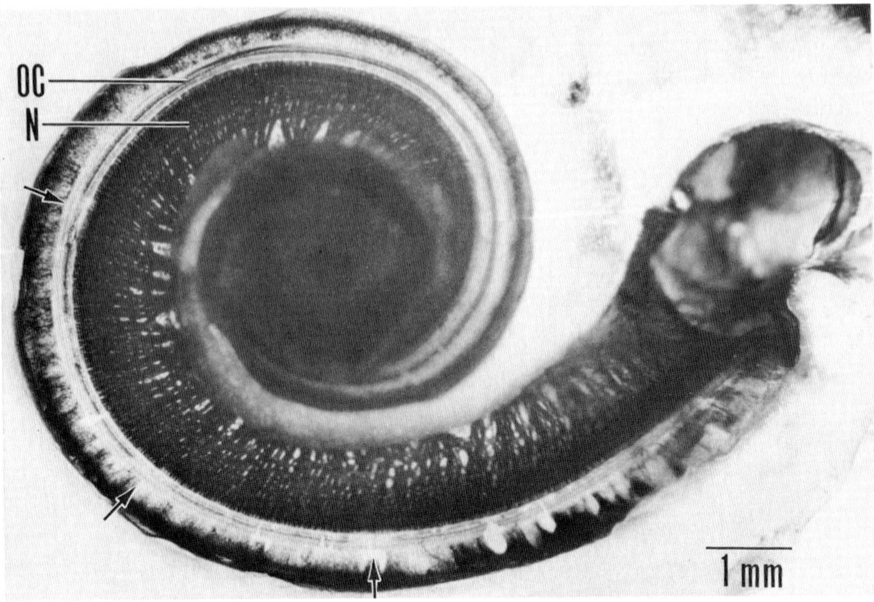

Figure 27-1. Left cochlea from case 3, showing network of myelinated nerve fibers (N) of normal density in osseous spiral lamina. Three areas of patchy degeneration (arrows) of Corti's organ (OC) are seen in the basal turn. In the adjacent regions, the distal ends of the nerve fibers have degenerated, giving the border of nerve fiber bundles a nibbled appearance (cf. Fig. 27-3). OsO_4.

times daily for 4 days, then 120 mg every 3 hours for 1 week. A third, 9-day course of gentamicin, 100 mg 3 times daily, was given about 1 month before death. Apparently her hearing had deteriorated during the course of the treatments. The audiogram obtained about 3 weeks before death showed a rather flat hearing loss of 20 to 30 dB.

HISTOPATHOLOGY

Only the right temporal bone was examined. The cytocochleogram for this ear showed slight scattered hair cell loss throughout the cochlea. The third row contained the largest number of missing outer hair cells. The loss was most severe in the most basal 8 mm of the cochlear duct and at the apex. This pattern of sensory cell degeneration also occurs in most individuals with aging [18]. Since the average number of hair cells in the normal population of this age group is not known, it is impossible to say to what extent aging contributed to the hair cell degeneration in this case. Only a slight nerve degeneration confined to the "hook" area was found, such as occurs also in "normal" specimens from patients in this age group. The stria vascularis was poorly preserved and difficult to evaluate reliably. The thickness of the stria appeared to be reduced in all turns.

Case 2

HISTORY

The patient was a 52-year-old woman who died of a poorly differentiated lymphoma. About 3 months prior to death, she had received amikacin, 360 mg 3 times daily, for 4 days, followed by gentamicin, 100 mg 3 times daily, for 10 days. About 1½ months later, amikacin, 300 mg 3 times daily, was given again for 1 week. The dose level was increased to 400 mg for 1 day; then treatment was interrupted for 3 days. It was resumed at 300 mg per day until the patient died 4 days later. An audiogram obtained during treatment showed a 20-dB hearing loss, except for a bilateral loss of about 40 dB at 8 kHz. Since pre-treatment audiograms had been normal, the hearing loss was attributed to ototoxicity.

HISTOPATHOLOGY

Only the left temporal bone was examined. The pathologic changes in this specimen were similar to those in the previous case. The hair cell loss was somewhat more severe at the basal end. In the second and third rows, the number of outer hair cells began to decline toward the zero level at about 16 mm from the basal end. A slight nerve degeneration extended from the basal end or hook region of the cochlea to involve approximately the first 10 mm of the osseous spiral lamina.

The stria vascularis displayed unusual pathologic changes. Numerous small areas of relatively diffuse atrophy were scattered along its entire length. These changes differed from the common form of atrophy, which is most severe at the upper and lower margins of the stria and may cause complete disappearance of the stria in the middle and apical turns.

Case 3

HISTORY

The third case is that of a 23-year-old woman who died of peritonitis and pneumonia. Four months prior to death, the patient had a laparotomy because of mechanical bowel obstruction, with abscesses and adhesions. A long-term peritonitis and extensive bowel necrosis followed, and the patient subsequently underwent abdominal surgery with repeated bowel resections. At the time of death, she had a very large upper abdominal midline incision and approximately 1 foot of intestine remaining. She had been treated with several different antibiotics, including the following ototoxic drugs: tobramycin, 70 mg IV at 8-hour intervals for 11 weeks until the day of death; and gentamicin, started 4 months before death with a daily injection of 240 mg/day IM for 3 weeks, followed by 150 mg IM per day for 1 week and 60 mg IM per day for another week, when treatment was discontinued. In addition, the patient had received 4 single doses of streptomycin and kanamycin about 4 months prior to death. Blood urea nitrogen (BUN) and creatinine values were normal, and autopsy showed no obvious kidney damage. The hearing loss which the patient must have suffered was not mentioned in the hospital records.

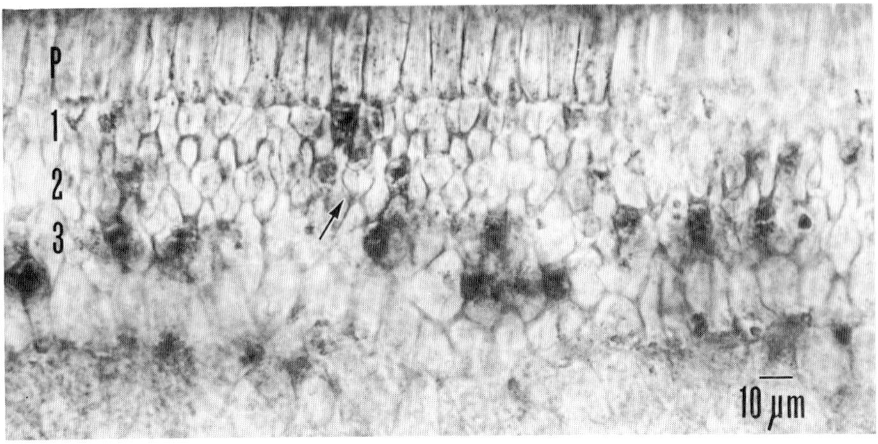

Figure 27-2. The surface of Corti's organ in the upper half of the basal turn in case 3, right ear. P designates head plates of inner pillar cells. Only about 16 scattered outer hair cells remain. Arrow points to a fresh phalangeal scar in the second row, with a Y-shaped figure inside the border. OsO_4, phase contrast.

HISTOPATHOLOGY

Hair cell degeneration was seen in both ears, but the degree of loss was markedly asymmetric (Figs. 27-1 through 27-4). The right ear showed severe to complete loss of outer hair cells throughout the cochlea. The largest number of sensory cells remained in an area between 10 and 20 mm from the basal end. A varying degree of inner hair cell loss was observed throughout the cochlea; the most severe loss occurred in the basal turn. In the left ear, an essentially complete loss of outer hair cells was limited to the basal 12 mm of the cochlea. Eighty to 90 percent of the inner hair cells had degenerated in the same area. Apical to this region, however, 60 to 80 percent of the sensory cells were present (Fig. 27-4). Several fresh phalangeal scars (Fig. 27-2) were seen in both ears, indicating that many of the hair cells had degenerated only recently.

An uneven or patchy degeneration of Corti's organ and its supporting elements was present in both ears. These changes were confined mainly to the lower half of the basal turn. Figure 27-1 shows that the two dark stripes on the basilar membrane representing the organ of Corti were disrupted in several small areas, where there was a more or less complete loss of sensory cells as well as supporting cells.

The density of the network of myelinated nerve fibers in the osseous spiral lamina was normal along the entire length of the cochlea. Nerve degeneration could be observed only peripherally in minute circumscribed areas, at the very distal end of the nerve fibers. These areas corresponded in size and location to regions on the basilar membrane where the supporting cells were missing. The nerve degeneration gave the appearance of small "cookie-bite" defects at the margin of the nerve network (Fig. 27-3) [20] along the normally smooth border formed at the habenula perforata, where the darkly stained myelin

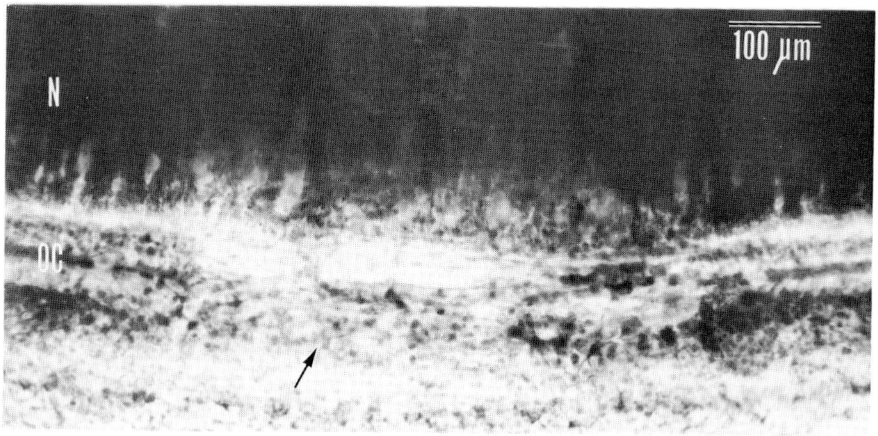

Figure 27-3. High-power view of the basilar membrane and the border of the nerve network (N) in Fig. 27-1, showing patchy degeneration of Corti's organ (OC) (arrow), with degeneration of the distal portions of the myelinated nerve fibers in the corresponding area. OsO_4, bright field.

sheaths normally terminate. When examined in sections of the modiolus, the ganglion cells of the basal turn exhibited no obvious pathologic changes.

Mild strial changes were observed in the middle and apical turns in both ears. Innumerable minute clear spots were present here, probably representing atrophy of the osmiophilic marginal cells. In the right ear, there was a small circumscribed area of severe strial atrophy in the apical turn.

Case 4

HISTORY

The patient was a 10-year-old boy who died of uremia several months after receiving a renal homotransplant. He had primary oxaluria (oxalosis), a rare inborn error of glyoxylic acid metabolism that leads to an overproduction of oxalic acid and deposition of calcium oxalate in the tissues. The disease is characterized by renal calculi, nephrocalcinosis, renal insufficiency, and recurrent urinary tract infection. The patient had developed *Pseudomonas* peritonitis for which peritoneal lavage was carried out with Inpersol containing neomycin, 50 mg/liter. The total amount of neomycin given appears to have been 400 to 600 mg. About 3 months after the perfusion, a severe progressive hearing loss was noted, which eventually stabilized at 55 to 65 dB for most frequencies. The state of his hearing immediately before death is not known.

HISTOPATHOLOGY

Only the right temporal bone was examined in the present study. The histologic findings in the left ear as seen in conventional sections have been described elsewhere [3]. Most of the hair cells had degenerated, except in the apical turn, where some outer hair cells were present (Figs. 27-5 and 27-6).

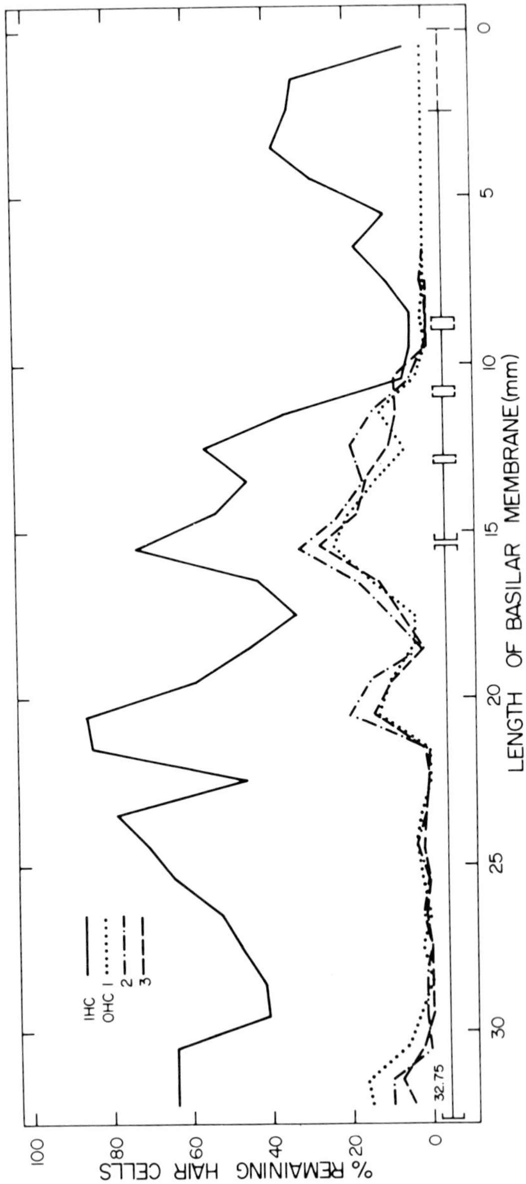
% REMAINING HAIR CELLS
0
20
40
60
80
100
LENGTH OF BASILAR MEMBRANE (mm)
0
5
10
15
20
25
30
32.75
IHC
OHC 1
2
3

A

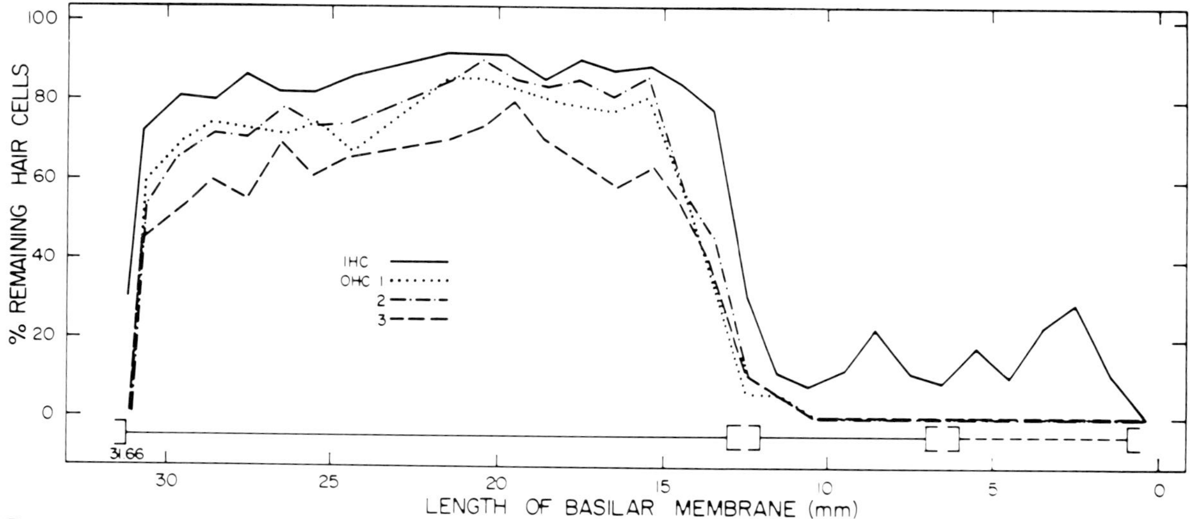

B

Figure 27-4. Cytocochleograms for case 3, showing distribution of remaining hair cells in (A) right ear and (B) left ear. Note the asymmetry of hair cell loss.

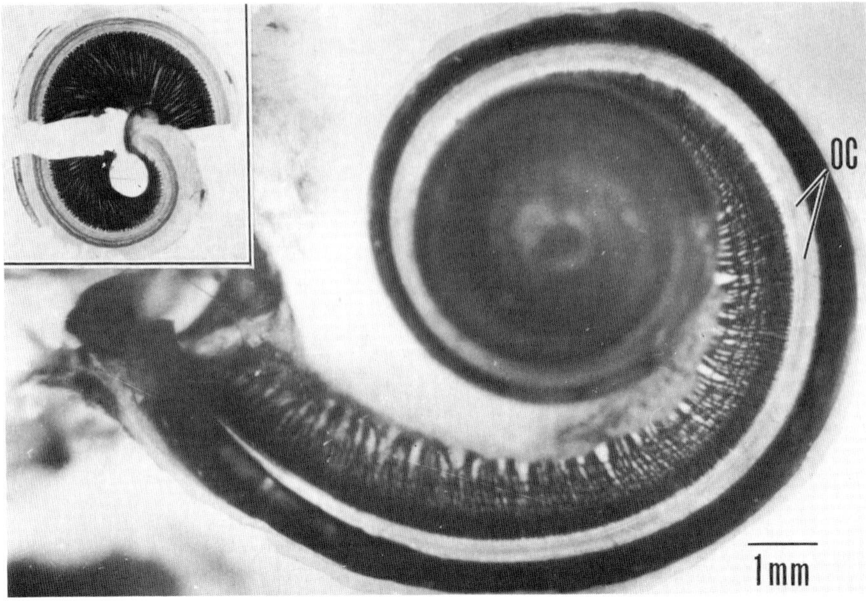

Figure 27-5. Right cochlea from case 4. A few outer hair cells were present, but only in the apical turn. Patchy loss of supporting cells (OC) and a long stretch of bare basilar membrane are seen in the upper half of the basal turn. In the corresponding area, the distal ends of myelinated fibers have degenerated (cf. Fig. 27-1). Inset: Upper half of middle turn and apical turn, with supporting cells present and no visible nerve degeneration.

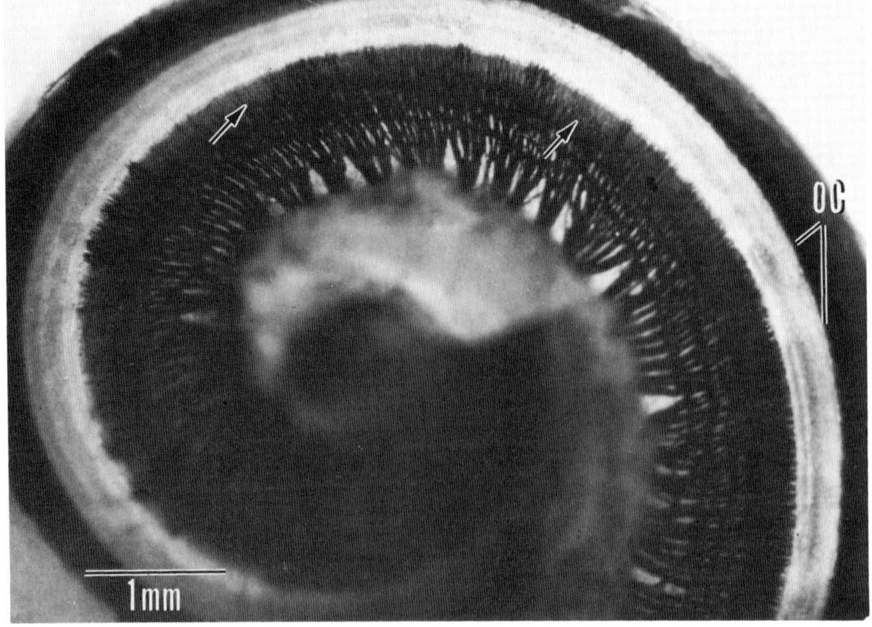

Figure 27-6. Close-up of the upper half of the basal turn in Fig. 27-5. Patchy degeneration of Corti's organ (OC), then complete loss extending throughout the turn. Note uneven degeneration of the distal ends of the nerve fibers in areas where the organ of Corti is completely absent (arrows). OsO_4.

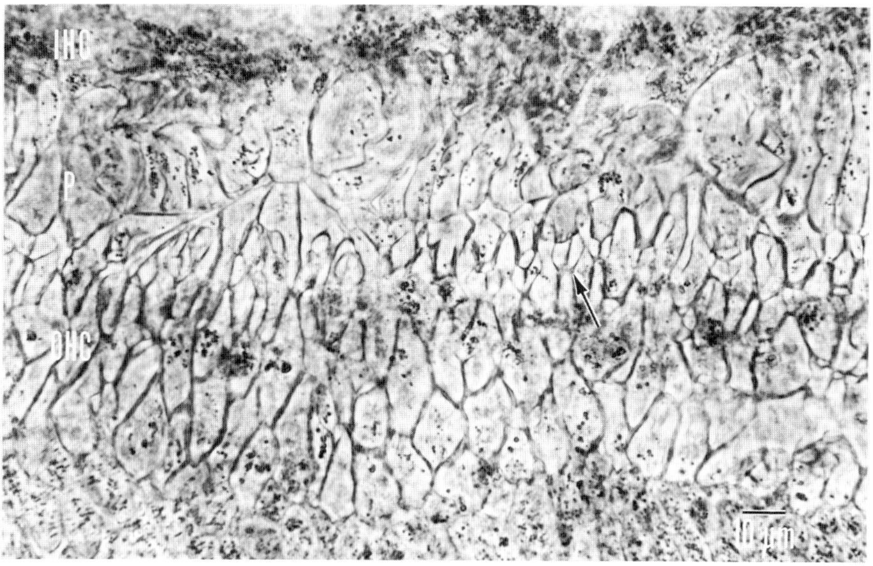

Figure 27-7. Reticular lamina in the middle turn of the cochlea shown in Figs. 27-5 and 27-6. All hair cells have degenerated. Arrow points to fresh phalangeal scar. Note the irregular arrangement of pillar cells, compared to that in Fig. 27-2. (IHC = site of inner hair cells; P = pillar cells; OHC = site of outer hair cells.) OsO_4, phase contrast. (Reproduced by permission from J. E. Hawkins, Jr., Drug Ototoxicity. In W. D. Keidel and W. D. Neff [Eds.], *Handbook of Sensory Physiology*. Heidelberg: Springer, 1976. Vol. V/3, p. 725.)

Several fresh phalangeal scars were seen, and the arrangement of the pillar cells was highly irregular (Fig. 27-7). The most severe damage occurred in the upper half of the basal turn, where there was a complete loss of supporting cells; islands and patches of supporting cells remained in the lower half. Adjacent to areas where the organ of Corti was completely missing and the basilar membrane was covered only with a thin epithelium, an uneven nerve degeneration was present, confined to the distal ends of the nerve fibers in the osseous spiral lamina (Figs. 27-5 and 27-6). Except in this region, the density of the nerve network was normal throughout the cochlea. The pattern of nerve degeneration in this specimen was similar to that observed in the previous case, but the degeneration was more severe and diffuse. The spiral ligament and stria vascularis were not evaluated systematically in this specimen.

Case 5

HISTORY

The patient, a 51-year-old woman, died of severe bleeding of the upper gastrointestinal tract. The pathologists felt that the underlying disorder was Hippel's disease or "blue rubber bleb nevus" syndrome. In addition to skin lesions, she had innumerable hemangiomata involving the gastrointestinal tract and the liver. The patient was hospitalized several times for gastrointestinal bleedings, anemia, and impending hepatic coma. For bowel sterilization and a reduced possibility of hepatic coma, the patient was given neomycin in 1969 with an oral dose averaging 2 g per day. Approximately a year later, BUN levels became high (65 mg percent); it was nevertheless decided that the neomycin treatment had to be continued, despite the obvious renal damage, because of the risk of hepatic coma. About 1 month later, a hearing deficit was noted; because of this and renal insufficiency, the neomycin therapy was discontinued. The BUN values subsequently became normal, and neomycin was again used sporadically. About 2 years after the initial neomycin treatment, the patient was completely deaf according to the hospital notes, but the exact time of onset of the hearing loss is not known. Bilateral tinnitus was also noted. There was no obvious history of dysequilibrium.

HISTOPATHOLOGY
No hair cells were visible in either ear. Supporting elements were completely absent in the first three quadrants [21] of the basal turn. A narrow strip of supporting cells extended from the upper half of the basal turn, gradually increasing in width toward the apical turn, where the largest number of supporting cells was seen. Similarly, the nerve fibers present in the osseous spiral lamina increased in number toward the apex, reaching their highest density in the middle and apical turns. There was good correlation between the presence of supporting cells and the presence of nerve fibers (Fig. 27-8). The general pattern of sensorineural degeneration in both ears was more or less symmetric, although the nerve degeneration in the basal turn was somewhat more severe in the left ear. Sections of the modiolus showed that, although most of the distal processes had degenerated in the basal turn, the corresponding ganglion cells and their proximal processes were still present (Figs. 27-9 and 27-10). Slight bilateral strial atrophy was observed, but it was no more severe than usually seen in specimens from this age group.

In this case, the neuroepithelia of the vestibular organs were examined by scanning electron microscopy. All showed extensive hair cell loss, as indicated by a greatly reduced number of stereociliary tufts in both ears (Fig. 27-11). On the maculae of the saccule and utricle, the type I cells located along the striola line were affected more severely than the surrounding type II cells. As a result, there appeared to be a path going through the center of the maculae.

Comments

The findings reported here are similar in many respects to those reported by previous observers [2, 27, 28, 30]. The technique used in this investigation, however, revealed some new aspects of inner ear pathology, particularly in relation to the pattern of nerve degeneration in the osseous spiral lamina.

The degree of hair cell loss in case 3, that of the patient treated with tobramycin and gentamicin, differed markedly in the two ears. This finding is in agreement with clinical studies in which at least nine cases of permanent or reversible unilateral hearing loss have been reported [32, 50]; in several of these patients, the vestibular organs were also involved. These findings are of some clinical interest; conceivably, a case of gentamicin or tobramycin

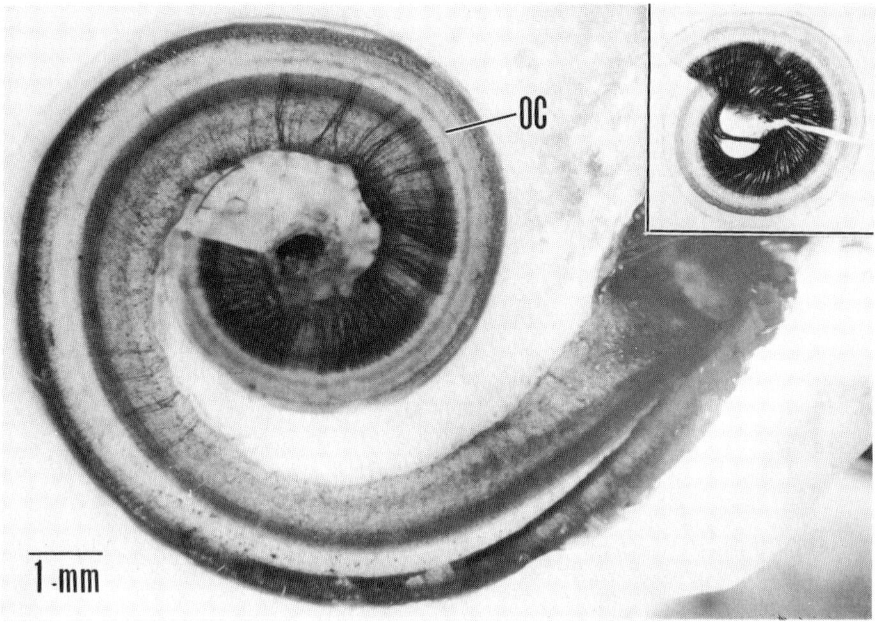

Figure 27-8. Left cochlea from case 5, showing severe secondary nerve degeneration about 6 years after initial oral neomycin medication. Remaining supporting cells are seen as a dark band (OC) on the basilar membrane. Inset: Upper half of middle and apical turns. Note the increasingly wide stripe of supporting cells and the increasing number of nerve fibers. OsO_4.

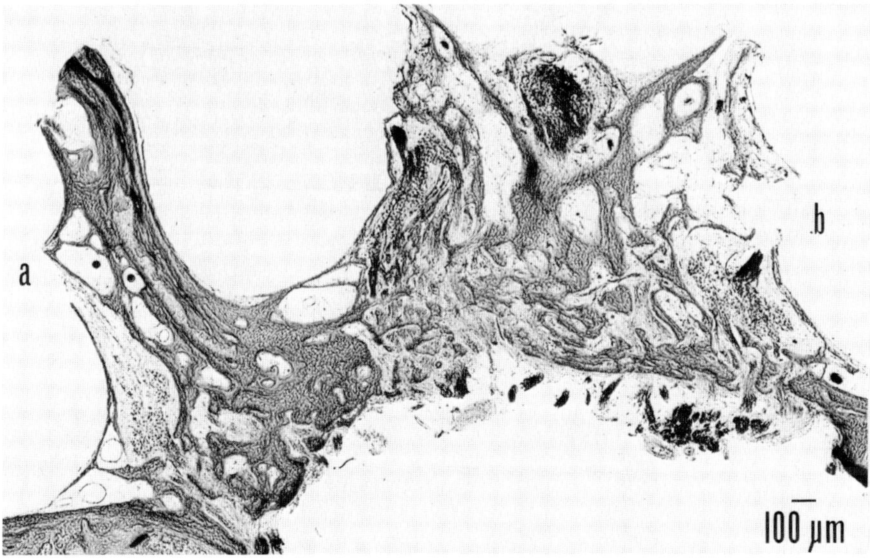

Figure 27-9. Midmodiolar section of the cochlea in Fig. 27-7 after Corti's organ and osseous spiral lamina have been dissected out. (The auditory nerve had been evulsed from the internal canal during autopsy.) The photomicrographs in this and the next illustration are printed so that their orientation is the same as that of the corresponding photomicrograph of the cochlear spiral (*a*). Note at *b* numerous ganglion cells with proximal (axonal) fibers and a thick black bundle of distal (dendritic) fibers. At *a*, fewer ganglion cells are present. There is a bundle of proximal fibers, but only a few distal fibers are seen. OsO_4, sections subsequently stained with H&E.

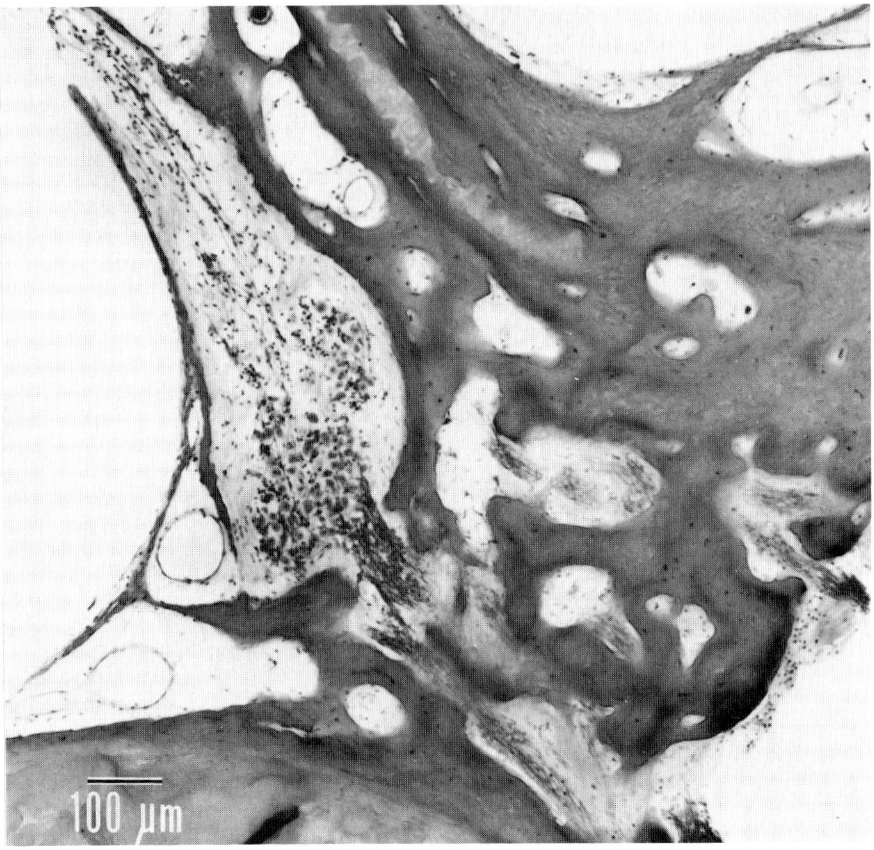

Figure 27-10. High-power view of remains of spiral ganglion at *a* in Fig. 27-8. Note numerous ganglion cells, with a thick bundle of proximal fibers and only a few distal fibers. OsO_4, stained with H&E.

ototoxicity with unilateral hearing loss and dizziness could mimic some of the symptoms and signs caused by an acoustic neurinoma.

In general, however, aminoglycoside-induced hearing loss tends to be symmetric in man [1, 10, 23, 36, 44] as well as in experimental animals [43]. In our material, we did not find the selective inner hair cell degeneration described previously in a case of neomycin ototoxicity [27]. Only outer hair cells remained in a small segment of the apical turn in case 3, but in both case 3 and case 4, the hair cell loss was much too severe at the time of death to reveal any generalized selective inner hair cells loss that may have existed earlier.

We had previously observed the irregular arrangements of the pillar cells and the phalangeal scars shown in Fig. 27-7 in primates treated with neomycin [43]. Presumably, this pattern of scarring of the reticular membrane reflects sudden, massive loss of hair cells and supporting cells and is characteristic of severe ototoxicity, such as that of neomycin.

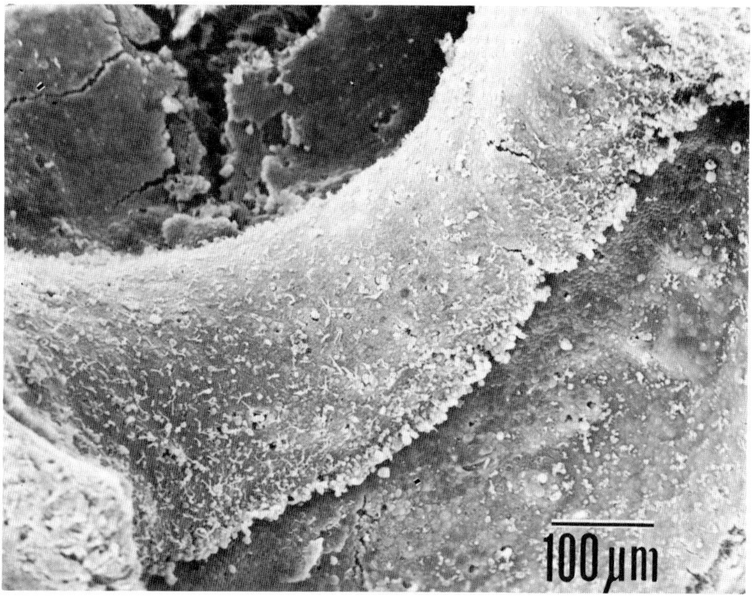

A

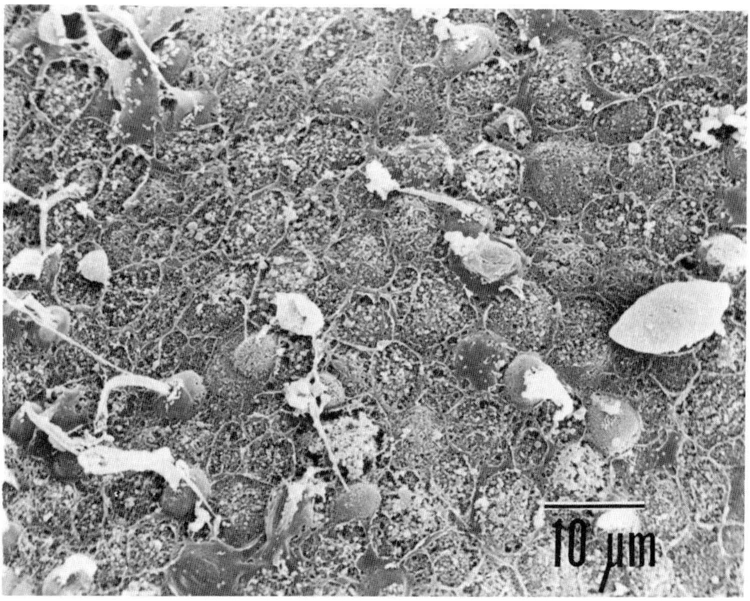

B

Figure 27-11. Scanning electron micrograph (case 5); crista of horizontal canal and ampulla. A. Low-power view of entire crista. B. High-power view of a small area. Note the scarcity of ciliary tufts.

Ever since cochlear prostheses were first introduced, the survival of nerve fibers in cases of ototoxic deafness has been of particular interest. In such devices, implanted electrodes are intended to stimulate the nerve fibers directly in patients who suffer from profound deafness [16, 33, 40]. They can provide such patients with a primitive sort of auditory sensation, and they have been reported to improve lipreading (and speaking) in the postlingually deaf [4]. Patients recently deafened by ototoxic drugs appear to be among the most promising candidates for implantation surgery. It is assumed that they have a larger population of nerve fibers than that of individuals with long-term deafness, who are known to have extensive nerve degeneration.

From this limited material, we cannot draw any general conclusions as to the usefulness of cochlear implants. Our previous [20] and present findings have shown that the population of nerve fibers in the osseous spiral lamina remains dense for a time, despite severe hair cell loss, as seen in case 5. In a few years, however, the secondary nerve degeneration can become so severe that tonotopical stimulation of the distal processes of cochlear neurons in the osseous spiral lamina of the basal turn becomes impossible (Fig. 27-7). Our study also confirms the well-known fact [20, 21, 35, 38, 41] that the presence of the supporting cells effectively delays secondary nerve degeneration (cf. Figs. 27-1, 27-3, 27-6, 27-7).

The earliest and most discrete degenerative changes that we have been able to discern in the first-order neurons appeared in the distal end of their processes in the osseous spiral lamina, in regions corresponding closely to segments of the basilar membrane where supporting elements were absent (cases 3 and 4). This gave the margin of the nerve network in the osseous spiral lamina a characteristic "nibbled" appearance (Figs. 27-1, 27-3, 27-5, 27-6). Covell and Noble [9] reported a similar degeneration pattern in conventional sections from rats with B_1 avitaminosis, stained with a chlorate-osmic-formalin mixture. We have found this type of degeneration pattern also in monkeys treated with ototoxic drugs [20], as well as in these two cases. It has also been observed in a case of ototoxicity caused by lividomycin, a new aminoglycoside [8, 48]. In the specimen from this patient, the distal half of the nerve fibers in the osseous spiral lamina had degenerated in portions of the basal turn [8, 48]. This form of nerve degeneration is probably characteristic of acute, severe ototoxicity. It appears to result from destruction of sensory and supporting cells, which deprives the unmyelinated portion of the cochlear neurons of the trophic and protective influence of the supporting cells. Insufficient repair of the reticular lamina may also accelerate sensory cell loss [5] and cause damage to the unmyelinated segments of the nerve fibers within Corti's organ. According to Spoendlin [42], injury to the unmyelinated portion of the nerve fiber initiates degeneration; such an injury, in an extreme form, appears to be responsible for the characteristic degeneration pattern seen in our two cases.

The findings in this study, as well as previous observations [22], indicate that the dendritic or distal process of the first-order neuron tends to degenerate much earlier than the axonal or proximal process (Figs. 27-8 and 27-9). Similar observations have been made by other investigators both in man [11, 35] and in experimental animals [24, 25]. Recently, Ylikoski et al. [51] demonstrated a fairly normal ultrastructure in surgical samples from the auditory nerves of four patients with long-term deafness. (The distal process could not be sampled.) A great number of the proximal processes with their ganglion cells thus seem capable of surviving for many years even if the corresponding distal processes have degenerated completely. It appears that such fibers can be stimulated electrically [25]. Changes in the ends of the proximal processes at the level of the cochlear nucleus would tend to go unnoticed with the techniques normally used for temporal bone histology. Recent studies of degeneration patterns following hair cell damage in animals by noise suggest, however, that early pathologic changes do occur in the ends of the proximal processes [34].

It is difficult to determine the degree and the precise location of degenerative changes in the first-order cochlear neurons in man from the study of conventional sections alone. The distal processes are poorly seen at best, and subtle, circumscribed changes such as those demonstrated in the specimens in Figs. 27-1, 27-3, 27-5, and 27-6 easily go unrecognized. Presumably, the degeneration seen in the right ear in case 4 was bilateral (Fig. 27-5); yet the conventional sections of the left ear did not reveal such changes. Sections do permit an estimate of the number of ganglion cells present, but cell bodies and their nuclei appear to be more susceptible to autolysis than their processes, and it is difficult to evaluate changes in their cytoplasm and nuclei. In fact, it appears that the earliest change in the cochlear neurons that can be seen in light microscopy of human specimens after ototoxic injury with aminoglycosides is the retrograde degeneration of the distal processes. Simultaneous or earlier degenerative changes may well occur in the cell body. Animal experiments indicate that, although the initial response to destruction of Corti's organ is visible in the distal process, changes also appear in the ganglion cells and the proximal processes within days or weeks after the insult to the hair cells [24, 46]. Such changes in man, if they occur, would be difficult to detect. We therefore believe that osmium-stained surface preparations of the osseous spiral lamina, which display the distal processes so clearly, reflect the condition of the neurons and the location of possible neuronal damage in man better than do conventional serial sections. A combination of the two techniques as used in this study probably provides the best way of evaluating cochlear nerve pathology.

A small fraction of neomycin can be absorbed when the drug is administered orally, or even topically. Reports of new cases of neomycin-induced deafness following such treatment continue to appear in the literature [29, 47]. Ballantyne [1] reported 13 patients who had received neomycin orally. Six of these patients developed sensorineural hearing loss. The incidence of deafness had little relationship to the dosage used. Neomycin obviously was absorbed by our two patients who received oral and topical administration. The absorption may well have been enhanced by the presence of intestinal hemangiomata in case 5, creating exceptionally high serum neomycin levels. This could, in part, explain the degeneration of vestibular sensory cells in this individual, which was so severe that it could not have been caused by aging alone. The fact that the type I sensory cells were affected more than the type II cells also supports the notion that the sensory cell loss was the result of ototoxicity [26], even though neomycin is not usually thought to be vestibulotoxic. There is evidence that neomycin in large doses can injure the vestibular neuroepithelia in the cat [15] and can affect the calcium metabolism of otoconia in the guinea pig [31].

We have previously suggested that the strial atrophy observed in various forms of deafness, including aminoglycoside-induced deafness in laboratory animals, may play an important role in sensory cell degeneration [19]. This notion could not be confirmed in the present study, although some strial changes were found that were thought to be unrelated to or atypical of aging and therefore presumably were secondary to the aminoglycoside treatment. Case 5, which showed severe long-term sensorineural degeneration caused by neomycin treatment, had a normal-appearing stria vascularis. In cases 1 and 2, on the other hand, which represented short-term and much milder ototoxic injury, an unusual form of diffuse strial atrophy was present in all turns. Apical strial atrophy was found in the specimens from case 3 with more severe, acute injury. This observation raises the question whether the striae damaged during aminoglycoside treatment can recover at a later stage. Repair of the stria after injury by noise has been reported in chinchillas [37], but that finding may or may not have a bearing on the present question. No definite causal relationship between strial injury and hair cell degeneration has yet been established.

References

1. Ballantyne, J. Iatrogenic deafness. *J. Laryngol. Otol.* 84:967, 1970.
2. Benitez, J. T., Schuknecht, H. F., and Brandenburg, J. H. Pathologic changes in human ear after kanamycin. *Arch. Otolaryngol.* 75:192, 1962.
3. Bergstrom, L., Jenkins, P., Sando, I., and English, G. M. Hearing loss in renal disease: Clinical and pathological studies. *Ann. Otol. Rhinol. Laryngol.* 82:555, 1973.
4. Bilger, R. C., et al. Evaluation of subjects presently fitted with implanted auditory prostheses. *Ann. Otol. Rhinol. Laryngol.* [Suppl. 38], 1977.
5. Bohne, B. A. Mechanisms of Noise Damage in the Inner Ear. In D. Henderson, R. P. Hamernik, D. S. Dosanjh, and J. H. Mills (Eds.), *Effects of Noise on Hearing.* New York: Raven, 1967. Pp. 41–68.
6. Bredberg, G., Engström, H., and Ades, H. W. Cellular pattern and nerve supply of the human organ of Corti. *Arch. Otolaryngol.* 82:462, 1965.
7. Bredberg, G. Cellular pattern and nerve supply of the human organ of Corti. *Acta Otolaryngol. (Stockh.)* [Suppl. 236], 1968.
8. Conraux, C. Discussion in Comptes Rendus des Séances, Société Française d'Oto-Rhino-Laryngologie et de Pathologie Cervico-Faciale, 75e Congrès Français, Paris, Sept. 1978, Librarie Arnette, Paris, p. 149.
9. Covell, W. P., and Noble, L. The significance of myelin sheath degeneration for the cochlear nerve. *Ann. Otol. Rhinol. Laryngol.* 46:895, 1937.
10. Dayal, V. S., Whitehead, G. L., and Smith, E. L. Gentamicin—progressive cochlear toxicity. *Can. J. Otolaryngol.* 4:348, 1975.
11. Egami, T., Sando, I., and Sobel, J. Noise-induced hearing loss: A human temporal bone case report. *Ann. Otol. Rhinol. Laryngol.* 87:868, 1978.
12. Graf, K. Histologische Veränderungen des Innenohres nach Behandlung der Meningitis tuberculosa mit Streptomycin. *Acta Otolaryngol. (Stockh.)* 39:121, 1951.

13. Hawkins, J. E., Jr. Drug Ototoxicity. In W. D. Keidel and W. D. Neff (Eds.), *Handbook of Sensory Physiology.* Heidelberg: Springer, 1976. Vol. V/3, pp. 707–748.
14. Hawkins, J. E., Jr., and Johnsson, L-G. Microdissection and Surface Preparations of the Inner Ear. In C. A. Smith and J. A. Vernon (Eds.), *Handbook of Auditory and Vestibular Research Methods.* Springfield, Ill.: Thomas, 1975. Pp. 5–52.
15. Hawkins, J. E., Jr., and Lurie, M. The ototoxicity of dihydrostreptomycin and neomycin in the cat. *Ann. Otol. Rhinol. Laryngol.* 62:1128, 1953.
16. House, W. F., et al. Cochlear implants. *Ann. Otol. Rhinol. Laryngol.* [Suppl. 27], 1976.
17. Johnsson, L-G., and Hawkins, J. E., Jr. A direct approach to cochlear anatomy and pathology in man. *Arch. Otolaryngol.* 85:599, 1967.
18. Johnsson, L-G., and Hawkins, J. E., Jr. Sensory and neural degeneration with aging, as seen in microdissections of the human inner ear. *Ann. Otol. Rhinol. Laryngol.* 81:179, 1972.
19. Johnsson, L-G., and Hawkins, J. E., Jr. Strial atrophy in clinical and experimental deafness. *Laryngoscope* 83:1105, 1972.
20. Johnsson, L-G. Sequence of degeneration of Corti's organ and its first-order neurons. *Ann. Otol. Rhinol. Laryngol.* 83:294, 1974.
21. Johnsson, L-G., and Hawkins, J. E., Jr. Degeneration patterns in human ears exposed to noise. *Ann. Otol. Rhinol. Laryngol.* 85:725, 1976.
22. Johnsson, L-G. Human inner ear pathology as seen in microdissections and surface preparations. University of Helsinki Thesis, 1979.
23. Jørgensen, M. B., and Schmidt, M. R. The ototoxic effect of kanamycin. *Acta Otolaryngol. (Stockh.)* 55:537, 1962.
24. Kellerhals, B., Engström, H., and Ades, H. W. Die Morphologie des Ganglion spirale Cochleae. *Acta Otolaryngol. (Stockh.)* [Suppl. 226], 1967.
25. Liberman, M. C., and Kiang, N. Y. S. Acoustic trauma in cats: Cochlear pathology and auditory-nerve activity. *Acta Otolaryngol. (Stockh.)* [Suppl. 358], 1978.
26. Lindeman, H. H. Regional differences in sensitivity of the vestibular sensory epithelia to ototoxic antibiotics. *Acta Otolaryngol. (Stockh.)* 67:177, 1969.
27. Lindsay, J. R., Proctor, L. R., and Work, W. P. Histopathologic inner ear changes in deafness due to neomycin in a human. *Laryngoscope* 70:382, 1960.
28. Lowry, L. D., May, M., and Pastore, P. Acute histopathologic inner ear changes in deafness due to neomycin: A case report. *Ann. Otol. Rhinol. Laryngol.* 82:876, 1973.
29. Manuel, M. A., Kurtz, I., Saiphoo, C. S., and Schacht, J. Nephrotoxicity and ototoxicity following irrigation of wounds with neomycin. *Can. J. Surg.* 22:274, 1979.
30. Matz, G. J., Wallace, T. H., and Ward, P. H. The ototoxicity of kanamycin. A comparative histopathological study. *Laryngoscope* 75:1690, 1965.
31. Mechigian, I., Preston, R. E., Johnsson, L-G., et al. Incorporation of radioactive calcium into otolithic membranes of the guinea pig after aminoglycoside treatment. *Acta Otolaryngol. (Stockh.)* 88:56, 1979.
32. Meyers, R. M. Ototoxic effects of gentamicin. *Arch. Otolaryngol.* 92:160, 1970.
33. Michelson, R. P. The results of electrical stimulation of the cochlea in human sensory deafness. *Ann. Otol. Rhinol. Laryngol.* 80:914, 1971.
34. Morest, D. K., and Bohne, B. A. Differential degeneration in the brain of chinchillas following inner and outer hair cell damage by cochlear stimulation. Abstracts of the 3rd Midwinter Research Meeting, Association for Research in Otolaryngology, St. Petersburg Beach, Florida, January 1980.
35. Otte, J., Schuknecht, H. F., and Kerr, A. G. Ganglion cell populations in normal and pathological human cochleae. Implications for cochlear implantation. *Laryngoscope* 88:1231, 1978.
36. Ranta, L. J. Acoustic and vestibular disturbances following streptomycin-treated tuberculosis meningitis in children. *Acta Otolaryngol. (Stockh.)* [Suppl. 136], 1958.

37. Santi, P. A., and Duvall, A. J. Stria vascularis pathology and recovery following noise exposure. *Otolaryngology* 86:354, 1978.
38. Schuknecht, H. F. Lesions of the organ of Corti. *Trans. Am. Acad. Ophthalmol. Otolaryngol.* 57:366, 1953.
39. Schuknecht, H. F. *Pathology of the Ear.* Cambridge: Harvard University Press, 1974.
40. Simmons, F. B. Electrical stimulation of the auditory nerve in man. *Arch. Otolaryngol.* 84:24, 1966.
41. Spoendlin, H. H., and Gacek, R. R. Electronmicroscopic study of the efferent and afferent innervation of the organ of Corti in the cat. *Ann. Otol. Rhinol. Laryngol.* 72:660, 1963.
42. Spoendlin, H. The Afferent Innervation of the Cochlea. In R. A. Naunton and C. Fernández (Eds.), *Evoked Electrical Activity in the Auditory Nervous System.* New York: Academic, 1978. Pp. 21–41.
43. Stebbins, W. C., Miller, J. M., Johnsson, L-G., et al. Ototoxic hearing loss and cochlear pathology in the monkey. *Ann. Otol. Rhinol. Laryngol.* 78:1007, 1969.
44. Tsuki, T., and Murai, S. Familial incidence of streptomycin hearing loss and hereditary weakness of the cochlea. *Audiology* 10:315, 1971.
45. Ward, P. H., and Gussen, R. Preparation of the Temporal Bone for Histopathological Study. In C. A. Smith and J. A. Vernon (Eds.), *Handbook of Auditory and Vestibular Research Methods.* Springfield, Ill.: Thomas, 1975. Pp. 53–71.
46. Webster, D. B., and Webster, M. Cochlear nerve projections following organ of Corti destruction. *Otolaryngology* 86:342, 1978.
47. Weinstein, A. J., McHenry, M. C., and Gavan, T. L. Systemic absorption of neomycin irrigating solution. *J.A.M.A.* 238:152, 1977.
48. Weiss, J-M. Ototoxicité des aminoglycosides. Université Louis Pasteur, Faculté de Médecine de Strasbourg, Thesis, 1978.
49. Whetnall, E. M., and Lucas, H. A. Changes in the internal ear and VIII nerve in fatal cases of tuberculosis meningitis treated by streptomycin and dihydrostreptomycin. *Proc. R. Soc. Med.* 45:779, 1952.
50. Winkel, O., Mørk Hansen, M., Kaaber, K., and Rozarth, K. A prospective study of gentamicin ototoxicity. *Acta Otolaryngol. (Stockh.)* 86:212, 1978.
51. Ylikoski, J., Collan, Y., and Palva, T. Pathologic features of the cochlear nerve in profound deafness. *Arch. Otolaryngol.* 104:202, 1978.

28. Histopathology of Human Aminoglycoside Ototoxicity

Joseph B. Nadol, Jr.

The interpretation of temporal bone histopathology for patients who suffered ototoxic injury is hampered by several inherent limitations: Postmortem alteration of specimens; admixture of other pathology, such as acoustic trauma, presbycusic degeneration, and genetically determined alterations; variable and uncertain drug dosages; and variable time intervals between exposure to an ototoxic substance and death limit the degree of specificity that can be ascribed to the findings. Nevertheless, examination of human specimens is of fundamental importance in the study of ototoxic drug effects for several reasons. Human specimens offer the most direct histopathologic correlation with clinically observed ototoxicity; furthermore, they allow validation of the applicability of animal data to the human situation. Finally, data from studies of man offer a histopathologic foundation for developing rational treatment, especially in those patients with profound hearing loss in whom cochlear implantation or cochlear nerve stimulation may become generally feasible. Eight cases of aminoglycoside toxicity and the associated histopathologic findings from the Temporal Bone Collection of the Massachusetts Eye and Ear Infirmary are presented.

Streptomycin

Streptomycin was the first of the aminoglycoside drugs to be introduced [28], and ototoxic side effects were described soon thereafter [8, 15]. Vestibular dysfunction is the first clinical sign of ototoxicity caused by streptomycin.

Case 1

This man underwent mitral valvulotomy at age 47 and received streptomycin postoperatively. This was administered intramuscularly, 1 g per day in 4 di-divided doses, for a total of 10 days. The patient's renal function was normal.

Within days following cessation of therapy, the patient became severely

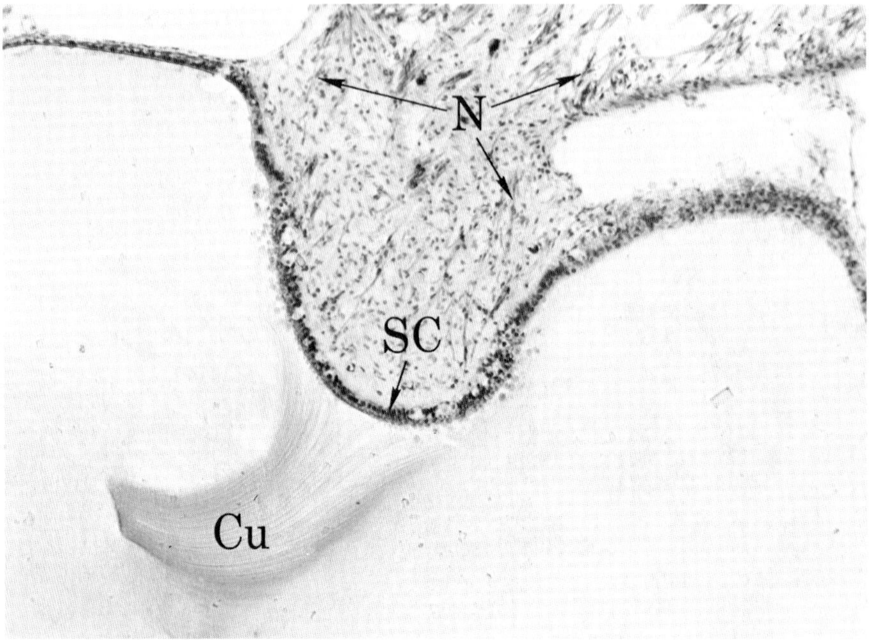

Figure 28-1. Case 1. Streptomycin ototoxicity. The crista of the posterior semicircular canal is normal except for loss of hair cells, which is most marked at the crest. The cupula (Cu), supporting cells (SC), and nerve fibers (N) appear normal. (Magnification ×175.)

ataxic, especially in the dark. He felt unable to drive his automobile. He experienced no hearing loss. Ice-water caloric stimulation showed no vestibular response in either ear. The Romberg test with eyes closed was markedly positive. His vestibular symptoms slowly improved, but did not disappear in the 4-year interval between drug administration and death.

HISTOPATHOLOGY

The cochlear hair cells, stria vascularis, and cochlear neuronal population were normal bilaterally. In the vestibular end organ there was a loss of approximately 75 percent of hair cells in all 3 cristae of both ears (Fig. 28-1). The hair cell loss was more marked at the crests, or more central aspect, of the cristae (Fig. 28-2) than at the "shoulders," or more peripheral aspect.

There appeared to be some loss of hair cells in the macula utriculi, but none in the saccule. The vestibular neuronal population appeared normal.

Case 2

This 55-year-old man developed vertigo and ataxia while being treated for advanced pulmonary tuberculosis with an unknown dosage of streptomycin. The patient's renal function was normal at the start of streptomycin treatment. Otologic examination revealed normal tympanic membranes and a positive

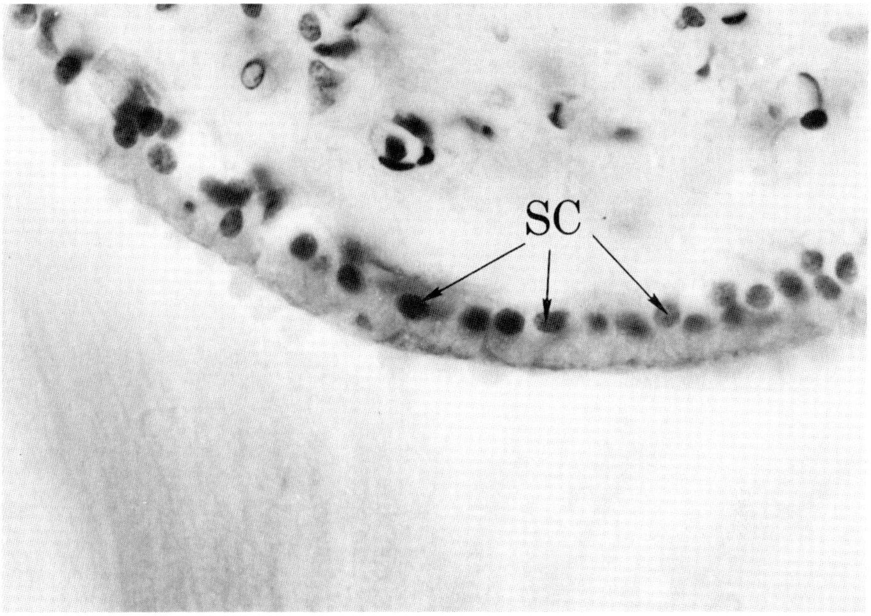

Figure 28-2. Case 1. Streptomycin ototoxicity. At the crest of the crista ampullaris of the posterior semicircular canal, a single row of supporting cells (SC) remains. There are no hair cells, which would appear as a separate row of nuclei external to the row of supporting cells. (Magnification ×1,285.) (Courtesy of Dr. Harold F. Schuknecht.)

Romberg sign, but no spontaneous nystagmus. An audiogram done one month before death revealed a bilateral mild high-frequency hearing loss considered consistent with presbycusis. The patient died of cardiac failure and a pulmonary embolus.

Histologic findings in both ears were similar. The hair cells of the organ of Corti were normal bilaterally. There was a loss of 30 to 50 percent of the cochlear neurons in the basal turn of both ears, consistent with primary neural degeneration of presbycusis. The maculae of the utricle and saccule were normal in both ears. In the cristae, however, there was a severe loss of hair cells (Fig. 28-3), which was complete at the crests and nearly complete on the slopes. The supporting cells were normal in all cristae.

Comment

Animal experimentation has demonstrated that the principal ototoxic effect of streptomycin is loss of hair cells of the vestibular end organs, primarily in the cristae, with little or no loss in the maculae [2, 6]. Furthermore, in animals, type I vestibular hair cells appear to be more susceptible to the ototoxic effect of streptomycin than type II cells, so that the crests of the cristae are more depopulated of hair cells than the shoulders [23, 33, 34]. The human histopathologic findings are in good agreement with the animal data. In addi-

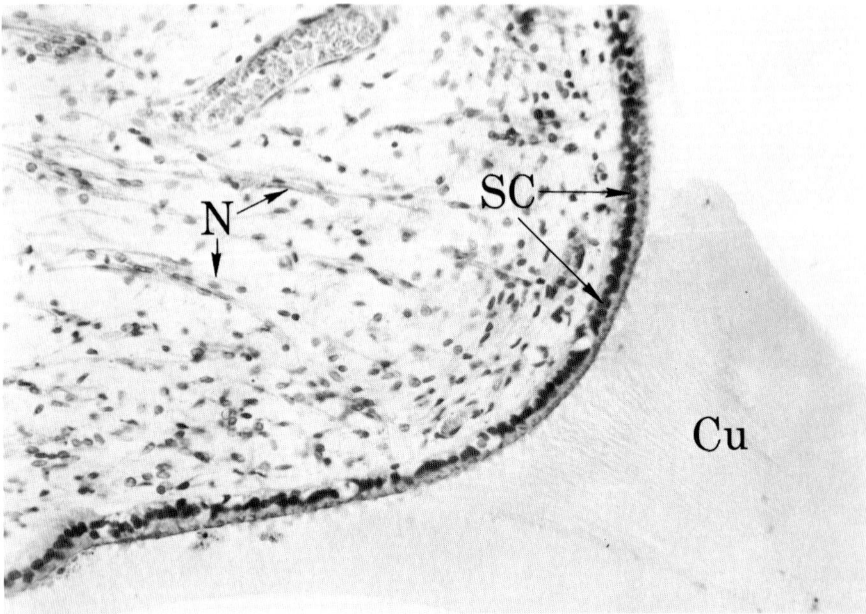

Figure 28-3. Case 2. Streptomycin ototoxicity. There is complete loss of hair cells at the crest of the crista ampullaris of the lateral semicircular canal. A few hair cells may remain at the shoulders of the crista. The cupula (Cu), supporting cells (SC), and neurons (N) appear normal. (Magnification ×390.)

tion, case 1 illustrates that, at least in some individuals, vestibular toxicity may result from a relatively small dose. This individual suffered permanent ataxia and some vestibular hair cell loss after a total dose of 10 g of streptomycin. Such individual variability in sensitivity was pointed out by Cawthorne and Ranger [7] and may involve a genetic predisposition [30]. In the absence of renal insufficiency, streptomycin ototoxicity is not common at a dose of 1 g or less per day even when continued for several weeks, whereas at a dose of 2 g per day more than 50 percent of all patients will develop vestibular abnormalities when therapy is continued for 9 to 12 weeks [4]. The selective vestibular toxicity of streptomycin has been employed successfully in the treatment of the vestibular symptoms of Menière's disease [29].

Neomycin

The clinical observation of severe ototoxicity caused by neomycin was made shortly after its introduction in 1949 [31]. Ototoxicity has been observed following oral administration [1, 3, 12, 13, 22], colonic irrigation [9], wound irrigation [5, 18], and intrapleural instillation [26]. Furthermore, the ototoxic effect is not strictly dose-related, since absorption from these sites is unpredictable.

Case 3

This 86-year-old woman developed osteomyelitis as a complication of fracture of the femur. This was treated by constant irrigation with a solution containing 1 g of neomycin, 50,000 units of bacitracin, and 50 mg of polymyxin in 1 liter of normal saline. The irrigation was administered at a rate of 50 ml per hour (1.2 g of neomycin per 24 hours) for 18 days. Hearing loss was first noticed during treatment and progressed after termination of the irrigation. The patient was profoundly deaf at the time of her death 6 months later. Although autopsy examination of the kidneys revealed mild nephrosclerosis, her renal function was normal during life.

HISTOPATHOLOGY

The pathologic findings in both inner ears were similar and consisted of loss of hair cells and, to a lesser extent, of cochlear neurons, most severe in the basal turn (Figs. 28-4 and 28-5). There were no remaining hair cells in the basal 25 mm of the cochleae (Fig. 28-6). In the basal turn of both ears, the height of the organ of Corti was decreased, suggesting damage to supporting cells as well as hair cells in these regions. There was a loss of 15 to 75 percent of spiral ganglion cells in the basal 15 mm of both cochleae (Fig. 28-7). The hair cell and neuronal populations of the vestibular labyrinths were normal.

Case 4

This man developed hepatic encephalopathy secondary to severe Laennec's cirrhosis at age 57. Starting at age 64 he was treated with oral neomycin at a dosage of 2 g per day. After 4 years of treatment, the dosage was increased to 4 g per day and continued for the next year until death. During this period, he complained of bilateral progressive hearing loss. An audiogram 6 months before death demonstrated a severe bilateral downward-sloping sensorineural loss with a speech discrimination of 70 percent. Neomycin therapy was continued. An audiogram 3 months before death demonstrated further hearing loss, particularly of speech discrimination (Fig. 28-8). He died at age 69 of hepatic and acute renal failure. Autopsy findings demonstrated acute tubular necrosis secondary to sepsis. Renal function was not a clinical problem during treatment with neomycin.

HISTOPATHOLOGY

The pathologic findings in both ears were identical. There was marked atrophy of several structures of the cochleae. Reissner's membrane was missing in the basal turn (Figs. 28-9 and 28-10). Atrophy of the stria vascularis and organ of Corti was seen in all turns (Figs. 28-9 and 28-10). No hair cells could be recognized, and, in addition, the supporting elements were reduced to a thin layer or low mound of epithelial cells. There was marked loss of cochlear neurons, particularly in the basal turn (Fig. 28-9). In contrast, the hair cells and neurons of the vestibular labyrinth appeared normal (Fig. 28-11).

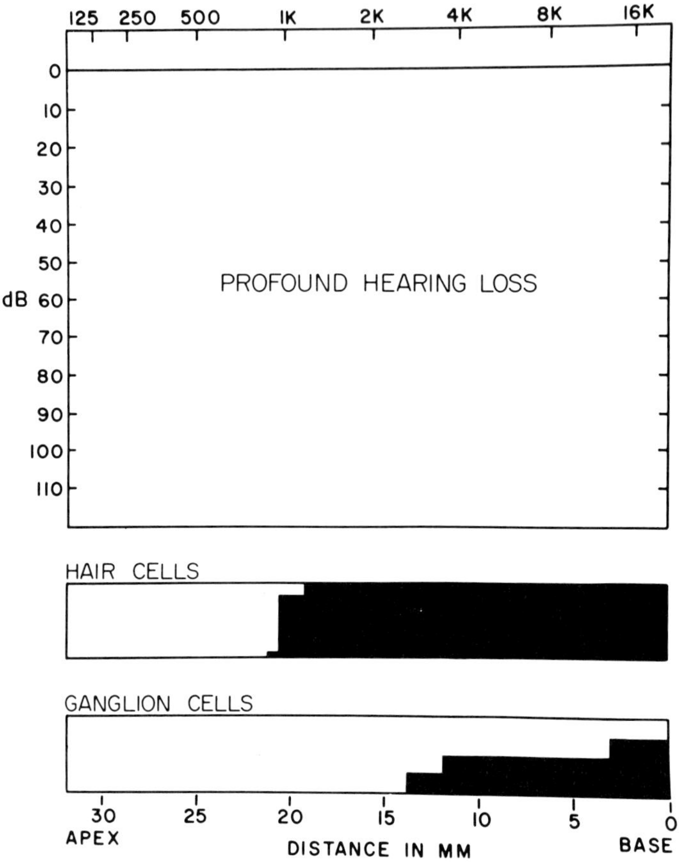

Figure 28-4. Case 3. Neomycin ototoxicity. Histogram of cellular loss, estimated as percentage of cells missing (shown in black), in left ear.

Case 5

This 53-year-old woman was treated with neomycin administered orally at a dose of 2 g per day for hepatic dysfunction. The neomycin treatment was continued to within a few days of death at age 54. Within weeks after starting neomycin therapy, she noticed a bilateral hearing loss. Audiograms done 6 months (Fig. 28-12) and 18 months (Fig. 28-13) after the beginning of therapy demonstrated a progressive bilateral sensorineural hearing loss with a marked decrement of discrimination. She died of intraventricular hemorrhage 2 weeks after the last audiogram. Although mild nephrosclerosis was noted at autopsy, renal function was normal during life.

HISTOPATHOLOGY

The pathologic findings were similar in both ears. There was loss of approximately 50 percent of inner and outer hair cells in the basal turn and of 20 per-

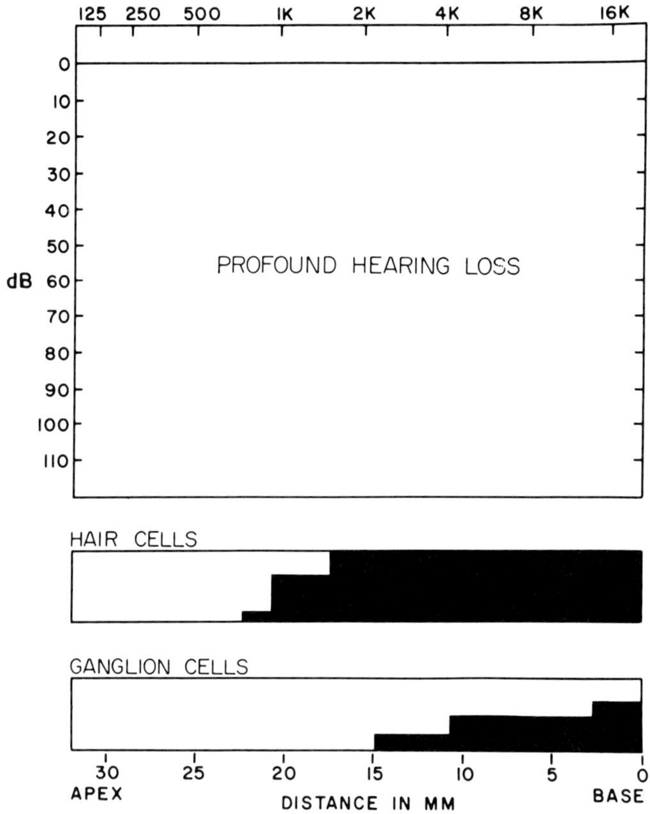

Figure 28-5. Case 3. Neomycin ototoxicity. Histogram of cellular loss, estimated as percentage of cells missing (shown in black), in right ear. (Courtesy of Dr. Harold F. Schuknecht.)

cent of hair cells in the middle turn of the cochlea (Figs. 28-14 and 28-15). In addition, a loss of about 50 percent of the cochlear neurons was noted in the basal and middle turns (Fig. 28-14). There was also marked atrophy of the stria vascularis in some regions of the middle and basal turns. In contrast, the hair cells and neurons of the vestibular system appeared normal.

Comment

These three cases demonstrate ototoxicity caused by neomycin administered orally or by wound irrigation. The hearing loss, when not total, was most severe at the high frequencies, and severe loss of speech discrimination was uniformly present. The primary histopathologic findings were loss of hair cells and, to a lesser extent, of cochlear neurons, most marked in the basal turns. The loss of speech discrimination seemed greater than would be expected from the loss of sensory or neural elements, suggesting severe dysfunction among surviving

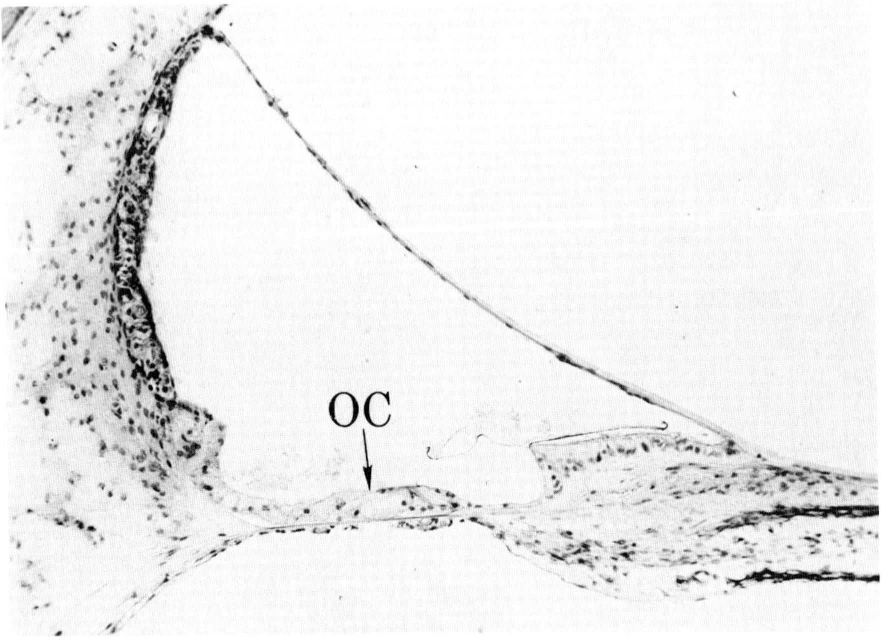

Figure 28-6. Case 3. Neomycin ototoxicity. Basal turn of the organ of Corti of the right ear. There are no remaining hair cells in the somewhat flattened organ of Corti (OC). (Magnification ×195.) (Courtesy of Dr. Harold F. Schuknecht.)

cells. Primary cochlear hair cell loss was also described in a human case by Lindsay et al. [24], and in guinea pigs by Kohonen [20]. In the animal study, the external hair cells of the basal turn were the first affected, followed by progression of loss in an apical direction. With increasing severity of the ototoxic effect, inner hair cells were lost, first in the apical turn, and then progressively in a basal direction.

Kanamycin

The primary ototoxic effect of kanamycin is auditory, and hearing loss is frequently preceded by tinnitus [11, 27]. Unlike the ototoxic effect of neomycin, the progression of hearing loss may be arrested, or, in a few patients, reversed, by termination of kanamycin therapy after the first signs of ototoxicity have been observed [11]. As with other aminoglycosides, impaired renal function potentiates the ototoxic effect of kanamycin [10], and in patients with renal compromise the ototoxic effect of this drug may continue after cessation of treatment [11].

Kanamycin can be used orally for bowel sterilization. Although less than 1 percent of orally administered dosage is absorbed, blood levels comparable to those seen with parenteral therapy may be achieved in patients with renal compromise [21].

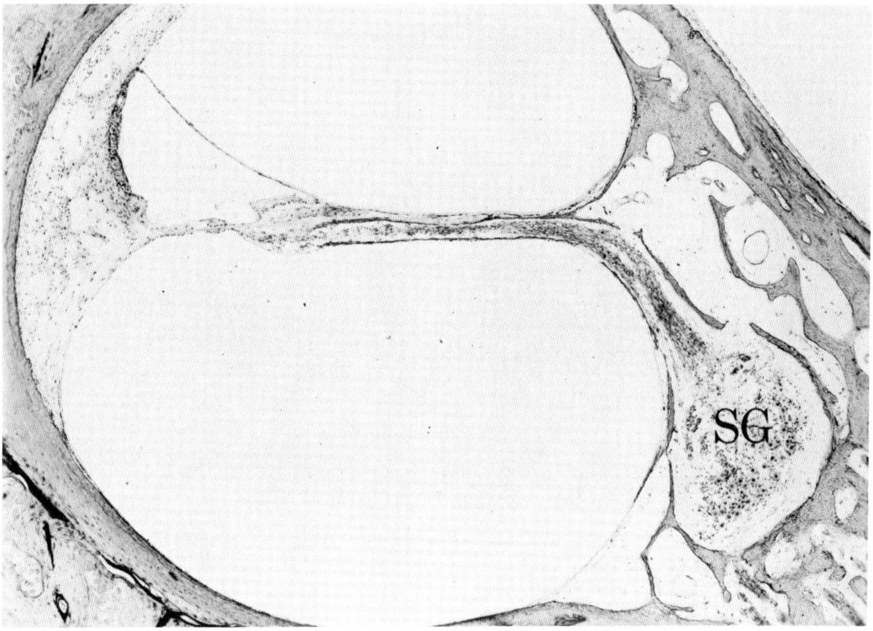

Figure 28-7. Case 3. Neomycin ototoxicity. Basal turn of the organ of Corti of the right ear. Approximately 30 percent of the normal population of spiral ganglion cells (SG) remains in Rosenthal's canal. (Magnification ×66.)

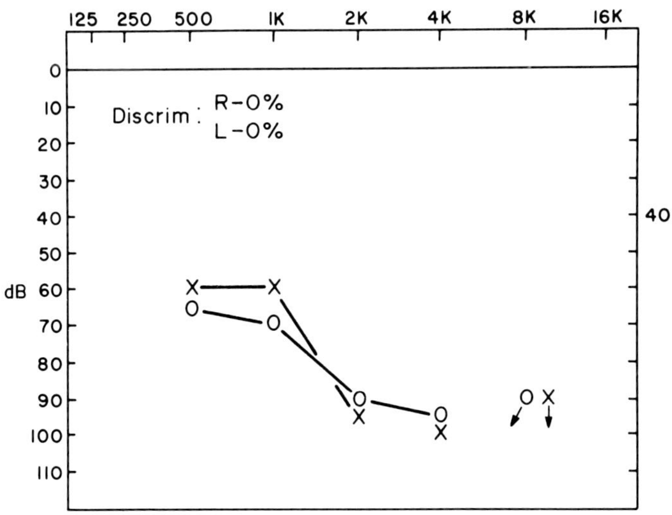

Figure 28-8. Case 4. Neomycin ototoxicity. Audiogram 3 months before death. (○ = right ear; × = left ear.)

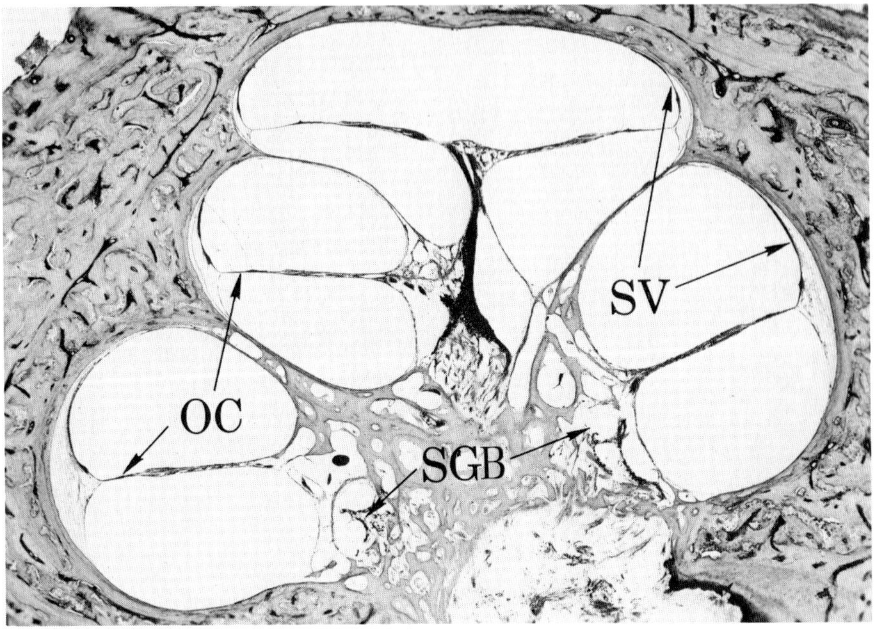

Figure 28-9. Case 4. Neomycin ototoxicity. Midmodiolar section of the right cochlea. There is marked atrophy of all components of the cochlear duct, including the organ of Corti (OC), stria vascularis (SV), and spiral ganglion, particularly in the basal turn (SGB). (Magnification ×28.)

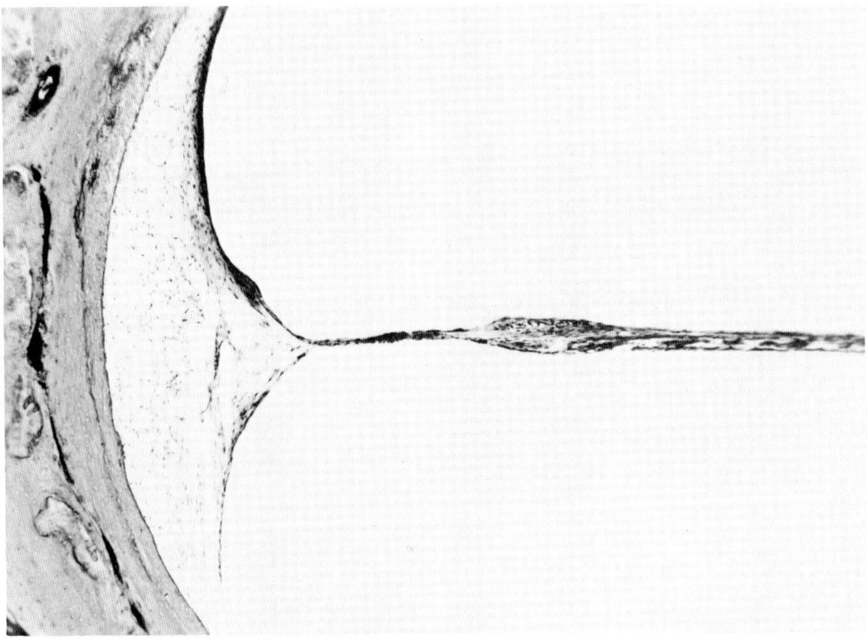

Figure 28-10. Case 4. Neomycin ototoxicity. Basal turn of the right cochlea. The organ of Corti is completely absent, and Reissner's membrane is missing. (Magnification ×90.)

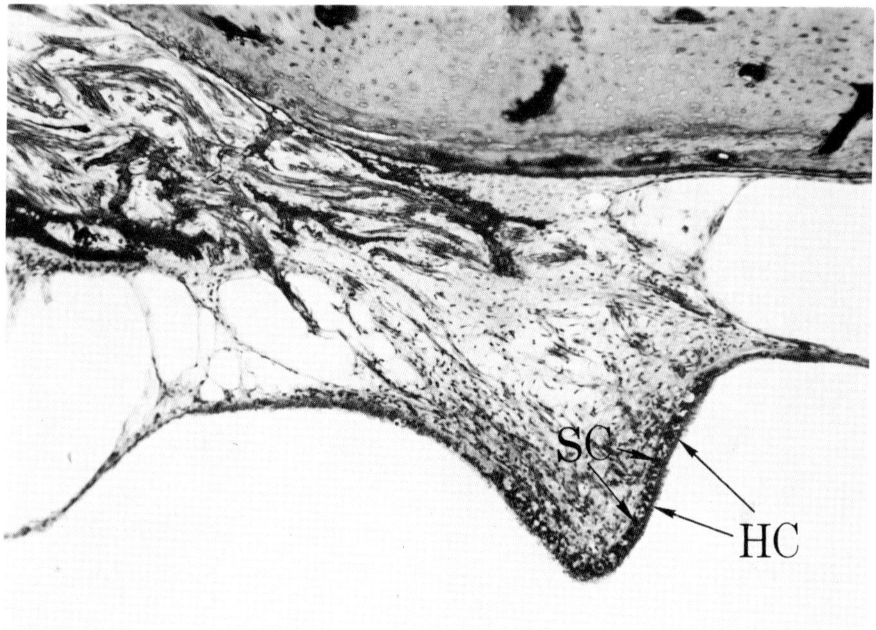

Figure 28-11. Case 4. Neomycin ototoxicity. The crista ampullaris of the lateral semicircular canal is normal, including supporting cells (SC) and hair cells (HC). (Magnification ×120.)

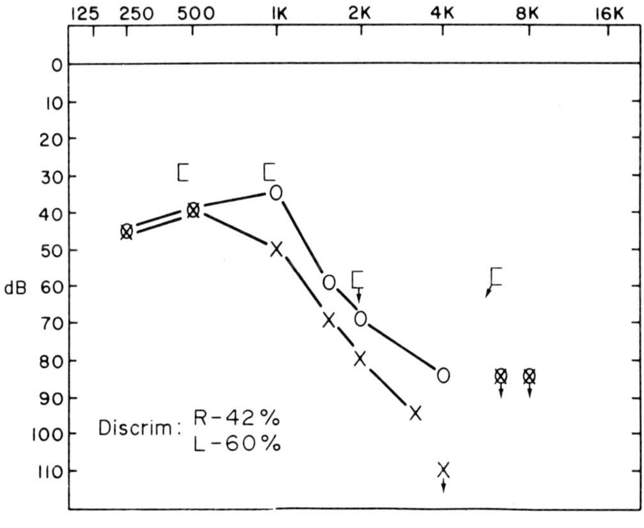

Figure 28-12. Case 5. Neomycin ototoxicity. Audiogram 6 months after beginning of neomycin therapy. (○ = right ear; × = left ear; [= bone conduction, right ear.)

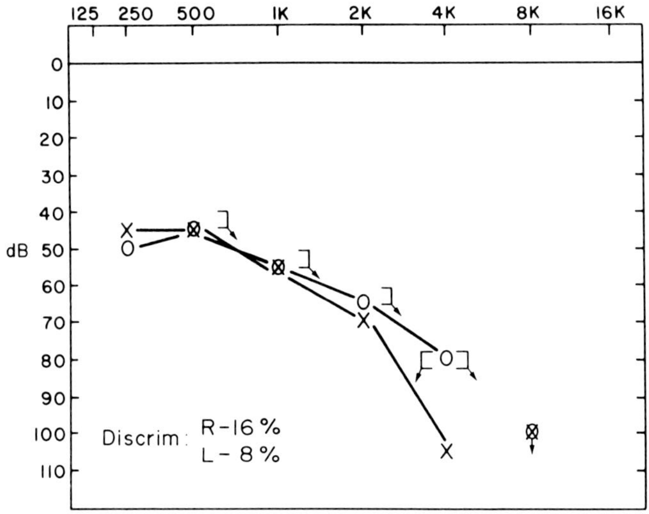

Figure 28-13. Case 5. Neomycin ototoxicity. Audiogram 18 months after beginning of neomycin therapy and 2 weeks before death. (○ = right ear; × = left ear;] = bone conduction, left ear.)

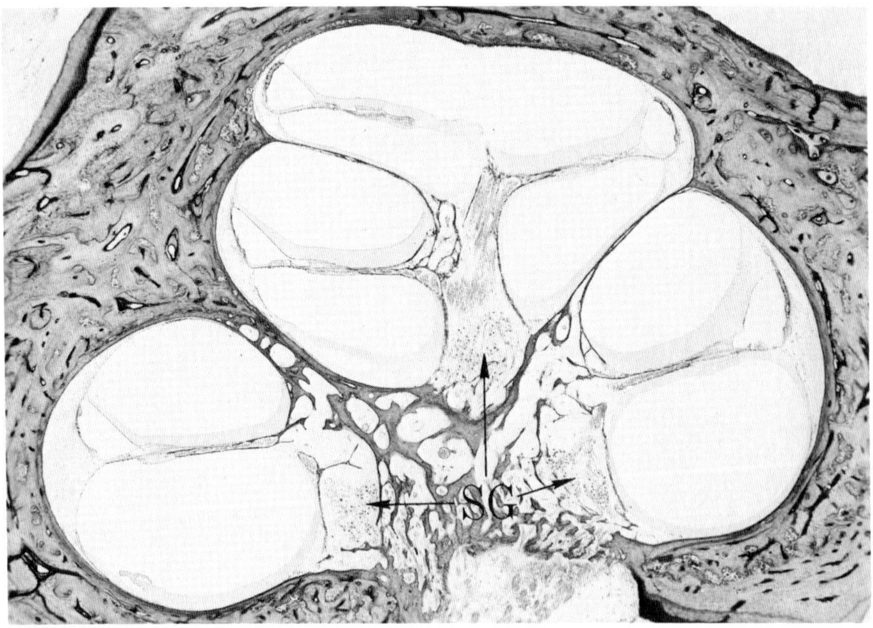

Figure 28-14. Case 5. Neomycin ototoxicity. Midmodiolar section of right inner ear. There has been loss of approximately 50 percent of spiral ganglion cells (SG.) The precipitate in the scalae vestibuli and tympani is probably caused by the terminal subarachnoid hemorrhage. (Magnification ×25.)

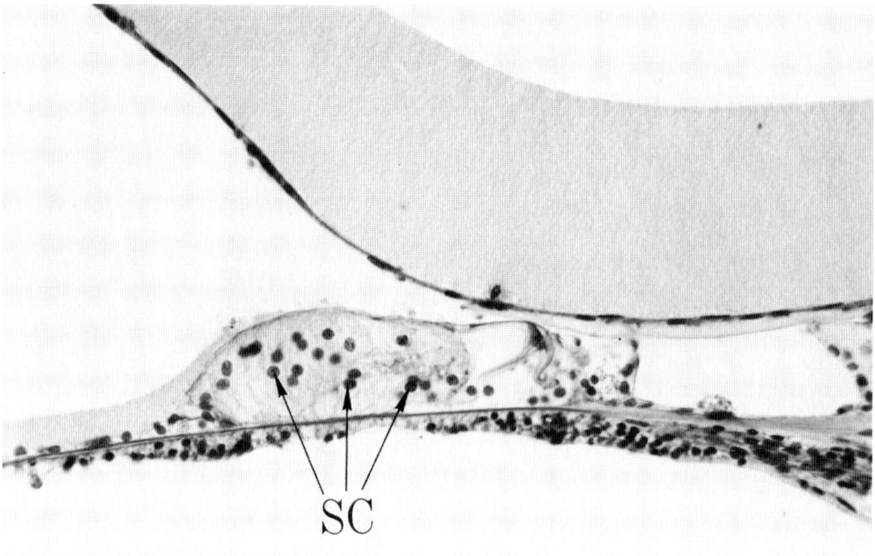

Figure 28-15. Case 5. Neomycin ototoxicity. Middle turn of the organ of Corti. There has been loss of inner and outer hair cells. The supporting cells (SC) appear normal. (Magnification ×450.)

Case 6

This 50-year-old woman with renal failure was treated for severe pyelonephritis with 1 g of kanamycin administered intramuscularly every 12 hours for 14 days. Within 3 days after the drug was stopped, a profound bilateral hearing loss was discovered. The patient had no vestibular symptoms. No improvement of hearing occurred between termination of therapy and her death 1 week later.

HISTOPATHOLOGY

The pathologic findings were similar in both ears. There was marked loss of hair cells in all turns (Fig. 28-16). In the basal 10 mm of both cochleae, the loss of inner and outer hair cells was almost complete. Between 10 and 14 mm, some inner hair cells remained, and between 14 and 27 mm, about half of the hair cells were missing. The hair cells were normal in the most apical 5 mm. The spiral ganglion cell population appeared normal throughout (Fig. 28-17). In areas of hair cell loss, the supporting structures of the organ of Corti usually appeared normal (Figs. 28-17 and 28-18), but in limited areas there was some loss of supporting elements (Fig. 28-19).

Case 7

This 49-year-old woman required a right nephrostomy tube to bypass ureteral obstruction secondary to adenocarcinoma of the cervix. She developed pyelonephritis and mild renal failure and was treated with kanamycin administered intramuscularly at a dosage of 1.5 g per day for 8 days. During the course of this treatment, she required pressors for maintenance of blood pres-

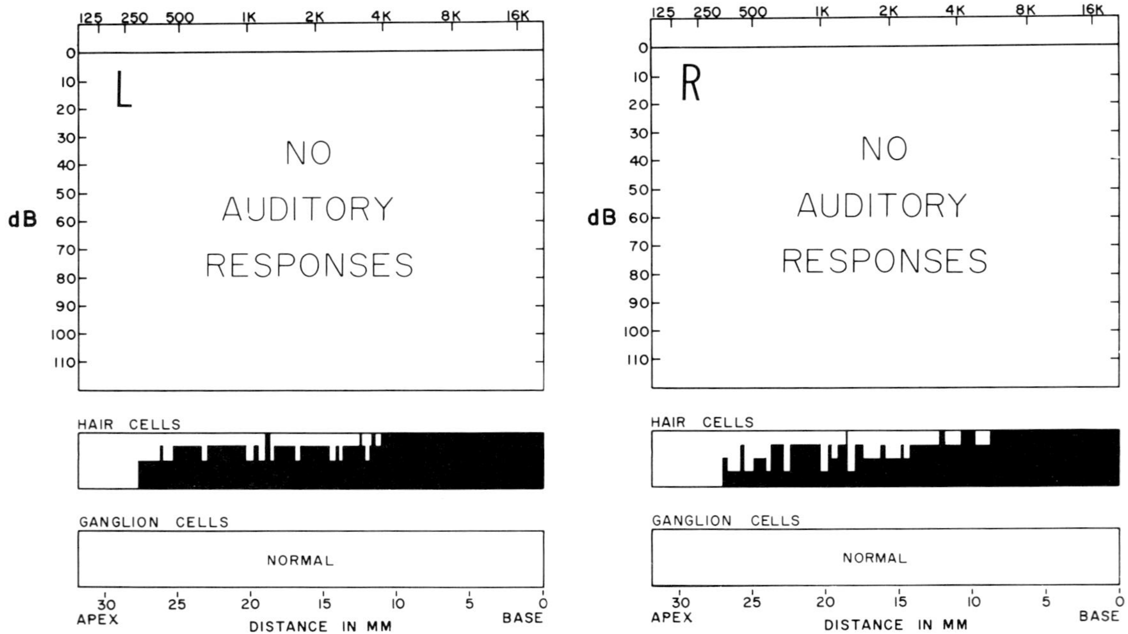

Figure 28-16. Case 6. Kanamycin ototoxicity. Histogram of cellular loss, estimated as percentage of cells missing (shown in black), in organ of Corti. (L = left ear; R = right ear.)

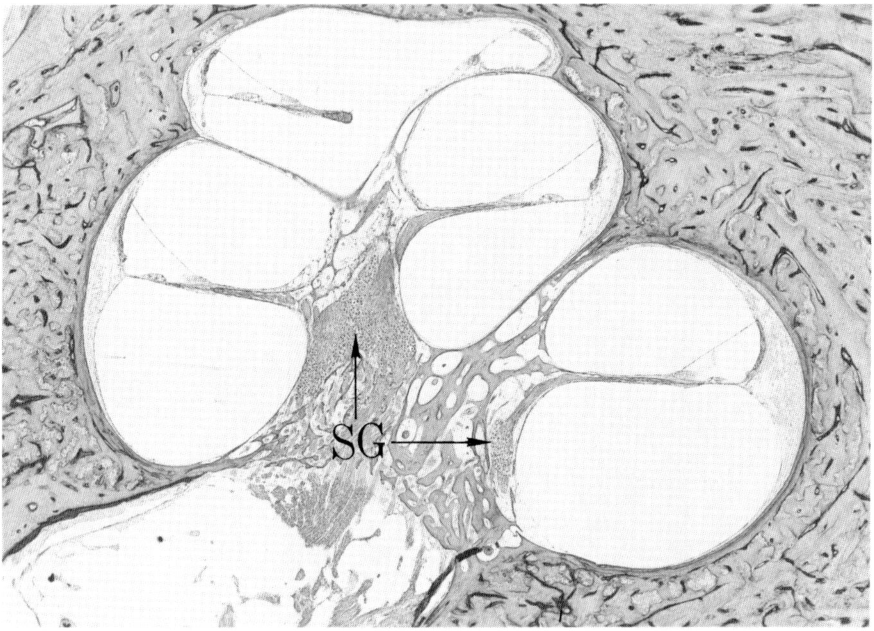

Figure 28-17. Case 6. Kanamycin ototoxicity. Midmodiolar section of right inner ear. The spiral ganglion cell population (SG) appears normal. (Magnification ×27.)

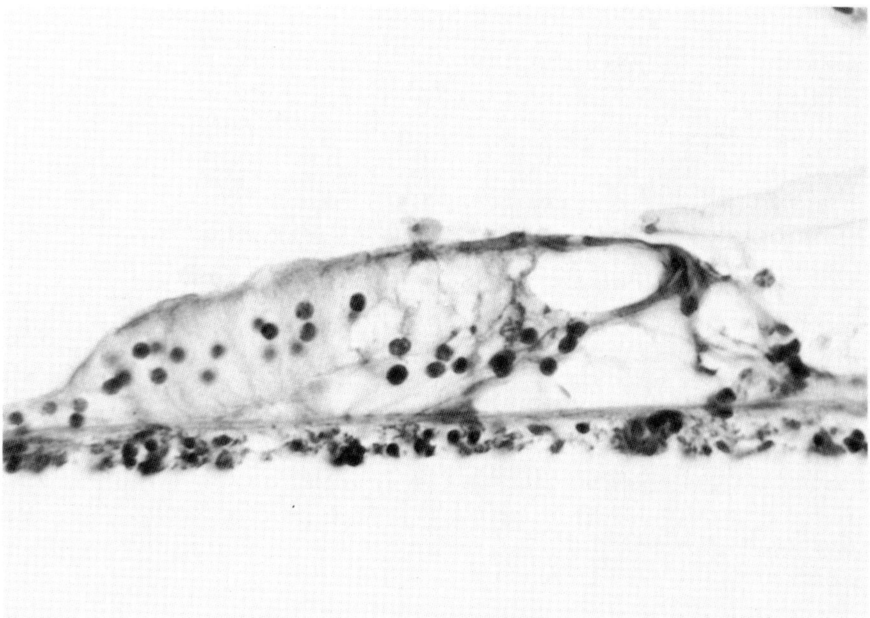

Figure 28-18. Case 6. Kanamycin ototoxicity. Left middle turn of cochlea. The supporting elements of the organ of Corti remain, but there has been complete loss of inner and outer hair cells. (Magnification ×685.)

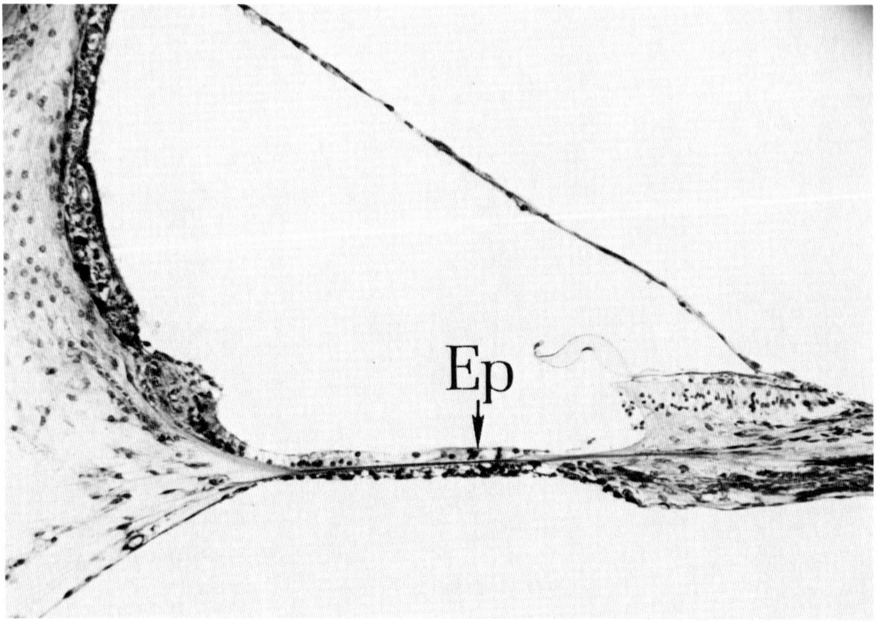

Figure 28-19. Case 6. Kanamycin ototoxicity. Basal turn of right cochlea. The organ of Corti has been lost completely and replaced by a thin layer of epithelial cells (Ep). (Magnification ×130.)

sure. On the last day of therapy, severe hearing loss was noted. The hearing loss progressed and became profound within several days. She died 3 months later. This case was previously reported by Igarashi and Yoshinobu [16].

HISTOPATHOLOGY

There was total loss of inner and outer hair cells in the left ear (Fig. 28-20) and of more than 90 percent of the hair cells in the right ear (Fig. 28-21). The supporting elements of the organ of Corti (Fig. 28-22) and the cochlear neuronal population (Figs. 28-23 and 28-24) were normal. The vestibular sensory and neuronal structures were normal (Figs. 28-25 and 28-26).

Case 8

This 27-year-old woman with abruptio placentae and eclampsia developed renal failure and required hemodialysis until the time of her death 2 months later. She received an initial dose of 1 g of kanamycin, followed by 0.25 g every second day for a total of 3 g in 18 days. Therapy was discontinued when an audiogram showed a bilateral high-frequency hearing loss. Subsequent audiograms demonstrated only a slight deterioration of hearing at termination of therapy. The last audiogram performed, 14 days after termination of treatment and 20 days before death (Figs. 28-27 and 28-28), showed no change in pure-tone thresholds through 1,000 Hz. At 2,000 Hz there had been a 20-dB deterioration on the right and 30-dB deterioration on the left, despite termi-

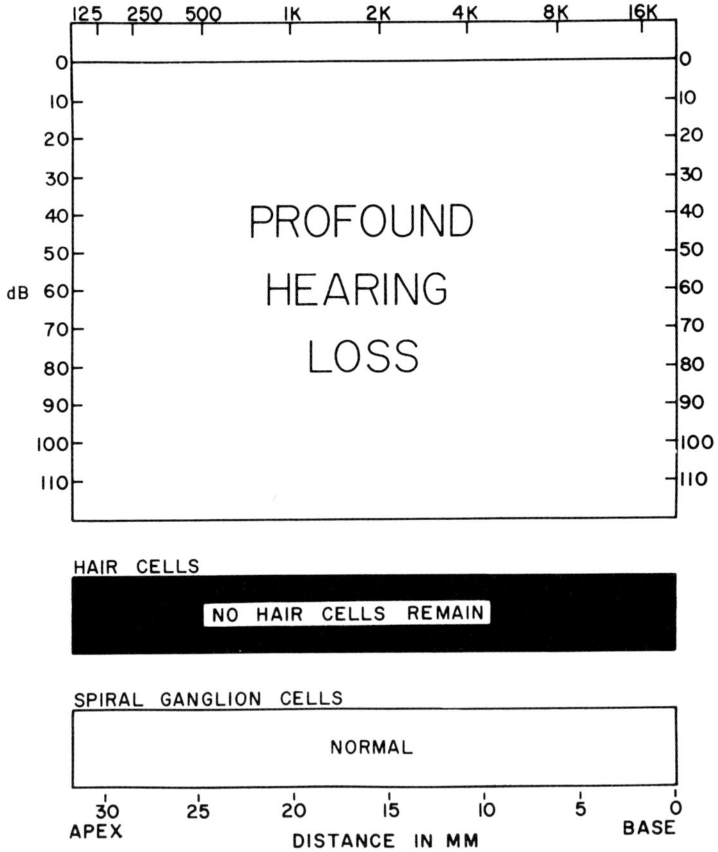

Figure 28-20. Case 7. Kanamycin ototoxicity. Histogram of cell loss, estimated as percentage of cells missing (shown in black), in left cochlea. (From M. Igarashi and T. Yoshinobu, Kanamycin deafness: A human temporal bone report. *Otolaryngol Clin. [Kyoto]* 56:301, 1968. Reprinted by permission.)

nation of kanamycin treatment. In addition, at 4,000 Hz there had been a 30-dB deterioration in the left ear only.

HISTOPATHOLOGY

There was nearly total loss of inner and outer hair cells in the basal 15 mm of both cochleae (Figs. 28-27 and 28-28). In the 12- to 15-mm region, the remaining cells were predominantly inner hair cells. The cochlear neurons and the supporting structures of the organ of Corti (Figs. 28-29 and 28-30) as well as the vestibular sensory and neuronal structures (Fig. 28-31) were normal.

Comment

These three cases demonstrate that, in man, the primary acute pathologic finding of kanamycin ototoxicity is loss of hair cells, most severe in the basal

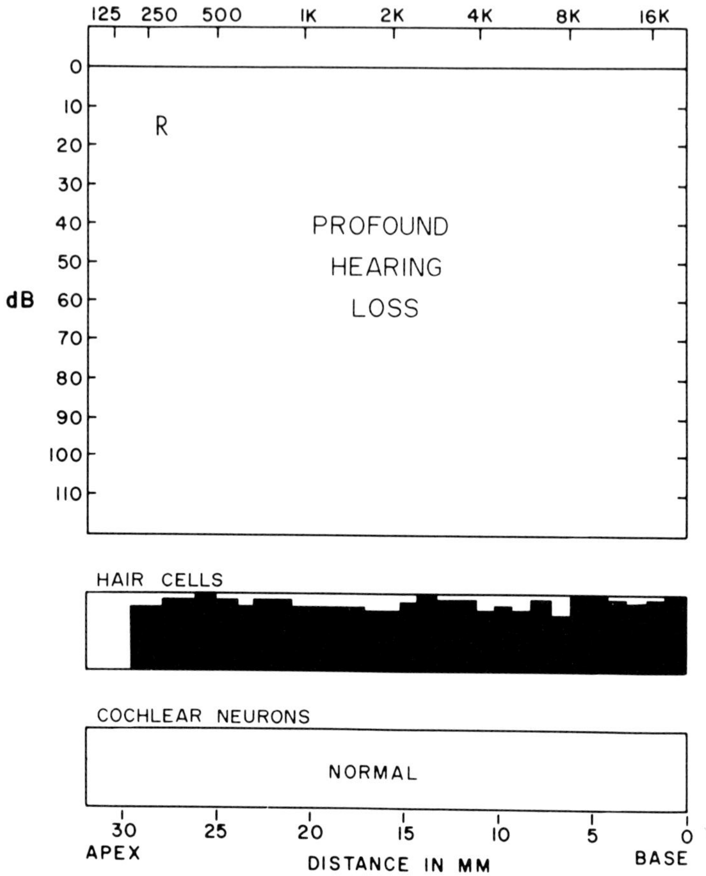

Figure 28-21. Case 7. Kanamycin ototoxicity. Histogram of cell loss, estimated as percentage of cells missing (shown in black), in right cochlea. (From M. Igarashi and T. Yoshinobu, Kanamycin deafness: A human temporal bone report. *Otolaryngol. Clin. [Kyoto]* 56:301, 1968. Reprinted by permission.)

turn. The cochlear neuronal population was uniformly preserved. Similarly, in animal experiments there seemed to be a selective effect on the hair cells of the organ of Corti, with the outer hair cells of the basal turn showing the most severe loss [14, 23, 25, 32]. In animals there were also ototoxic effects in the vestibular system, but these were less severe than those in the auditory apparatus. Type I cells on the crests of the cristae and stria of the utricle showed the greatest damage, but very little effect was found in the saccule. Although the primary acute effect in man and animals is loss of auditory hair cells, there is some evidence that kanamycin ototoxicity may eventually result in loss of cochlear neurons as well. Ishii et al. [17] demonstrated decreased lysosomal enzymatic activity in both hair cells and cochlear neurons prior to cell death in guinea pigs treated with kanamycin. Loss of activity was noted first in external

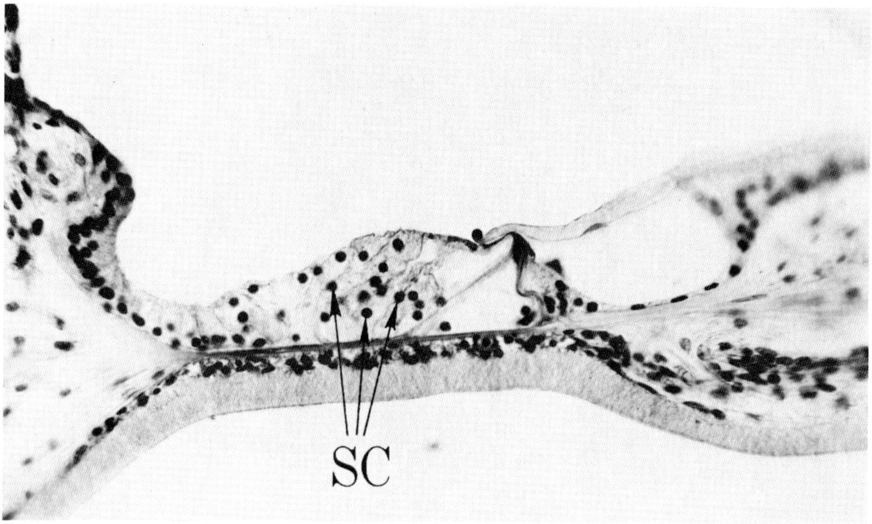

Figure 28-22. Case 7. Kanamycin ototoxicity. Basal turn of left cochlea. The supporting structures and supporting cells (SC) are normal. No inner or outer hair cells remain. (Magnification ×220.) (From N. Igarashi and T. Yoshinobu, Kanamycin deafness: A human temporal bone report. *Otolaryngol. Clin.* [*Kyoto*] 56:301, 1968. Reprinted by permission.)

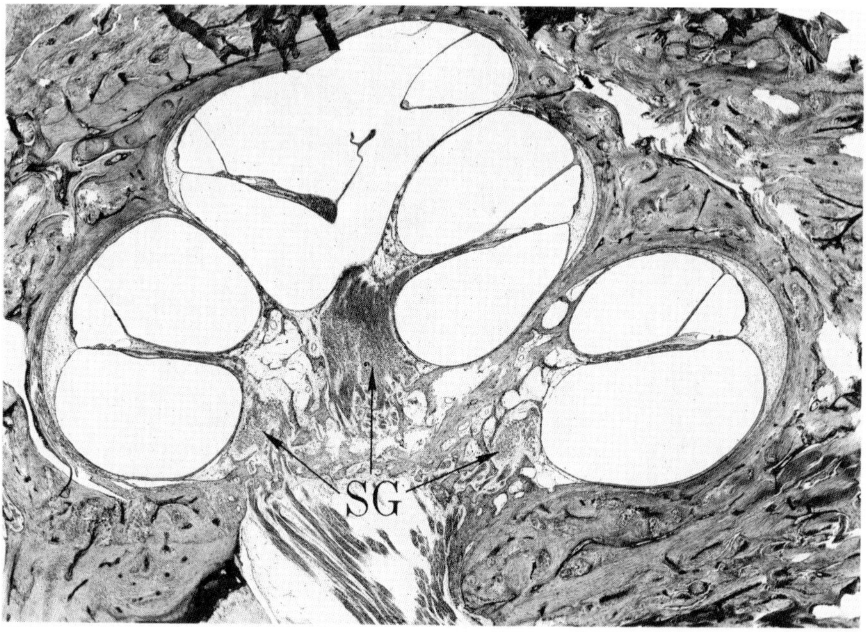

Figure 28-23. Case 7. Kanamycin ototoxicity. Midmodiolar section of left cochlea. The spiral ganglion cell population (SG) appears normal. (Magnification ×27.)

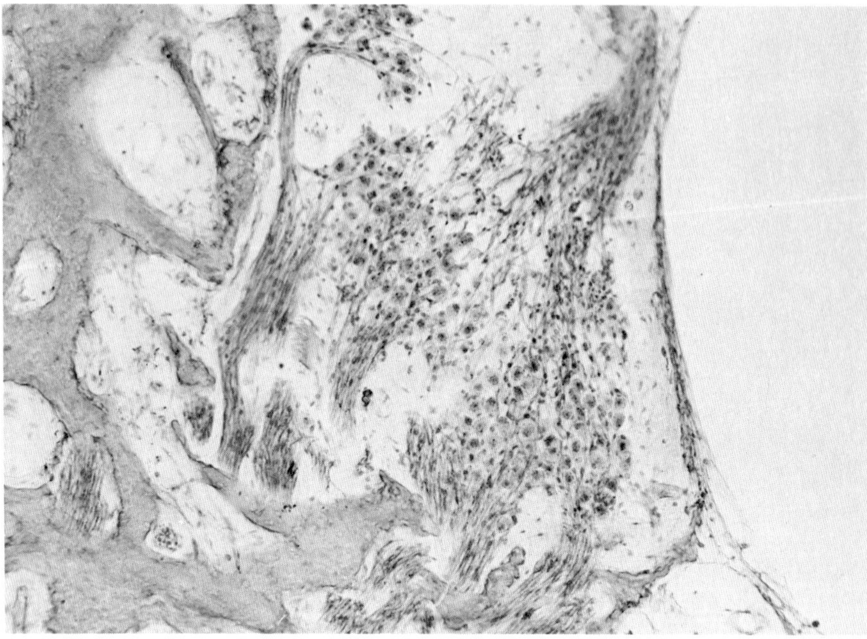

Figure 28-24. Case 7. Kanamycin ototoxicity. Rosenthal's canal of upper basal turn of right cochlea. The spiral ganglion cells appear normal in number and structure. (Magnification ×130.) (From M. Igarashi and T. Yoshinobu, Kanamycin deafness: A human temporal bone report. *Otolaryngol. Clin.* [*Kyoto*] 56:301, 1968. Reprinted by permission.)

Figure 28-25. Case 7. Kanamycin ototoxicity. The crista ampullaris of the posterior semicircular canal contains normal numbers of hair and supporting cells. (Magnification ×90.) (From M. Igarashi and T. Yoshinobu, Kanamycin deafness: A human temporal bone report. *Otolaryngol. Clin.* [*Kyoto*] 56:301, 1968. Reprinted by permission.)

Figure 28-26. Case 7. Kanamycin ototoxicity. The hair and supporting cell populations of the right macula sacculi are normal. (Magnification ×160.) (From M. Igarashi and T. Yoshinobu, Kanamycin deafness: A human temporal bone report. *Otolaryngol. Clin.* [*Kyoto*] 56:301, 1968. Reprinted by permission.)

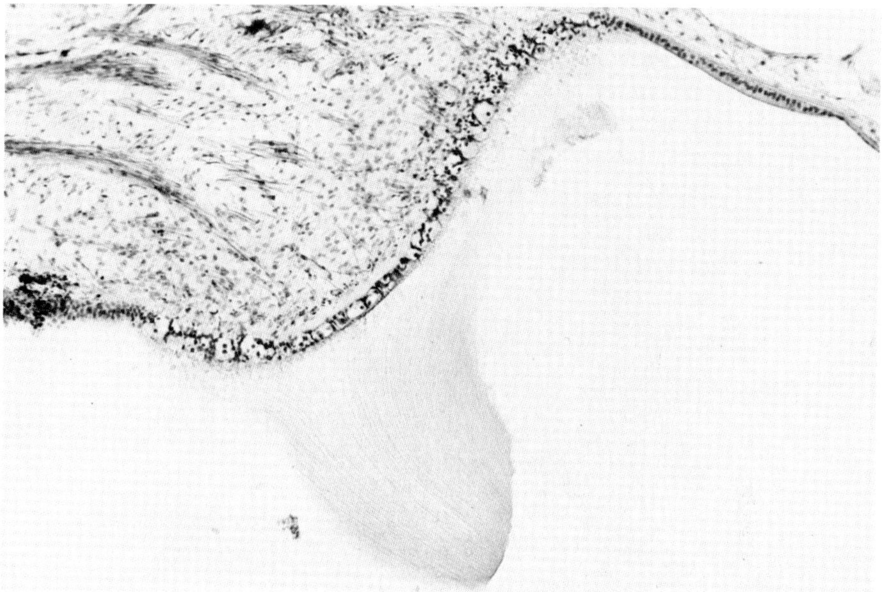

28-25

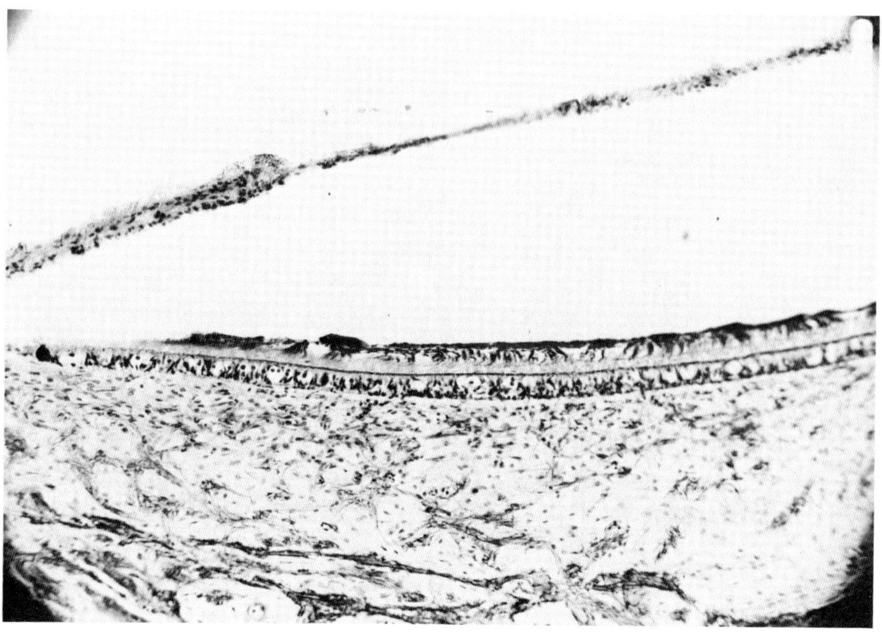

28-26

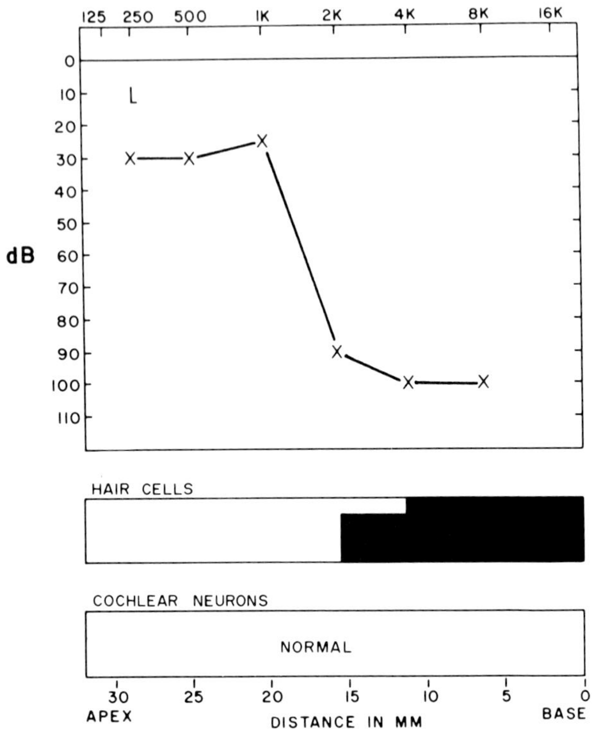

Figure 28-27. Case 8. Kanamycin ototoxicity. Audiogram 7 weeks before death, and histogram of cell loss, estimated as percentage of cell loss (shown in black), in left cochlea.

hair cells of the basal turn, with progression in an apical direction. The apical cochlear neurons were the first to be involved, with progression in the basal direction. Furthermore, Kiang et al. [19] found that, despite nearly total loss of inner and outer hair cells in cats treated with kanamycin, the neuronal population was normal in number and responded to electrical stimulation for several months after treatment. When the survival time after drug administration was extended to 4 or 5 years, however, there was marked loss of cochlear neurons in addition to hair cell loss. Significant loss of primary cochlear neurons would clearly have an adverse effect on the prospects for successful use of direct cochlear neuronal stimulation.

Figure 28-28. Case 8. Kanamycin ototoxicity. Audiogram 7 weeks before death, and histogram of cell loss, estimated as percentage of cell loss (shown in black), in right cochlea.

Figure 28-29. Case 8. Kanamycin ototoxicity. Midmodiolar section of left cochlea. The spiral ganglion cell population (SG) appears normal. (Magnification ×23.)

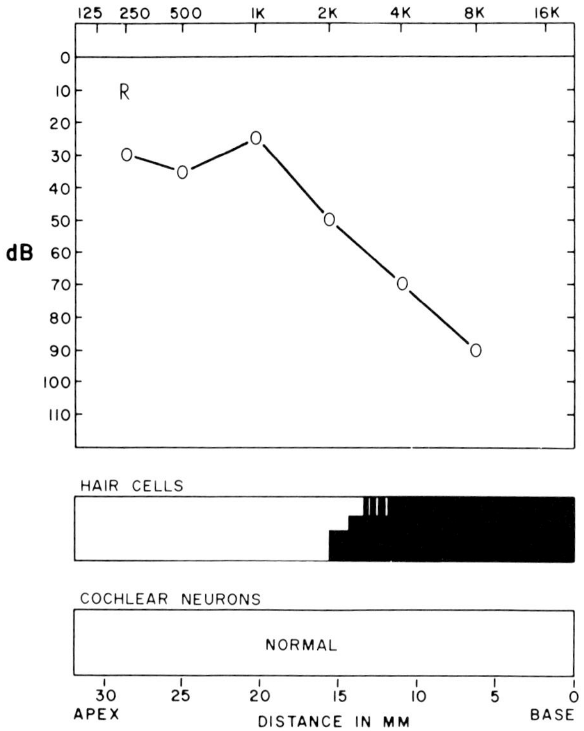
125
250
500
1K
2K
4K
8K
16K
dB
0
10
20
30
40
50
60
70
80
90
100
110
R
HAIR CELLS
COCHLEAR NEURONS
NORMAL
30
25
20
15
10
5
0
APEX
DISTANCE IN MM
BASE

28-28

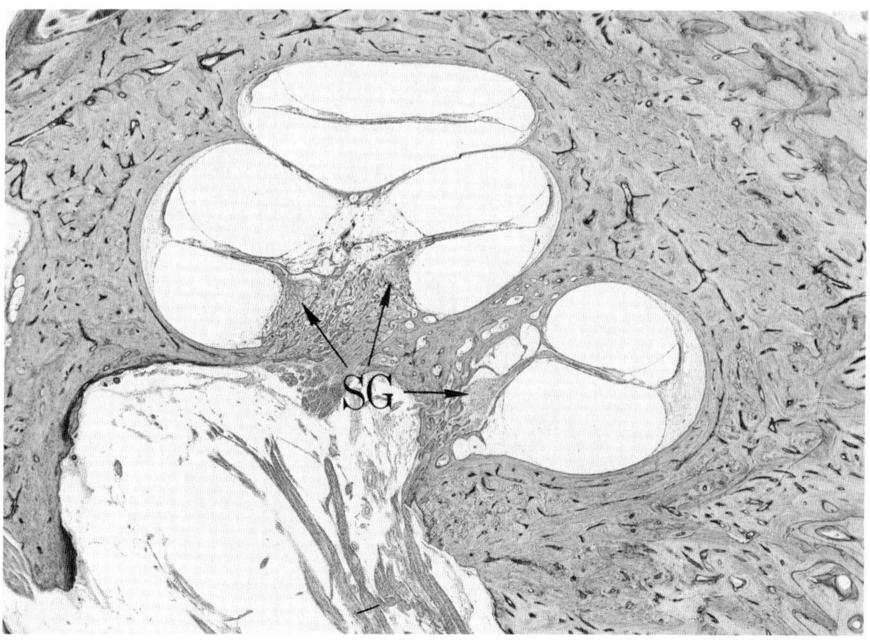
SG

28-29

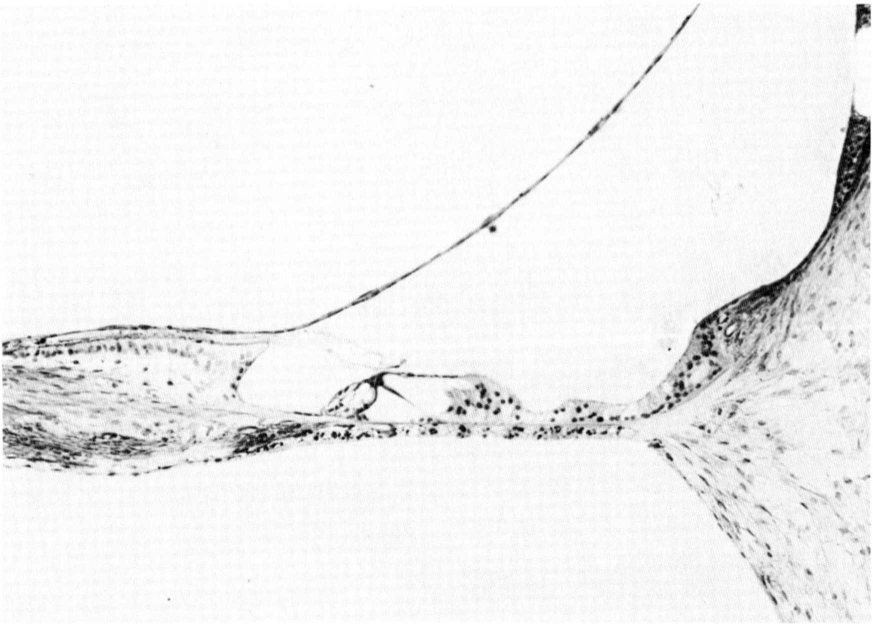

Figure 28-30. Case 8. Kanamycin ototoxicity. Basal turn of left cochlea. No inner or outer hair cells remain. Supporting elements appear normal. (Magnification ×220.)

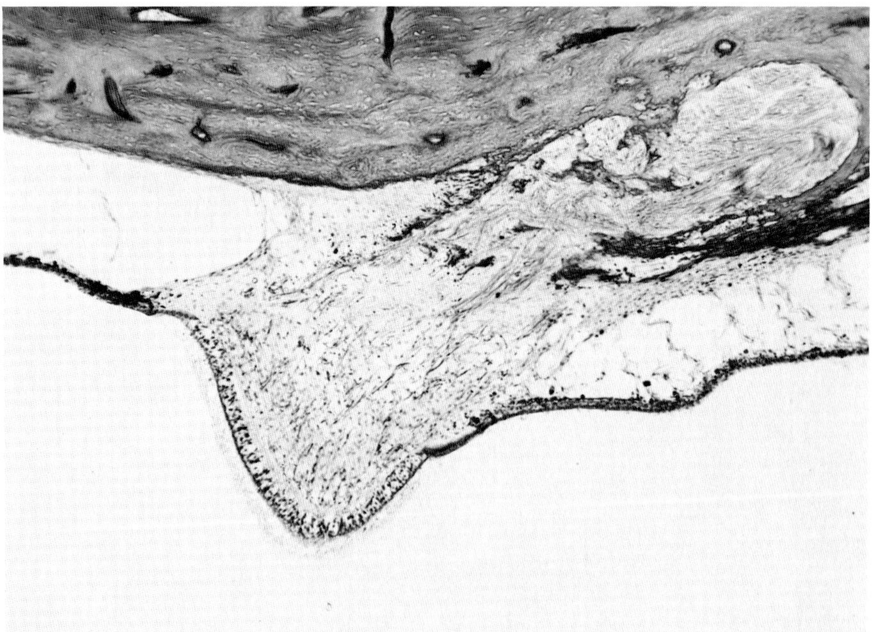

Figure 28-31. Case 8. Kanamycin ototoxicity. The hair and supporting cells and neurons of the crista ampullaris of the lateral semicircular canal appear normal. (Magnification ×120.)

Conclusion

Despite the limitations inherent in the study of human postmortem material, the histopathologic findings in eight cases of human ototoxicity caused by streptomycin, neomycin, and kanamycin correlate well with experimental animal data. The primary histopathologic alteration in cases of streptomycin toxicity is loss of hair cells of the vestibular system, and in cases of neomycin and kanamycin toxicity, loss of hair cells of the organ of Corti. In addition, neomycin seems to cause severe neuronal loss and dysfunction early in the course of degeneration, whereas after kanamycin ototoxicity, there is nearly complete preservation of the first-order neurons, despite severe hair cell loss early in the course of degeneration. In the cat, however, neuronal degeneration may progress for several years following cessation of kanamycin administration.

References

1. Ballantyne, J. Iatrogenic deafness. *J. Laryngol. Otol.* 84:967, 1970.
2. Berg, K. The toxic effect of streptomycin on the vestibular and cochlear apparatus. *Acta Otolaryngol. (Stockh.)* [Suppl. 97], 1951.
3. Berk, D. P., and Chalmers, T. Deafness complicating antibiotic therapy of hepatic encephalopathy. *Ann. Intern. Med.* 73:393, 1970.
4. Bignall, J. R., Crofton, J. W., and Thomas, J. A. B. Effect of streptomycin on vestibular function. *Br. Med. J.* 1:554, 1951.
5. Campanelli, P. A., Grimes, E., and West, M. L. Hearing loss in a child following neomycin irrigation. *Med. Ann. DC* 35:541, 1966.
6. Caussé, R. Action toxique vestibulaire et cochléaire de la streptomycine au point de vue expérimental. *Ann. Otolaryngol.* 66:518, 1949.
7. Cawthorne, T., and Ranger, D. Toxic effect of streptomycin upon balance and hearing. *Br. Med. J.* 1:1444, 1957.
8. Farrington, R., Hull-Smith, H., Bunn, P., and McDermott, W. Streptomycin toxicity. Reactions to highly purified drug on long-continued administration to human subjects. *J.A.M.A.* 134:679, 1947.
9. Fields, R. L. Neomycin ototoxicity: Report of a case due to rectal and colonic irrigations. *Arch. Otolaryngol.* 79:67, 1964.
10. Finland, M. Summary of the monograph on the basic and clinical research of the new antibiotic, kanamycin. *Ann. N.Y. Acad. Sci.* 76:391, 1958.
11. Frost, J. O., Hawkins, J. E., and Daly, J. F. Kanamycin. II. Ototoxicity. *Am. Rev. Respir. Dis.* 82:23, 1960.
12. Gibson, W. S., Jr. Deafness due to orally administered neomycin. *Arch. Otolaryngol.* 86:163, 1967.
13. Halpern, E. B., and Heller, M. F. Ototoxicity of orally administered neomycin: Report of a case. *Arch. Otolaryngol.* 73:675, 1961.
14. Hawkins, J. E., Jr. The ototoxicity of kanamycin. *Ann. Otol. Rhinol. Laryngol.* 68:698, 1959.
15. Hinshaw, H., and Feldman, W. Streptomycin in treatment of clinical tuberculosis: A preliminary report. *Proc. Staff Meet. Mayo Clin.* 20:313, 1945.
16. Igarashi, M., and Yoshinobu, T. Kanamycin deafness: A human temporal bone report. *Otolaryngol. Clin. (Kyoto)* 56:301, 1968.
17. Ishii, T., Ishii, D., and Balogh, K., Jr. Lysosomal enzymes in the inner ears of kanamycin-treated guinea pigs. *Acta Otolaryngol. (Stockh.)* 65:449, 1968.
18. Kelly, D. R., Nilo, E. R., and Berggren, R. B. Brief recording: Deafness after topical neomycin wound irrigation. *N. Engl. J. Med.* 280:1338, 1969.

19. Kiang, N. Y., Liberman, M. C., and Levine, R. A. Auditory-nerve activity in cats exposed to ototoxic drugs and high-intensity sounds. *Ann. Otol. Rhinol. Laryngol.* 85:752, 1976.
20. Kohonen, A. Effect of some ototoxic drugs upon the pattern and innervation of cochlear sensory cells in the guinea pig. *Acta Otolaryngol. (Stockh.)* [Suppl. 208], 1965.
21. Kunin, C. M., and Finland, M. Restrictions imposed on antibiotic therapy by renal failure. *Arch. Intern. Med.* 104:1030, 1959.
22. Last, P. M., and Sherlock, S. Systemic absorption of orally administered neomycin in liver disease. *N. Engl. J. Med.* 262:385, 1960.
23. Lindeman, H. H. Regional differences in sensitivity of the vestibular sensory epithelia to ototoxic antibiotics. *Acta Otolaryngol. (Stockh.)* 67:177, 1969.
24. Lindsay, J. R., Proctor, L. R., and Work, W. P. Histopathologic inner ear changes in deafness due to neomycin. *Laryngoscope* 70:382, 1960.
25. Matz, G. J., Wallace, T. H., and Ward, P. H. The ototoxicity of kanamycin: A comparative histopathological study. *Laryngoscope* 75:1690, 1965.
26. Myerson, M., Knight, H., Gambarini, A., et al. Intrapleural neomycin causing ototoxicity. *Ann. Thorac. Surg.* 9:483, 1970.
27. Naunton, R. F., and Ward, P. H. The ototoxicity of kanamycin sulfate in the presence of compromised renal function. *Arch. Otolaryngol.* 69:398, 1959.
28. Schatz, A., Bugie, E., and Waksman, S. Streptomycin, a substance exhibiting antibiotic activity against gram-positive and gram-negative bacteria. *Proc. Soc. Exp. Biol. Med.* 57:244, 1944.
29. Schuknecht, H. F. Ablation therapy with management of Menière's disease. *Acta Otolaryngol. (Stockh.)* [Suppl. 132], 1957.
30. Tsuiki, T., and Murai, S. Familial incidence of streptomycin hearing loss and hereditary weakness of the cochlea. *Audiology* 10:315, 1971.
31. Waisbren, B., and Spink, W. A clinical appraisal of neomycin. *Ann. Intern. Med.* 33:1099, 1950.
32. Ward, P. H., and Fernandez, C. The ototoxicity of kanamycin in guinea pigs. *Ann. Otol. Rhinol. Laryngol.* 70:132, 1961.
33. Watanuki, K. Pathology of the vestibular sensory epithelia in streptomycin and kanamycin ototoxicosis. *Jpn. J. Otol.* 74:52, 1971.
34. Wersäll, J., and Hawkins, J. E., Jr. The vestibular sensory epithelia in the cat labyrinth and their reactions in chronic streptomycin intoxication. *Acta Otolaryngol. (Stockh.)* 54:1, 1962.

Discussion of Chapters 27 and 28

Dr. Hinojosa: We recently had the opportunity to examine the temporal bones of a young man who died after developing asymptomatic auditory toxicity due to gentamicin. This 28-year-old patient with acute lymphoblastic leukemia received gentamicin, 100 mg (1.54 mg/kg body weight) intravenously every 8 hours, in several courses over a total of 54 days during his 75-day terminal hospitalization. His serum creatinine remained normal throughout. The highest peak concentration of gentamicin in serum, assayed at least twice a week during therapy, was 7.7 μg/ml. The patient did not receive ethacrynic acid, furosemide, vancomycin, or *cis*-platinum. His hearing was normal except for a 30- to 40-dB deficit at 8.0 kHz in the right ear seen in repeated audiograms obtained up to 36 days before his death. Although he had no auditory symptoms of toxicity, an audiogram performed 1 day before death showed bilateral sensorineural hearing loss, as depicted in Figs. D-1A and D-2A.

Twenty-micron sections of decalcified temporal bones were stained with hematoxylin and eosin. Every tenth section was studied, and the organ of Corti and the spiral ganglion cells were reconstructed. The counts of ganglion cells are shown in Figs. D-1B and D-2B. These graphs show that the numbers of ganglion cells in this patient were reduced from those of five normal controls. Overall, our patient had 20,415 and 22,163 ganglion cells in the left and right ears, respectively, compared with a mean of 34,147 in the controls. In contrast, the hair cells of the organ of Corti were normal. Fig. D-3 shows a midmodiolar section with a reduced number of ganglion cells and normal hair cells. Thus, in this case, contrary to the usual picture of diminished hair cells in aminoglycoside auditory toxicity, our patient's ganglion cells were diminished in number, whereas the hair cells had remained normal.

Dr. Hawkins: I would like to ask the speakers if they have ever seen degeneration of Scarpa's ganglion cells after aminoglycoside treatment.

A

B

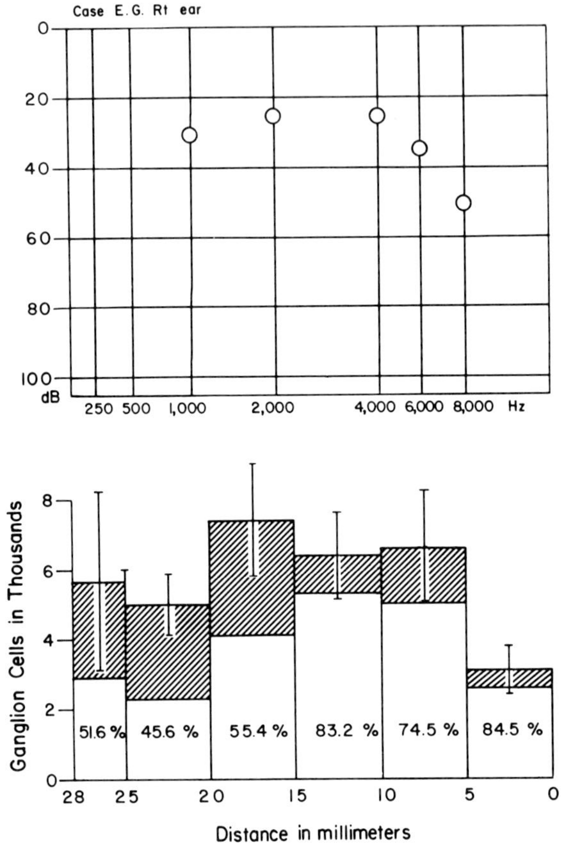

Figure D-1. Right ear. A. The audiogram shows a mild sensorineural hearing loss. Frequencies on the audiogram correspond to the positions on the histogram (B). B. The histogram shows ganglion cells counted in each of six 5-mm areas along the organ of Corti from base to apex. The standard deviation in each area is indicated by a vertical marker. The number of surviving ganglion cells is indicated in percentage of normal by a clear area at the base of each 5-mm section. (Shaded areas represent cell loss.) The basal coil is represented approximately by three 5-mm areas from right to left, the middle coil by the fourth and fifth areas, and the apical coil by the last area on the left.

A

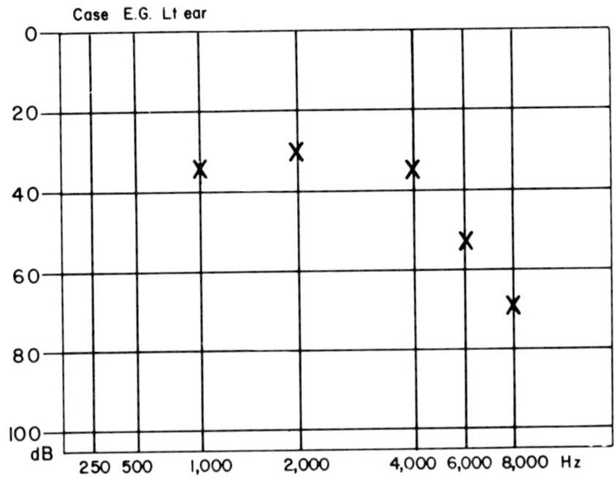

B

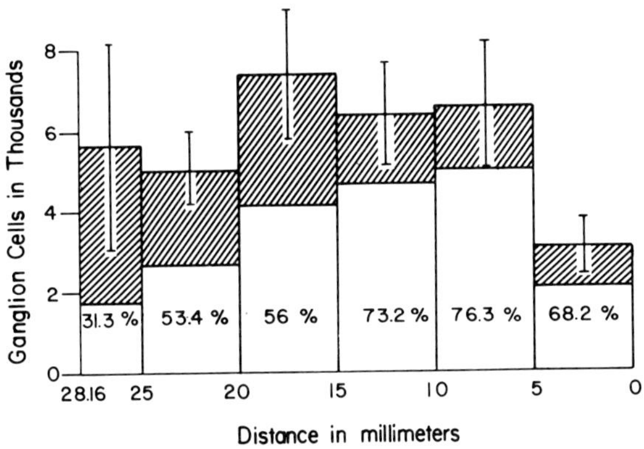

Figure D-2. Left ear. A. The audiogram shows a mild sensorineural hearing loss. B. The percentage of ganglion cells remaining is indicated in the histogram in each of the 5-mm regions along the organ of Corti. The number of remaining cells is lower than that in the right ear.

Dr. Nadol: We have not seen any decrease in the number of cells of Scarpa's ganglion even in the few cases of streptomycin treatment in which the hair cells have degenerated. The neuronal population of myelinated nerve fibers also appeared to be normal.

Dr. Hinojosa: We haven't counted the vestibular ganglion cells in order to demonstrate any loss of neurons. I think that this would be the only way of determining whether there is such a loss.

Dr. Anniko: It is easy to quantify the presence or absence of cochlear hair cells, but this is more difficult to do for vestibular hair cells. Under normal conditions of aging, a 40 percent loss of vestibular hair cells could occur. Therefore, it may be very difficult to separate effects of the ototoxic hair cell

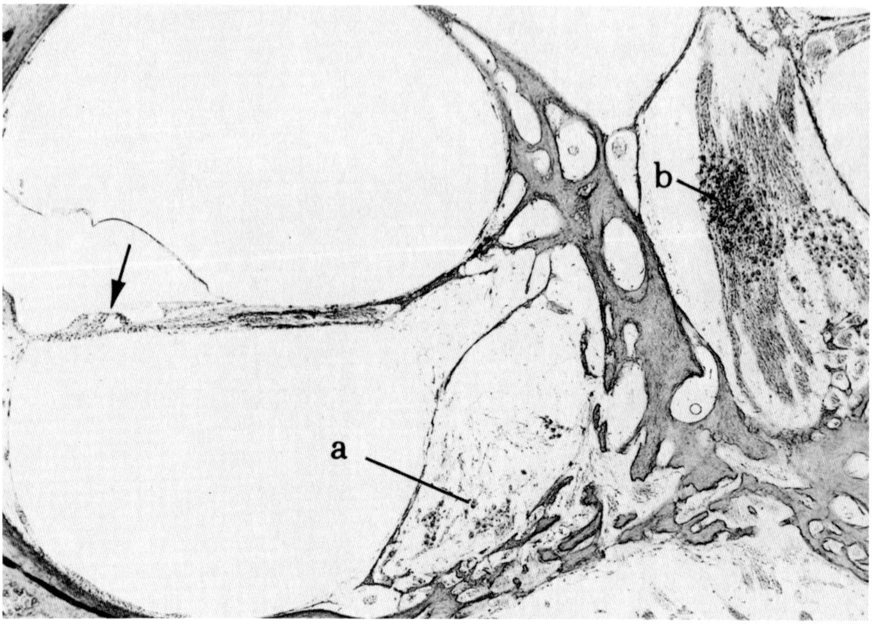

Figure D-3. Portion of midmodiolar section illustrating the reduction of ganglion cells in the basal (a) and second (b) turns. The organ of Corti (arrow) is well preserved, without pathologic changes. (Magnification ×46.)

damage from degeneration due to the normal aging process. Have any of you tried to separate these two factors?

Dr. Nadol: We are counting vestibular neurons and have found a decrease in neuronal fibers coincident with aging. I would say that the changes which we observe due to ototoxicity are much more obvious than what one sees simply with aging. The patient who received streptomycin clearly had vestibular symptoms. It is true that hair cell loss and first-order vestibular neuronal loss can occur with the aging process.

Dr. Brummett: A question I raise not just to Dr. Hinojosa, but to all of the speakers this afternoon, is: If the drug had in fact caused the Scarpa's ganglion cells to degenerate, would you expect to see any cells at all? What would you expect to see in the ganglion cells if they were dying from the effect of the drug?

Dr. Johnsson: I think it is extremely difficult to evaluate the state of the ganglion cells in human temporal bones. You can evaluate their numbers, but to judge their functional state is difficult. I think the only way to observe early neuronal changes in the human temporal bone is by using a surface preparation method and looking at the distal process, where you are likely to find the earliest changes. Most of the temporal bones I showed you are now being processed for sectioning, by surface preparation, but I am almost sure that, in cross section, the number of ganglion cells will be close to normal, and very little will be seen in the conventional celloidin H&E-stained sections.

Dr. Nadol: I want to emphasize that cochlear neurons degenerate, especially with neomycin. The exact initiating factor is still open to question—whether it is a primary neuronal degeneration due to toxic effects or whether it is a secondary effect.

Regarding Dr. Johnsson's comments, the "dying-back" phenomenon is seen also in other forms of degeneration. For example, it is seen in either primary or secondary cochlear neuronal degeneration with aging. It seems that the most distal dendritic fibers show earlier changes and degeneration, which is consistent with the central neural pathology, the dying-back phenomenon.

Dr. Hawkins: Dr. Igarashi, do you have any comment on the vestibular ganglion cells?

Dr. Igarashi: I have no comment on that. However, I have one interesting case that is similar to what Dr. Hinojosa has reported. The patient underwent cardiac surgery. Postoperatively, she received 80, 120, or 160 mg of gentamicin intravenously per day for a total dose of 4,540 mg in 7 weeks. The patient became very dizzy. The attending physician stopped the gentamicin and, after 25 days, the symptom disappeared. The patient died 3 months later, and the temporal bone findings were similar to what Dr. Hinojosa has reported. There was no hair cell loss in the cristae ampullares, maculae, or cochlea.

Dr. Wersäll: Dr. Nadol described two temporal bones that showed that the number of ganglion cells was normal. How much time elapsed between aminoglycoside administration and temporal bone fixation? Did you determine the number of ganglion cells relative to the normal number?

Dr. Nadol: We process these temporal bones by semiserial section. We do about 450 horizontal sections. Every tenth section is examined, and an estimate of ganglion cells is made. Therefore, our process is qualitative and not quantitative. It might be reported as 70 to 80 percent of normal; however, what is a normal number of spiral ganglion cells in man is open to question.

Dr. Hawkins: Let me urge all of you to send any interesting, well-fixed human temporal bones that you can find and acquire either to the "banks" of the Huron in Ann Arbor or to those of Lake Michigan or of the Charles River in Boston.

Index

Index